Dengue Virus: Diagnosis and Treatment

Dengue Virus: Diagnosis and Treatment

Edited by Walter Cameron

STATES
ACADEMIC PRESS
www.statesacademicpress.com

States Academic Press,
109 South 5th Street,
Brooklyn, NY 11249, USA

Visit us on the World Wide Web at:
www.statesacademicpress.com

ISBN: 978-1-63989-147-4

Cataloging-in-Publication Data

Dengue virus : diagnosis and treatment / edited by Walter Cameron.
p. cm.
Includes bibliographical references and index.
ISBN 978-1-63989-147-4
1. Dengue viruses. 2. Dengue. 3. Dengue--Diagnosis. 4. Dengue--Treatment. I. Cameron, Walter.
RC137 .D46 2022
616.921--dc23

Table of Contents

Preface

This book aims to highlight the current researches and provides a platform to further the scope of innovations in this area. This book is a product of the combined efforts of many researchers and scientists, after going through thorough studies and analysis from different parts of the world. The objective of this book is to provide the readers with the latest information of the field.

Dengue fever is a disease caused by dengue virus and spread by mosquitoes. The symptoms of the disease generally start three to four days after the infection. These may be headache, muscle and joint pain, fever, vomiting, and a characteristic skin rash. It usually takes two to seven days for the patient to recover. In some cases, the disease may develop into a more severe condition, known as dengue hemorrhagic fever, which results in low levels of blood platelets, bleeding and blood plasma leakage. It may also develop into dengue shock syndrome which results in dangerously low blood pressure. Female mosquitoes of several species of Aedes genus can spread dengue. This book unfolds the unexplored aspects of dengue fever and the dengue virus that causes it. Its aim is to present researches that have transformed the diagnosis and treatment of this disease. Those in search of information to further their knowledge will be greatly assisted by this book.

I would like to express my sincere thanks to the authors for their dedicated efforts in the completion of this book. I acknowledge the efforts of the publisher for providing constant support. Lastly, I would like to thank my family for their support in all academic endeavors.

Editor

1

Cellular Control of Dengue Virus Replication: Role of Interferon-Inducible Genes

Hirotaka Takahashi and Youichi Suzuki

Abstract

Dengue, one of the most common mosquito-borne viral infectious diseases in the world, is caused by the dengue virus (DENV). This enveloped RNA virus has immunologically distinct serotypes that increase the risk of life-threatening diseases, such as dengue haemorrhagic fever. However, no effective antiviral therapy against DENV infection has yet been established. As seen in other RNA viruses, various cellular factors have been reported to participate in efficient DENV replication. On the other hand, increasing recent evidence demonstrates that host cells harbour inhibitory factors that limit the DENV replication. In particular, it is well known that the response of interferons (IFNs), the first line of a host defence system against invading pathogens, evokes the expression of a number of genes that negatively regulate various steps of virus replication. This set of inhibitory genes, called interferon-stimulated genes (ISGs), is considered to be a central force in IFN-mediated antiviral responses. In this chapter, we focus our attention on the cellular factors involved in DENV infection, particularly to those that modulate DENV replication through their association with viral RNA. In addition, we also summarize general experimental approaches for identifying the host factors of RNA viruses, including DENV.

Keywords: dengue virus, cellular factors, RNA untranslated regions, interferon-stimulated genes, identification systems

1. Introduction

Dengue virus (DENV) is an enveloped and positive-strand RNA virus that belongs to the genus *Flavivirus* of the Flaviviridae family [1]. An important characteristic of the Flavivirus is that this genus consists of a large number of arthropod-borne viruses, many of which are transmitted by mosquitoes and ticks. In addition, flavivirus infection often causes life-threatening diseases in humans, such as haemorrhagic fever, encephalitis, and meningitis [2]. Recently, the Zika virus (ZIKV), a member of the flavivirus family that has spread explosively throughout the Americas, is reported to be associated with neurological complications [3, 4]. Flaviviruses, therefore, have significant clinical as well as economic impacts on modern society.

DENV is a mosquito-borne virus widely distributed in the tropical and subtropical areas of the world. This flavivirus infection is transmitted to humans via the bite of infected mosquitos. The primary vector of DENV infection is *Aedes aegypti*, while *Aedes albopictus*, which originated in Asia but has extended its range to other regions of the world, is also capable of spreading a dengue outbreak. DENV has four antigenically distinct serotypes (from DENV-1 to DENV-4). Primary infection with one of the serotypes is often asymptomatic or causes self-limiting dengue fever (DF). However, secondary infection of different serotypes increases the risk of more serious forms of DENV infection, such as dengue haemorrhagic fever (DHF) and dengue shock syndrome (DSS), due to the presence of non- or sub-neutralizing antibodies generated during the primary infection. Therefore, dengue is a significant threat to humans, yet there is currently no specific antiviral available for DENV infection [1, 5]. However, it should be noted that a live attenuated vaccine against DENV developed by Sanofi Pasteur (Dengvaxia) has been licensed for use in a limited number of countries, including Mexico and the Philippines, although the efficacy of the DENV vaccine in endemic countries is still under investigation [6].

2. Brief overview of DENV replication

DENV infection begins with its entry into a permissive cell via receptor-mediated endocytosis (**Figure 1**). So far, various types of human cells, such as macrophages, lymphocytes, hepatocytes, and endothelial cells, are reportedly susceptible to DENV infection. Among them, monocyte lineage cells (i.e., dendritic cells [DCs] and macrophages) are thought to be the primary targets of DENV in humans. As the entry receptors of DENV, several cellular proteins, including C-type lectin receptors (e.g., DC-SIGN/CD209, mannose receptor/CD206) and phosphatidylserine receptors (e.g., TIM, TAM), have been demonstrated [7].

Upon entry into the cell, a membrane fusion between DENV envelope (E) glycoprotein and endosomal vesicle occurs, leading to the release of viral RNA into the cytoplasm. The DENV genome is a single-stranded positive-sense RNA and is approximately 10-kb long. The viral RNA contains a single long open reading frame (ORF) flanked by highly structured 5′ and 3′ untranslated regions (UTRs), with a type 1 cap (m7GpppAmp) at the 5′ terminus and no poly(A) tract at the 3′ terminus [8]. The single ORF is translated to a large polyprotein, which is subsequently cleaved co- and post-translationally into three structural (capsid [C], pre-membrane [prM], and E) and seven non-structural (NS) proteins (NS1, NS2A, NS2B, NS3, NS4A, NS4B, and NS5) by viral (NS3) and host proteases (**Figure 1A**). Of the NS proteins, NS5, the largest viral protein, functions as an RNA-dependent RNA polymerase (RdRp), which synthesizes a complementary minus-strand RNA template and, in turn, produces many copies of

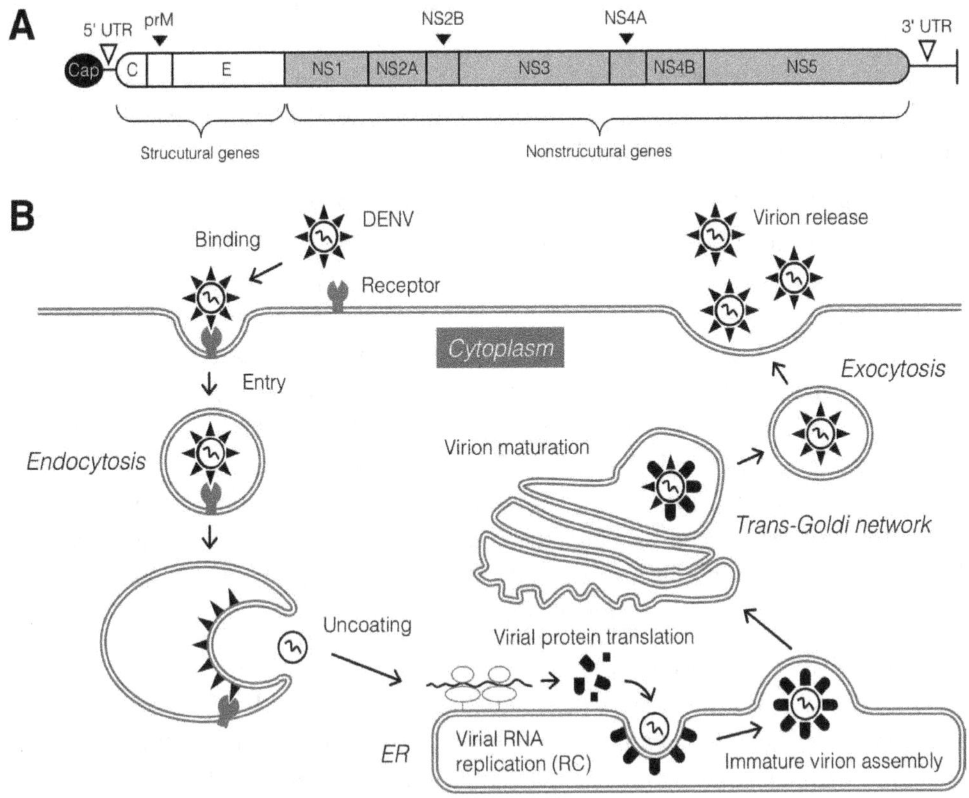

Figure 1. The genome structure and replication cycle of DENV.

positive-strand viral genomic RNA. Viral RNA replication takes place in the so-called replication complexes (RCs) composed of viral RNA and proteins as well as hypothetical cellular proteins, which are formed on the endoplasmic reticulum (ER) membrane. This membrane structure, rearranged by DENV infection, is also the place of viral RNA translation, protein processing, and progeny virion assembly [9]. The immature particles then bud into the ER lumen and are transported through the secretion pathway of the trans-Golgi network, in which progeny virions undergo a maturation process via a conformational change of prM and E proteins on the virion surface. Finally, mature, infectious virions egress from infected cells by exocytosis (**Figure 1B**) [5, 8].

3. Cellular factors involved in DENV replication: interaction with viral RNA untranslated regions

As seen in other RNA and DNA viruses, flaviviruses, including DENV, have been shown to utilize biological processes of the host to replicate efficiently in infected cells through the interaction between viral and cellular proteins. Although the biological relevance of many of the host interactors in *in vivo* replication and the pathogenicity of DENV remain unclear, those virus-host interactions could serve as attractive targets of antiviral drugs [2]. In addition to the entry receptors, intracellular factors implicated in the replication cycle of DENV have been comprehensively reviewed elsewhere [2, 8, 10, 11]. Meanwhile, it is becoming apparent that various cellular cofactors are recruited into the 5′ and 3′ UTRs of DENV RNA, which results in enhanced virus replication [12].

The DENV 5′ and 3′ UTRs are approximately 100 and 350–700 nucleotides long, respectively (**Figure 1A**). The primary sequences located within or adjacent to the UTRs have been shown to be essential for virus replication [8]. For instance, complementary sequences, termed CS (cyclization sequence) elements, found in the ORF of capsid and the 3′ UTR and UAR (upstream of the AUG region) elements, found in the 5′ and 3′ UTRs, are reported to physically anneal to mediate DENV genome cyclization. This cyclization is likely to recruit the DENV RdRp at the 5′ end of the viral genome and then likely to facilitate viral RNA amplification [13]. Additionally, DENV UTRs form stable secondary and tertiary structures, and these structural integrities are thought to be important for the regulation of viral RNA synthesis and translation process. Therefore, albeit the sequences are diverse, UTR secondary structures are highly conserved among flaviviruses [8]. Furthermore, these regions have been demonstrated to contain several cellular proteins [12].

An early study that employed an *in vitro*-formed nucleoprotein complex of synthesized DENV 3′ UTR and mosquito cell extracts identified some RNA-binding proteins—the La autoantigen, translation elongation factor-1α (EF-1α), and polypyrimidine tract-binding protein (PTB)—as the DENV UTR-associated cellular factors in cells [14]. Subsequent studies have also revealed that human La protein binds not only with the DENV 3′ UTR but also with the 5′ UTR [15, 16]. Interestingly, interactions of La protein with viral proteins NS3 and NS5 were shown, suggesting that the La protein is somehow involved in the function of RC in infected cells [15]. The La autoantigen is reported to associate with RNA polymerase III transcription; interestingly, this RNA-binding protein has also been shown to stimulate the translation of viral and cellular mRNAs by binding with their UTRs [17]. As with mosquito EF-1α, its human homologue (i.e., EF1A) has been reported to specifically recognize the conserved 3′-terminal stem-loop (SL) in the 3′ UTR of West Nile virus (WNV) RNA [18]. Given the colocalization of EF-1α with the DENV RC in the infected cell [19], it can be suggested that this cellular protein also plays an important role in the function of flaviviral RNA. However, the precise step of flaviviral replication in which EF-1α is involved remains to be elucidated [19].

PTB is a ubiquitous RNA-binding protein known to be involved in splicing, polyadenylation, stability, and translation of cellular mRNA [20]. With regard to its role in virus infection, PTB has been shown to bind to the UTRs of picornaviruses [21, 22] and the hepatitis C virus (HCV) [23]; it functions as an internal ribosome entry site, (IRES)-trans-acting factor, to activate viral translation [24, 25]. On the other hand, several studies have raised questions about the involvement of PTB in the translation process of those RNA viruses [26–28]. Interestingly, both La and PTB were implicated in HCV replication [29]. In the case of DENV infection, PTB is reportedly required for efficient replication. Furthermore, PTB interacted with a DENV protein, NS4, as well as viral RNA, suggesting that PTB associates with DENV RCs [30]. Although it remains unclear whether PTB regulates DENV RNA simplification or the translation process (or another step of virus infection), PTB may function as a molecular chaperone to stabilize the structured viral RNA [30, 31]. In addition to the host factors mentioned above, recent studies using tobramycin RNA aptamer affinity chromatography identified DDX6 (DEAD-box RNA helicase) and ERI3 (putative 3′–5′ RNA exonuclease) as DENV UTR-binding cellular proteins that promote DENV replication [32, 33].

The genome of flaviviruses, including DENV, encodes enzymes required for viral RNA synthesis (i.e., RdRp and helicase) and viral protein processing (i.e., protease); however, the viral protein translation process must rely fully on the translational machinery of the host [34], except for the methyltransferase activity conferred by NS5, which adds a type 1 7-methylguanosine cap to the 5′ terminus of viral RNA. It is, therefore, not surprising that cellular factors are associated with DENV RNA during viral translation [8, 35]. At the initiation step of eukaryotic mRNA translation, a 5′ cap structure is first recognized by a eukaryotic initiation factor, eIF4E, which, in turn, leads to the recruitment of eIF4G. eIF4G serves as a scaffold protein that binds the DEAD-box RNA helicase eIF4A and also the poly(A)-binding protein (PABP), resulting in the circularization of mRNA [8]. This complex formation induces the association of the 43S ribosomal subunit through the binding of the eIF3 complex. Finally, the 60S ribosomal subunit joins the initiation complex that enables the elongation process of translation [8]. In the case of DENV, its genomic RNA is 5′ capped but lacks 3′-end poly(A) sequences [8]. Nevertheless, PABP is shown to interact with DENV 3′ UTR *in vitro* by recognizing the A-rich regions upstream of 3′ SL in the 3′ UTR [36]. Indeed, a study using chimeras reported that mRNA based on a cellular (globin) gene and DENV RNA revealed that DENV 3′ UTR exhibits functions similar to those of polyadenylated non-viral UTRs in enhancing translation rather than RNA stabilization [37]. Thus, it is plausible that as with cellular mRNA, translated DENV RNA also forms a closed-loop structure via association with host translation factors [38]. In addition, it is demonstrated that DENV RNA may be able to produce proteins by a 5′ cap-independent translation mechanism in certain cellular situations in which the eIF4E is starved and, thereby, canonical host translation is inhibited [39].

4. Experimental procedures for identifying the cellular factors

In the following sections, we summarize several general approaches to search for the cellular factors involved in virus infections.

4.1. Conventional methods using living cells

4.1.1. Gene expression analysis and proteomic analysis

Studies using a microarray system, quantitative RT-PCR analysis, and GeneChip analysis have revealed that the expression levels of many mRNAs in host cells are dramatically altered upon DENV infection [40–42]. It is highly possible that some of these DENV-responsible genes and their products function as crucial positive or negative regulators of DENV replication in cells. Indeed, tumour necrosis factor–related apoptosis-inducing ligand (TRAIL), whose mRNA expression level significantly increased with DENV infection, was found to be a negative regulator of DENV replication [42]. In addition to the analysis of the gene expression profile, the global host protein expression profile upon DENV infection was also investigated by comprehensive proteomic analysis. Conventionally, the total host proteins extracted from infected cells and control cells were separated by two-dimensional PAGE (2-D PAGE), and the proteins whose expression levels were altered by the viral infection were picked up, and their amino acid sequences were determined with mass spectrometry (MS) analysis. Previous studies have identified many host factors that respond to DENV infection [43, 44]. More recently, a proteomic analysis based on stable isotope labelling by amino acids in cell culture (SILAC), which overcame the limitations of sensitivity and resolution of 2-D PAGE, was developed and applied to DENV research [45, 46]. The technologies of high-throughput gene expression analysis and proteomic analysis are thought to be powerful tools for understanding the global cellular expression profile of host cells upon DENV infection, both at the gene and at the protein levels. From the results of these assays alone, however, it is difficult to distinguish whether DENV-responsible host factors that are identified are indeed involved in the regulation of viral replication. To understand the roles and functions of these hit factors requires further functional analysis.

4.1.2. RNAi screening

RNA interference (RNAi) is a well-known approach for identifying novel host factors in virus-infected cells. When the knockdown of a host gene by RNAi alters the efficiency of viral replication, it is highly possible that this gene works as a host factor of the virus. Currently, commercial siRNA pools that cover most human genes are available, and many genome-wide comprehensive screenings for many kinds of viruses have been performed thus far [47–49]. In studies of flaviviruses, hundreds of host factor proteins involved with the early steps of WNV infection have been identified by silencing more than 20,000 human genes from a small interfering RNA (siRNA) pool [50]. An additional bioinformatic study, followed by the siRNA screening, revealed that many of these hits were involved in the ubiquitin-proteasome pathway and the ER-associated degradation (ERAD) pathway, both of which are essential for many steps of viral replication. In addition to host factors in human cells, one study aimed to identify host factors from insect cells, another host of DENV [51]. In that study of DENV-adapted cells from *Drosophila melanogaster* and an siRNA pool targeting more than 20,000 genes of *Drosophila*, the proteins that accelerate or inhibit the replication of DENV in *Drosophila* cells were identified [51]. Then human analogues of hit genes in *Drosophila* cells were subsequently silenced in DENV-infected human cultured cells, and 42 of these were found to be common host factors in human and *Drosophila* cells [51]. It is noteworthy that RNAi screening can identify host factors that can affect viral replication either by direct interaction with viral components or by indirect interaction, such as the regulation of the IFN pathway.

4.1.3. Yeast two-hybrid analysis

For researchers attempting to identify host factors that directly interact with viral proteins, yeast two-hybrid (Y2H) analysis is a common and effective way; numerous host factors of many viruses, including DENV, have been identified using this system [52–58]. Taking advantage of good throughput, several large screenings were performed to build DENV host interactomes using human cDNA libraries. One study reported that a Y2H analysis using either partial or full-length DNA fragments encoding each DENV protein and the human liver cDNA library identified 105 viral-host interactions; further knockdown experiments using siRNAs revealed that six proteins were essential for the efficient viral replication of DENV [59]. Another study also carried out a Y2H assay using NS3 and NS5 proteins from DENV and other flaviviruses as bait, and 108 human proteins were identified as interacting with NS3 or NS5 or both [60]. In addition, Y2H assays were performed to identify DENV proteins interacting with host factors from human and mosquito cDNA libraries. They identified several common host factors conserved in both humans and mosquitos [61]. These studies identified many host proteins that interact with DENV proteins; however, few of the hits overlap in independent studies. Although this might be caused mainly by the fact that the assay in each study was performed in different conditions and with different cDNA libraries, it is also possible that each study includes many false positives and false negatives.

4.2. Wheat germ–based protein array system

4.2.1. Overview of the protein array technology

As described above, the living cell-based methods are powerful tools for identifying viral-host interactions since the assays could be carried out under physiological conditions, at least partially. However, these methods have several disadvantages. First, proteins whose expression levels are quite low or that show cytotoxicity are hard to analyse. Second, immunoprecipitation assays are commonly used to detect the interaction between a protein and a protein; however, the number of interactions that can be detected at one time is limited. Therefore, it is highly possible that many researchers have potentially overlooked important but difficult-to-detect interactions in their first screenings using living cells. To solve these problems, we recently developed a novel biochemical screening method based on a wheat germ cell–free protein synthesis system (wheat cell-free system) and high-throughput binding assay. The wheat cell-free system enables the synthesis of various kinds of eukaryotic proteins in a 96-well format [62]. So far, proteins having several transmembrane domains, relatively large molecular weights, and cytotoxic activity were successfully synthesized by this system [63, 64]. This robust protein synthesis system allows us to establish a "protein array", from which tens to thousands of recombinant proteins sorted by their functions were arrayed into each well of a 96-well plate [65]. The protein arrays currently available in our research group are shown in **Table 1** [65–70]. Based on these protein arrays, we have established a high-throughput binding assay for identifying proteins directly bound to target proteins from the array. To perform hundreds to tens of thousands of binding reactions, a luminescent-based binding assay, called AlphaScreen, was employed [65, 66, 71]. This assay is able to use crude translation products of wheat cell-free synthesis to detect binding reactions by mixing these crude proteins in a 384-well plate, followed by adding two beads and the antibody for detection. Because of its flexibility, AlphaScreen can be used not only as a binding assay but also as a protein cleavage assay for a viral protease. The principle of the assays is shown in **Figure 2**.

Protein array	Origin	Number of proteins	References
Protein kinase	Human and mouse	400	Masaki et al. [66], Miyakawa et al. [67], Kudoh et al. [68]
E3 ligase	Human and mouse	250	Takahashi et al. [65], Tan et al. [69]
Deubiquitinating enzyme	Human	85	Unpublished
Single transmembrane protein	Human and mouse	730	Unpublished
Auto-antigen protein	Human and mouse	2100	Matsuoka et al. [70]

Table 1. Wheat cell–free-based protein arrays currently available in our research group.

4.2.2. Practical applications for viral research

We and other research groups have done several assays using this technology to identify host proteins that interacted with viral proteins. In researching the HCV (a virus related to DENV), several protein kinases were found to bind directly with the HCV non-structural protein NS5A using the protein kinase array; by phosphorylating NS5A through additional functional analysis using a cultured cell system, one protein kinase, Casein kinase I-α, was found to regulate viral replication [66]. The protein kinase array was used to identify other host factors that

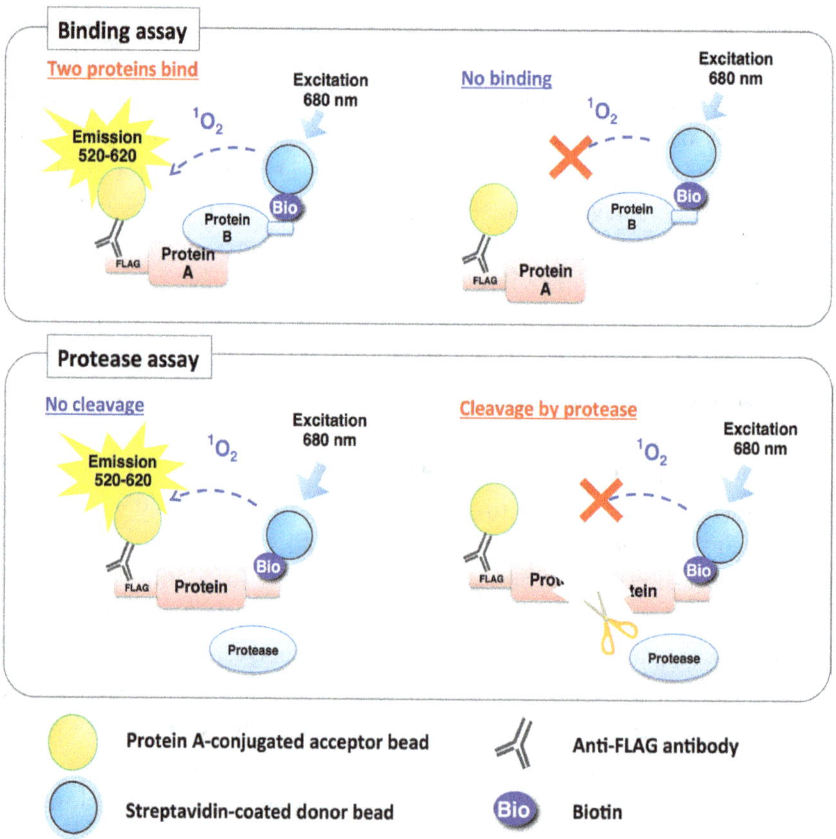

Figure 2. A schematic diagram of binding assay and protease assay based on AlphaScreen technology.

functionally interacted with human immunodeficiency virus (HIV) proteins [67, 68]. In the case of the protease assay, one research article demonstrated that a protease from xenotropic murine leukaemia virus-related virus (XMRV) and 24 cellular proteins that were target candidates of the viral protease were synthesized; *in vitro* cleavage assay revealed several novel substrates of XMRV protease [72], indicating the feasibility of using wheat cell–free-based protein array technology and high-throughput biochemical assay based on AlphaScreen.

4.2.3. *Wheat cell–free protein array for DENV research*

Thus far, NS3 and NS5 proteins of DENV have been considered difficult to synthesize as full-length active recombinant proteins using a conventional protein expression system, such as for *Escherichia coli*. We previously reported that the wheat cell-free system successfully synthesized full-length NS3 and NS5 proteins in a soluble form; some biochemical analyses revealed that both recombinant proteins possessed enzymatic activities [63], indicating the usefulness of the expression system for the preparation of DENV proteins. In addition to these soluble proteins, NS4B, a protein with at least three transmembrane domains, was synthesized with the wheat cell-free system (**Figure 3A**). Our preliminary study demonstrated that NS4B was

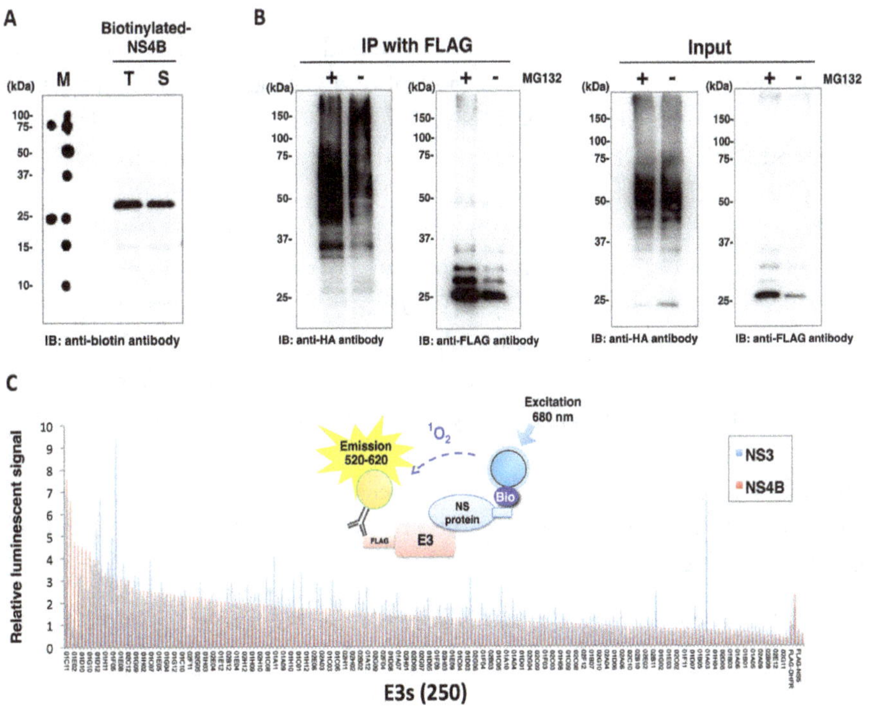

Figure 3. Identification of E3 ligases targeting DENV NS4B by wheat cell-free-based protein array system. (A) Expression of biotinylated NS4B with wheat cell-free system. The total translation products of NS4B (T) and supernatant (S) after centrifugation of the total translation product were subjected to SDS-PAGE, followed by immunoblot analysis using anti-biotin antibody. M is the molecular marker. (B) Ubiquitination of NS4B. HEK293T cells overexpressing FLAG-tagged NS4B and HA-tagged ubiquitin were treated with proteasomal inhibitor MG132, and FLAG-tagged NS4B was precipitated with anti-FLAG antibody. The NS4B and ubiquitin were detected by immunoblot analysis using anti-FLAG antibody and anti-HA antibody, respectively. (C) AlphaScreen assay to identify the E3s targeting DENV NS3 and NS4B proteins using the E3 protein array. Biotinylated NS3 and NS4B were used as bait, and biotinylated DHFR was used as negative control of NS proteins. The relative luminescent signal was calculated as follows: the value from E3 and NS4B/value from E3 and DHFR.

highly ubiquitinated when NS4B was overexpressed in HEK293T cells (**Figure 3B**), suggesting that the amount of NS4B expressed was regulated in host cells in a ubiquitin/proteasome-dependent manner. When a protein is ubiquitinated and, subsequently, degraded by the 26S proteasome, E3 is a determinant of the ubiquitination, as E3 specifically binds to the target protein and transfers activated ubiquitin from the ubiquitin conjugation enzyme, E2 [73]. Therefore, we screened NS4B-binding E3s from the E3 protein array using AlphaScreen, as we recently reported [65]. NS3 was used as control to determine the NS4B-specific E3s. As shown in **Figure 3C**, many E3s were found to bind with recombinant NS4B. Currently, additional functional analysis, such as *in vitro* ubiquitination assay and protein degradation assay in cells, is ongoing.

5. Restriction of DENV infection by cellular inhibitors

As previously mentioned, DENV hijacks the host's biological process for its efficient replication. Meanwhile, it has become apparent that DENV infection can be limited by cellular factors. In this sense, the innate immune response induced by IFN is considered to be the first line of defence against DENV [8]

Generally, RNA viruses that infect target cells are sensed by the pattern recognition receptors (PRRs), which specifically recognize a component of invading viruses. As for DENV infection, the membrane-bound Toll-like receptors (TLR3, TLR7, TLR8) and the cytosolic receptors (retinoic acid-inducible gene I [RIG-I], melanoma differentiation-associated gene 5 [MDA5]) are reported to be the PRRs for viral RNA [74–77]. These recognitions in turn activate adaptor molecules of the PRR, leading to the activation of a downstream phosphorylation cascade and the subsequent production of IFN and pro-inflammatory cytokines (**Figure 4**) [78]. Among the IFNs produced, type I IFNs, including IFNα, IFN-β, and IFN-ω, play an important role in antiviral immunity [79]. The type I IFN then binds to its receptors (IFNAR) on neighbouring cells and signals to induce the phosphorylation of signal transducers and the activators of transcriptions 1 and 2 (STAT1 and 2) in cytoplasm. This phosphorylation of STAT1/2 triggers the formation of IFN-stimulated gene factor 3 (ISGF3) with IFN-regulatory factor 9 (IRF9). Finally, the ISGF3 complex translocates to the nucleus and acts as a transcription activator for the expression of a number of genes by binding to the IFN-stimulated response elements (ISREs) on chromosomes (**Figure 4**) [80].

As seen above, IFN is considered to be an inducer of the antiviral state, and it has been well demonstrated that actual antiviral effector molecules in the IFN response are a subset of the genes upregulated by IFN, which are called IFN-stimulated genes (ISGs). Thus far, hundreds of genes have been classified as ISGs, and many of them are reported to have inhibitory effects on divergent families of viruses, including flaviviruses [80–83]. Importantly, several ISGs have also been shown to restrict DENV infection, and their suppressive effects are likely to be exerted at the multiple steps of virus replication, including virus entry (IFITMs [84, 85], ADAP2 [86]), viral RNA/protein synthesis (ISG20 [87], viperin [88, 89]), and infectious virion production (tetherin [90], ISG15 [91, 92]). In addition, a comprehensive study using an overexpression of a cDNA library derived from known ISGs demonstrates the involvement of

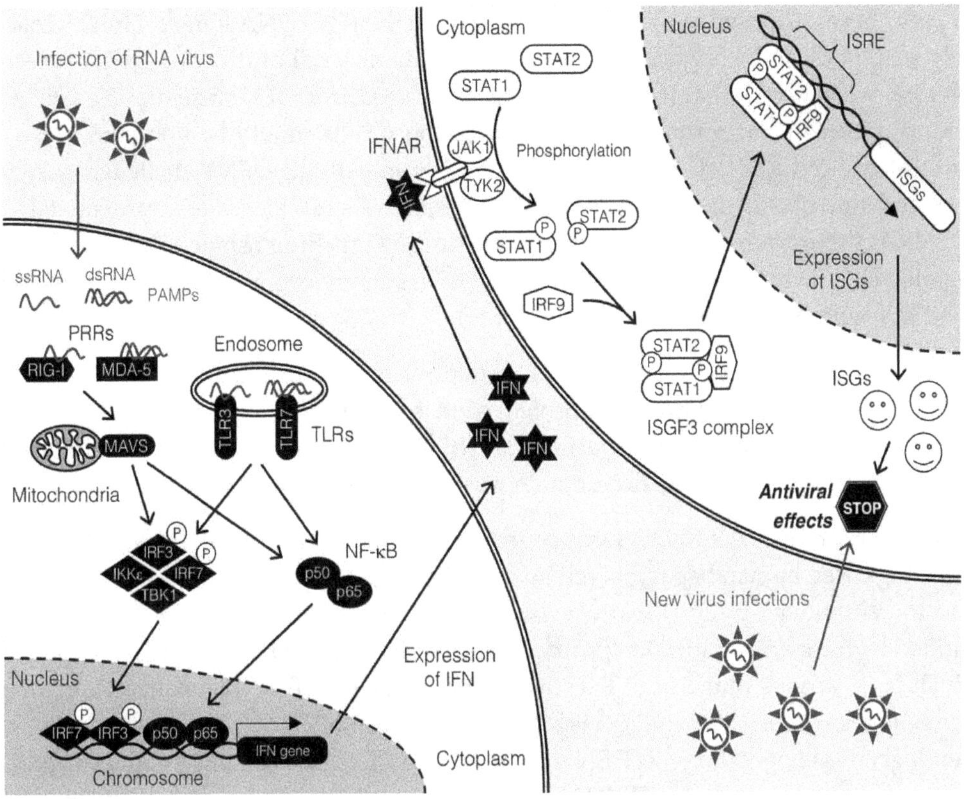

Figure 4. Intracellular recognition of RNA viruses and IFN responses (left). PRRs-sensing virus-specific nucleic acid structures (ssRNA and dsRNA) activate signalling cascades via phosphorylation of transcription factors (IRF3 and IRF7), which leads to the expression of IFN genes together with NF-κB (right). Binding of IFNs produced from virus-infected cells to type I IFN receptor (IFNAR) activates JAK1 and TYK2, which, in turn, phosphorylate STAT1 and STAT2. Phosphorylation of STAT1/2 induces the formation of ISGF3 complex with IRF9, and finally, ISGF3 translocated in nucleus binds to ISREs to induce ISG expressions. ssRNA, single-stranded RNA; dsRNA, double-stranded RNA; MAVS, mitochondrial antiviral-signalling protein; JAK1, Janus kinase 1; and TYK2, tyrosine kinase 2.

many more ISGs in the restriction of DENV [93]. However, the precise mechanisms of these ISG-mediated anti-DENV activities remain unclear, and we will have to wait for future studies for detailed analysis.

6. Identification of RyDEN/C19orf66 as novel anti-DENV ISG

It has been well demonstrated that a gain-of-function (i.e., overexpression) screen of cDNA is a powerful approach to identifying antiviral ISGs [82, 83, 93, 94]. In a recent study, we employed the gain-of-function strategy using a pool of cDNA library derived from type 1 IFN-treated cells to search for ISGs suppressing DENV replication in human cells [95]. In this approach, a human cervical carcinoma cell line, HeLa, was treated with type I IFN (a mixture of human IFN-α and -ω) for 24 hours at a concentration that had been reported to inhibit DENV infection *in vitro* [96], and mRNA from the IFN-treated HeLa cells was converted into a library of cDNA and transferred to a HIV-based lentiviral vector. Then, a human hepatoma cell line, Huh7.5, was exposed to the HIV vector carrying the IFN cDNA library. Huh7.5 cells are highly susceptible to DENV and, therefore, exhibit massive cell death upon DENV infection. Therefore, we expected that if anti-DENV genes derived from IFN-treated HeLa cells were introduced into DENV-permissive Huh7.5 cells, those cells should be non-permissive and survive DENV-induced cell death. As anticipated, even with the DENV challenge, surviving cell clones were obtained; subsequent sequencing analysis revealed that approximately half of DENV-resistant clones harboured an ORF of a gene on chromosome 19, *C19orf66*, in the integrated HIV vector genome [95]. Since *C19orf66* was a previously uncharacterized gene, we named this *r*epressor of *y*ield of *DEN*V (RyDEN).

The ORF of RyDEN (*C19orf66*) encodes a 291 amino acid protein, and the secondary structure prediction suggested that the RyDEN protein contained a nuclear localization signal (NLS) in the middle region and a nuclear export signal (NES) in the C-terminal region. Additionally, a characteristic glutamic acid (E)-rich domain was found in the C-terminus.

The anti-DENV activity of RyDEN was confirmed by creating stable cell lines that expressed epitope tag-fused human hepatoma cell lines, and all DENV serotypes (i.e., DENV-1–4) were found to be inhibited by RyDEN expressions. In line with the fact that this gene was first identified by the gain-of-function approach using an IFN-derived cDNA library, expressions of RyDEN in various human cell lines were upregulated by IFN treatment to a greater or lesser extent, indicating that RyDEN is a bona fide anti-DENV ISG. More importantly, when the endogenous expression of RyDEN mRNA was knocked down by RNAi, the suppressive activity of type I IFNs against DENV became less effective, suggesting that RyDEN was a major contributor of the IFN-mediated anti-DENV response [95].

One question to ponder: what is the molecular mechanism by which RyDEN suppresses DENV replication? Affinity purification-mass spectrometry analysis with affinity tag-fused RyDEN found that RyDEN interacted with two other cellular proteins, poly(A)-binding protein cytoplasmic 1 (PABPC1) and La motif-related protein 1 (LARP1). PABPC1 is a member of the PABP family; as described above, this protein bridges the 5′ and 3′ ends of mRNA by binding both the eIF4G and the poly(A) tail, which stimulates the initiation of translation [97]. LARP1 is also an RNA-binding protein and one of the LARPS, which shares the signature motif with the La autoantigen, called the La motif (LM). Therefore, Larp and La proteins are categorized as being in the same family [98]. Intriguingly, LARP1 is shown to interact with PABP to stimulate the mRNA translation process [99, 100]. Considering the positive effect of PABP on translation [97], the association of PABPC1 and LARP1 with RyDEN suggests that RyDEN might interfere with the translation of DENV RNA by inhibiting PABPC1 and LARP1 functions. Indeed, this speculation was supported by the following findings: (i) an RNAi-mediated knockdown of PABPC1 and LARP1 significantly reduced the level of DENV replication, (ii) PABPC1 interacted with DENV RNA in infected cells, (iii) the expression of RyDEN suppressed the expression of the reporter protein from a DENV-based sub-genomic RNA replicon that lacked structural (C, prM, E) genes, and (iv) the recruitment of RyDEN to the DENV RNA 3′ UTR was enhanced by the presence of PABPC1 *in vitro* [95]. Therefore, one could envisage that the anti-DENV activity of RyDEN, an antiviral ISG, is exerted during the translation of viral RNA by associating PABPC1/LARP1 with the 3′ UTR and somehow interfering with the function of the translation factors (**Figure 5**). Or another possibility is that

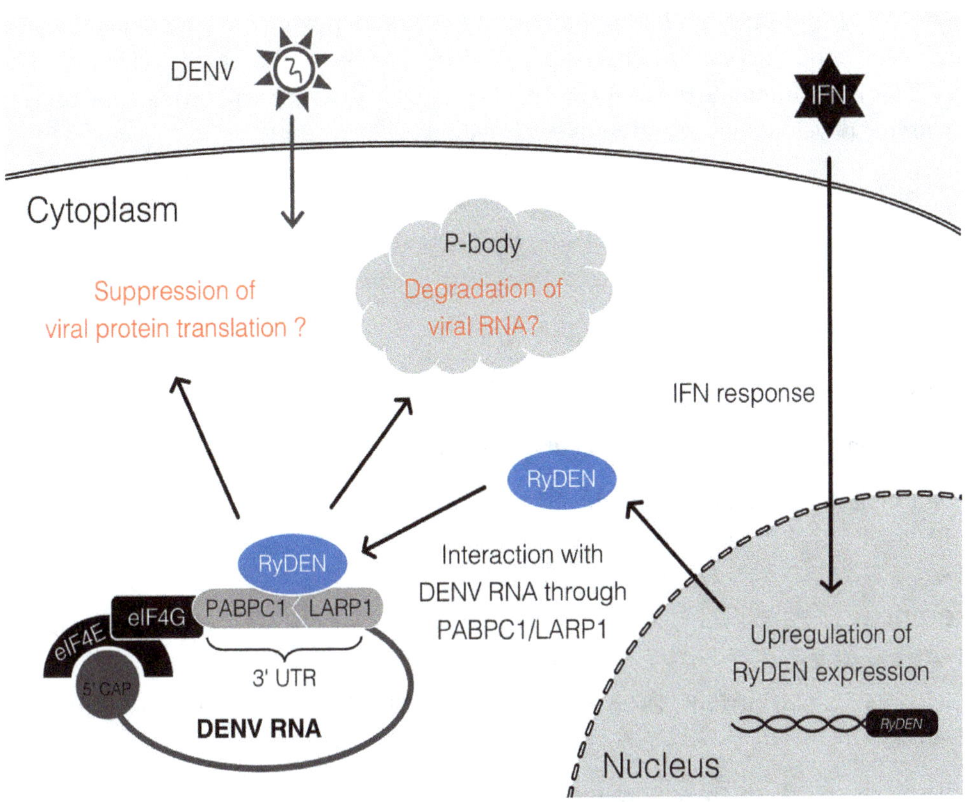

Figure 5. Possible mechanisms by which RyDEN restricts the function of DENV RNA. RyDEN, whose expression is upregulated by IFN, associates with DENV RNA through interaction with PABPC1 and LARP1 that are required for DENV replication. This association may result in (i) translational suppression or (ii) degradation of viral RNA in the cytoplasm.

RyDEN may facilitate the degradation of viral RNA, since PABPC1 and LARP1 have been reported to be involved in eukaryotic mRNA decay as processing body (P-body) and stress granule (SG) components (**Figure 5**) [99, 101]. In accordance with this notion, a recent study revealed that RyDEN (also referred to as FLJ11286 or IRAV) was colocalized with cytoplasmic P-bodies in IFN-treated cells [102]. Furthermore, it was noteworthy that RyDEN expression limited a diverse range of RNA and DNA viruses [83, 95, 102], indicating that RyDEN is a broad-spectrum antiviral ISG.

7. Concluding remarks

This chapter highlighted the molecular interactions between DENV and host factors, particularly focused on the cellular regulation of DENV replication. As is well known, IFN response is one of the host controls of DENV infection and pathogenesis [96, 103, 104]. Although the effector molecules in the IFN response that actually interfere with virus replication remain fully clarified, profound efforts have been made to identify the IFN-inducible cellular factors restricting RNA virus replication, including DENV [80]. It should be noted that antagonistic effects of DENV infection on IFN signalling and production, which are mediated by several means using viral factors, are observed [105–107]. However, the characterization of anti-DENV ISGs is to illuminate the "heel of Achilles" of DENV, which will provide the underpinnings for the development of antivirals against dengue.

Author details

Hirotaka Takahashi[1] and Youichi Suzuki[2]*

*Address all correspondence to: californiacircle@gmail.com

1 Proteo-Science Center, Ehime University, Matsuyama, Japan

2 Department of Microbiology and Infection Control, Osaka Medical College, Takatsuki, Japan

References

[1] Guzman MG, Harris E. Dengue. Lancet. 2015;**385**:453-465. doi:10.1016/S0140-6736(14) 60572-9

[2] Pastorino B, Nougairede A, Wurtz N, Gould E, de Lamballerie X. Role of host cell factors in flavivirus infection: implications for pathogenesis and development of antiviral drugs. Antiviral Research. 2010;**87**:281-294. doi:10.1016/j.antiviral.2010.04.014

[3] Basarab M, Bowman C, Aarons EJ, Cropley I. Zika virus. BMJ. 2016;**352**:i1049. doi: 10.1136/bmj.i1049

[4] Becker R. Missing link: animal models to study whether Zika causes birth defects. Nature Medicine. 2016;**22**:225-227. doi:10.1038/nm0316-225

[5] Diamond MS, Pierson TC. Molecular insight into dengue virus pathogenesis and its implications for disease control. Cell. 2015;**162**:488-492. doi:10.1016/j.cell.2015.07.005

[6] Villar L, Dayan GH, Arredondo-Garcia JL, Rivera DM, Cunha R, Deseda C, Reynales H, Costa MS, Morales-Ramirez JO, Carrasquilla G, Rey LC, Dietze R, Luz K, Rivas E, Miranda Montoya MC, Cortes Supelano M, Zambrano B, Langevin E, Boaz M, Tornieporth N, Saville M, Noriega F, Group CYDS. Efficacy of a tetravalent dengue vaccine in children in Latin America. New England Journal of Medicine. 2015;**372**:113-123. doi:10.1056/NEJMoa1411037

[7] Perera-Lecoin M, Meertens L, Carnec X, Amara A. Flavivirus entry receptors: an update. Viruses. 2013;**6**:69-88. doi:10.3390/v6010069

[8] Clyde K, Kyle JL, Harris E. Recent advances in deciphering viral and host determinants of dengue virus replication and pathogenesis. Journal of Virology. 2006;**80**:11418-11431. doi:10.1128/JVI.01257-06

[9] den Boon JA, Diaz A, Ahlquist P. Cytoplasmic viral replication complexes. Cell Host Microbe. 2010;**8**:77-85. doi:10.1016/j.chom.2010.06.010

[10] Fischl W, Bartenschlager R. Exploitation of cellular pathways by Dengue virus. Current Opinion in Microbiology. 2011;**14**:470-475. doi:10.1016/j.mib.2011.07.012

[11] Krishnan MN, Garcia-Blanco MA. Targeting host factors to treat West Nile and dengue viral infections. Viruses. 2014;**6**:683-708. doi:10.3390/v6020683

[12] Bidet K, Garcia-Blanco MA. Flaviviral RNAs: weapons and targets in the war between virus and host. Biochemical Journal. 2014;**462**:215-230. doi:10.1042/BJ20140456

[13] Villordo SM, Gamarnik AV. Genome cyclization as strategy for flavivirus RNA replication. Virus Research. 2009;**139**:230-239. doi:10.1016/j.virusres.2008.07.016

[14] De Nova-Ocampo M, Villegas-Sepulveda N, del Angel RM. Translation elongation factor-1alpha, La, and PTB interact with the 3′ untranslated region of dengue 4 virus RNA. Virology. 2002;**295**:337-347. doi:10.1006/viro.2002.1407

[15] Garcia-Montalvo BM, Medina F, del Angel RM. La protein binds to NS5 and NS3 and to the 5′ and 3′ ends of Dengue 4 virus RNA. Virus Research. 2004;**102**:141-150. doi:10.1016/j.virusres.2004.01.024

[16] Yocupicio-Monroy RM, Medina F, Reyes-del Valle J, del Angel RM. Cellular proteins from human monocytes bind to dengue 4 virus minus-strand 3′ untranslated region RNA. Journal of Virology. 2003;**77**:3067-3076.

[17] Bousquet-Antonelli C, Deragon JM. A comprehensive analysis of the La-motif protein superfamily. RNA. 2009;**15**:750-764. doi:10.1261/rna.1478709

[18] Blackwell JL, Brinton MA. Translation elongation factor-1 alpha interacts with the 3′ stem-loop region of West Nile virus genomic RNA. Journal of Virology. 1997;**71**:6433-6444.

[19] Davis WG, Blackwell JL, Shi PY, Brinton MA. Interaction between the cellular protein eEF1A and the 3′-terminal stem-loop of West Nile virus genomic RNA facilitates viral minus-strand RNA synthesis. Journal of Virology. 2007;**81**:10172-10187. doi:10.1128/JVI.00531-07

[20] Romanelli MG, Diani E, Lievens PM. New insights into functional roles of the polypyrimidine tract-binding protein. International Journal of Molecular Sciences. 2013;**14**:22906-22932. doi:10.3390/ijms141122906

[21] Hellen CU, Witherell GW, Schmid M, Shin SH, Pestova TV, Gil A, Wimmer E. A cytoplasmic 57-kDa protein that is required for translation of picornavirus RNA by internal ribosomal entry is identical to the nuclear pyrimidine tract-binding protein. Proceedings of the National Academy of Sciences of the United States of America. 1993;**90**:7642-7646.

[22] Jang SK, Wimmer E. Cap-independent translation of encephalomyocarditis virus RNA: structural elements of the internal ribosomal entry site and involvement of a cellular 57-kD RNA-binding protein. Genes and Development. 1990;**4**:1560-1572.

[23] Ito T, Lai MM. An internal polypyrimidine-tract-binding protein-binding site in the hepatitis C virus RNA attenuates translation, which is relieved by the 3′-untranslated sequence. Virology. 1999;**254**:288-296. doi:10.1006/viro.1998.9541

[24] Jang SK. Internal initiation: IRES elements of picornaviruses and hepatitis c virus. Virus Research. 2006;**119**:2-15. doi:10.1016/j.virusres.2005.11.003

[25] Martinez-Salas E, Pacheco A, Serrano P, Fernandez N. New insights into internal ribosome entry site elements relevant for viral gene expression. Journal of General Virology. 2008;**89**:611-626. doi:10.1099/vir.0.83426-0

[26] Aizaki H, Choi KS, Liu M, Li YJ, Lai MM. Polypyrimidine-tract-binding protein is a component of the HCV RNA replication complex and necessary for RNA synthesis. Journal of Biomedical Science. 2006;**13**:469-480. doi:10.1007/s11373-006-9088-4

[27] Choi KS, Huang P, Lai MM. Polypyrimidine-tract-binding protein affects transcription but not translation of mouse hepatitis virus RNA. Virology. 2002;**303**:58-68.

[28] Tischendorf JJ, Beger C, Korf M, Manns MP, Kruger M. Polypyrimidine tract-binding protein (PTB) inhibits Hepatitis C virus internal ribosome entry site (HCV IRES)-mediated translation, but does not affect HCV replication. Archives of Virology. 2004;**149**:1955-1970.

[29] Domitrovich AM, Diebel KW, Ali N, Sarker S, Siddiqui A. Role of La autoantigen and polypyrimidine tract-binding protein in HCV replication. Virology. 2005;**335**:72-86. doi:10.1016/j.virol.2005.02.009

[30] Anwar A, Leong KM, Ng ML, Chu JJ, Garcia-Blanco MA. The polypyrimidine tract-binding protein is required for efficient dengue virus propagation and associates with the viral replication machinery. Journal of Biological Chemistry. 2009;**284**:17021-17029. doi:10.1074/jbc.M109.006239

[31] Karakasiliotis I, Chaudhry Y, Roberts LO, Goodfellow IG. Feline calicivirus replication: requirement for polypyrimidine tract-binding protein is temperature-dependent. Journal of General Virology. 2006;**87**:3339-3347. doi:10.1099/vir.0.82153-0

[32] Ward AM, Bidet K, Yinglin A, Ler SG, Hogue K, Blackstock W, Gunaratne J, Garcia-Blanco MA. Quantitative mass spectrometry of DENV-2 RNA-interacting proteins reveals that the DEAD-box RNA helicase DDX6 binds the DB1 and DB2 3′ UTR structures. RNA Biology. 2011;**8**:1173-1186. doi:10.4161/rna.8.6.17836

[33] Ward AM, Calvert ME, Read LR, Kang S, Levitt BE, Dimopoulos G, Bradrick SS, Gunaratne J, Garcia-Blanco MA. The Golgi associated ERI3 is a flavivirus host factor. Scientific Reports. 2016;**6**:34379. doi:10.1038/srep34379

[34] Jackson RJ, Hellen CU, Pestova TV. The mechanism of eukaryotic translation initiation and principles of its regulation. Nature Reviews: Molecular Cell Biology. 2010;**11**:113-127. doi:10.1038/nrm2838

[35] Li MM, MacDonald MR, Rice CM. To translate, or not to translate: viral and host mRNA regulation by interferon-stimulated genes. Trends in Cell Biology. 2015;**25**:320-329. doi:10.1016/j.tcb.2015.02.001

[36] Polacek C, Friebe P, Harris E. Poly(A)-binding protein binds to the non-polyadenylated 3′ untranslated region of dengue virus and modulates translation efficiency. Journal of General Virology. 2009;**90**:687-692. doi:10.1099/vir.0.007021-0

[37] Chiu WW, Kinney RM, Dreher TW. Control of translation by the 5′- and 3′-terminal regions of the dengue virus genome. Journal of Virology. 2005;**79**:8303-8315. doi:10.1128/JVI.79.13.8303-8315.2005

[38] Edgil D, Harris E. End-to-end communication in the modulation of translation by mammalian RNA viruses. Virus Research. 2006;**119**:43-51. doi:10.1016/j.virusres.2005.10.012

[39] Edgil D, Polacek C, Harris E. Dengue virus utilizes a novel strategy for translation initiation when cap-dependent translation is inhibited. Journal of Virology. 2006;**80**:2976-2986. doi:10.1128/JVI.80.6.2976-2986.2006

[40] Liew KJ, Chow VT. Differential display RT-PCR analysis of ECV304 endothelial-like cells infected with dengue virus type 2 reveals messenger RNA expression profiles of multiple human genes involved in known and novel roles. Journal of Medical Virology. 2004;**72**:597-609. doi:10.1002/jmv.20034

[41] Warke RV, Xhaja K, Martin KJ, Fournier MF, Shaw SK, Brizuela N, de Bosch N, Lapointe D, Ennis FA, Rothman AL, Bosch I. Dengue virus induces novel changes in gene expression of human umbilical vein endothelial cells. Journal of Virology. 2003;**77**: 11822-11832.

[42] Warke RV, Martin KJ, Giaya K, Shaw SK, Rothman AL, Bosch I. TRAIL is a novel antiviral protein against dengue virus. Journal of Virology. 2008;**82**:555-564. doi:10.1128/JVI.01694-06

[43] Higa LM, Caruso MB, Canellas F, Soares MR, Oliveira-Carvalho AL, Chapeaurouge DA, Almeida PM, Perales J, Zingali RB, Da Poian AT. Secretome of HepG2 cells infected with dengue virus: implications for pathogenesis. Biochimica et Biophysica Acta. 2008;**1784**:1607-1616. doi:10.1016/j.bbapap.2008.06.015

[44] Kanlaya R, Pattanakitsakul SN, Sinchaikul S, Chen ST, Thongboonkerd V. The ubiquitin-proteasome pathway is important for dengue virus infection in primary human endothelial cells. Journal of Proteome Research. 2010;**9**:4960-4971. doi:10.1021/pr100219y

[45] Chiu HC, Hannemann H, Heesom KJ, Matthews DA, Davidson AD. High-throughput quantitative proteomic analysis of dengue virus type 2 infected A549 cells. PLoS One. 2014;**9**:e93305. doi:10.1371/journal.pone.0093305

[46] Viktorovskaya OV, Greco TM, Cristea IM, Thompson SR. Identification of RNA binding proteins associated with dengue virus RNA in infected cells reveals temporally distinct host factor requirements. PLoS Neglected Tropical Diseases. 2016;**10**:e0004921. doi:10.1371/journal.pntd.0004921

[47] Zhou H, Xu M, Huang Q, Gates AT, Zhang XD, Castle JC, Stec E, Ferrer M, Strulovici B, Hazuda DJ, Espeseth AS. Genome-scale RNAi screen for host factors required for HIV replication. Cell Host Microbe. 2008;**4**:495-504. doi:10.1016/j.chom.2008.10.004

[48] Brass AL, Dykxhoorn DM, Benita Y, Yan N, Engelman A, Xavier RJ, Lieberman J, Elledge SJ. Identification of host proteins required for HIV infection through a functional genomic screen. Science. 2008;**319**:921-926. doi:10.1126/science.1152725

[49] Tai AW, Benita Y, Peng LF, Kim SS, Sakamoto N, Xavier RJ, Chung RT. A functional genomic screen identifies cellular cofactors of hepatitis C virus replication. Cell Host Microbe. 2009;**5**:298-307. doi:10.1016/j.chom.2009.02.001

[50] Krishnan MN, Ng A, Sukumaran B, Gilfoy FD, Uchil PD, Sultana H, Brass AL, Adametz R, Tsui M, Qian F, Montgomery RR, Lev S, Mason PW, Koski RA, Elledge SJ, Xavier RJ, Agaisse H, Fikrig E. RNA interference screen for human genes associated with West Nile virus infection. Nature. 2008;**455**:242-245. doi:10.1038/nature07207

[51] Sessions OM, Barrows NJ, Souza-Neto JA, Robinson TJ, Hershey CL, Rodgers MA, Ramirez JL, Dimopoulos G, Yang PL, Pearson JL, Garcia-Blanco MA. Discovery of insect and human dengue virus host factors. Nature. 2009;**458**:1047-1050. doi:10.1038/nature07967

[52] Duan X, Lu X, Li J, Liu Y. Novel binding between pre-membrane protein and vacuolar ATPase is required for efficient dengue virus secretion. Biochemical and Biophysical Research Communications. 2008;**373**:319-324. doi:10.1016/j.bbrc.2008.06.041

[53] Shapira SD, Gat-Viks I, Shum BO, Dricot A, de Grace MM, Wu L, Gupta PB, Hao T, Silver SJ, Root DE, Hill DE, Regev A, Hacohen N. A physical and regulatory map of host-influenza interactions reveals pathways in H_1N_1 infection. Cell. 2009;**139**:1255-1267. doi:10.1016/j.cell.2009.12.018

[54] Falcon AM, Fortes P, Marion RM, Beloso A, Ortin J. Interaction of influenza virus NS1 protein and the human homologue of Staufen *in vivo* and *in vitro*. Nucleic Acids Research. 1999;**27**:2241-2247.

[55] Gao L, Tu H, Shi ST, Lee KJ, Asanaka M, Hwang SB, Lai MM. Interaction with a ubiquitin-like protein enhances the ubiquitination and degradation of hepatitis C virus RNA-dependent RNA polymerase. Journal of Virology. 2003;**77**:4149-4159.

[56] Taguwa S, Okamoto T, Abe T, Mori Y, Suzuki T, Moriishi K, Matsuura Y. Human butyrate-induced transcript 1 interacts with hepatitis C virus NS5A and regulates viral replication. Journal of Virology. 2008;**82**:2631-2641. doi:10.1128/JVI.02153-07

[57] Ambrosino C, Palmieri C, Puca A, Trimboli F, Schiavone M, Olimpico F, Ruocco MR, di Leva F, Toriello M, Quinto I, Venuta S, Scala G. Physical and functional interaction of HIV-1 Tat with E2F-4, a transcriptional regulator of mammalian cell cycle. Journal of Biological Chemistry. 2002;**277**:31448-31458. doi:10.1074/jbc.M112398200

[58] Kalpana GV, Marmon S, Wang W, Crabtree GR, Goff SP. Binding and stimulation of HIV-1 integrase by a human homolog of yeast transcription factor SNF5. Science. 1994;**266**:2002-2006.

[59] Khadka S, Vangeloff AD, Zhang C, Siddavatam P, Heaton NS, Wang L, Sengupta R, Sahasrabudhe S, Randall G, Gribskov M, Kuhn RJ, Perera R, LaCount DJ. A physical

interaction network of dengue virus and human proteins. Molecular & Cellular Proteomics. 2011;**10**:M111.012187. doi:10.1074/mcp.M111.012187

[60] Le Breton M, Meyniel-Schicklin L, Deloire A, Coutard B, Canard B, de Lamballerie X, Andre P, Rabourdin-Combe C, Lotteau V, Davoust N. Flavivirus NS3 and NS5 proteins interaction network: a high-throughput yeast two-hybrid screen. BMC Microbiology. 2011;**11**:234. doi:10.1186/1471-2180-11-234

[61] Mairiang D, Zhang H, Sodja A, Murali T, Suriyaphol P, Malasit P, Limjindaporn T, Finley RL, Jr. Identification of new protein interactions between dengue fever virus and its hosts, human and mosquito. PLoS One. 2013;**8**:e53535. doi:10.1371/journal.pone.0053535

[62] Sawasaki T, Ogasawara T, Morishita R, Endo Y. A cell-free protein synthesis system for high-throughput proteomics. Proceedings of the National Academy of Sciences of the United States of America. 2002;**99**:14652-14657. doi:10.1073/pnas.232580399

[63] Takahashi H, Takahashi C, Moreland NJ, Chang YT, Sawasaki T, Ryo A, Vasudevan SG, Suzuki Y, Yamamoto N. Establishment of a robust dengue virus NS3-NS5 binding assay for identification of protein-protein interaction inhibitors. Antiviral Research. 2012;**96**:305-314. doi:10.1016/j.antiviral.2012.09.023

[64] Takeda H, Ogasawara T, Ozawa T, Muraguchi A, Jih PJ, Morishita R, Uchigashima M, Watanabe M, Fujimoto T, Iwasaki T, Endo Y, Sawasaki T. Production of monoclonal antibodies against GPCR using cell-free synthesized GPCR antigen and biotinylated liposome-based interaction assay. Scientific Reports. 2015;**5**:11333. doi:10.1038/srep11333

[65] Takahashi H, Uematsu A, Yamanaka S, Imamura M, Nakajima T, Doi K, Yasuoka S, Takahashi C, Takeda H, Sawasaki T. Establishment of a wheat cell-free synthesized protein array containing 250 human and mouse E3 ubiquitin ligases to identify novel interaction between E3 ligases and substrate proteins. PLoS One. 2016;**11**:e0156718. doi:10.1371/journal.pone.0156718

[66] Masaki T, Matsunaga S, Takahashi H, Nakashima K, Kimura Y, Ito M, Matsuda M, Murayama A, Kato T, Hirano H, Endo Y, Lemon SM, Wakita T, Sawasaki T, Suzuki T. Involvement of hepatitis C virus NS5A hyperphosphorylation mediated by casein kinase I-alpha in infectious virus production. Journal of Virology. 2014;**88**:7541-7555. doi:10.1128/JVI.03170-13

[67] Miyakawa K, Sawasaki T, Matsunaga S, Tokarev A, Quinn G, Kimura H, Nomaguchi M, Adachi A, Yamamoto N, Guatelli J, Ryo A. Interferon-induced SCYL2 limits release of HIV-1 by triggering PP2A-mediated dephosphorylation of the viral protein Vpu. Science Signaling 2012;**5**:ra73. doi:10.1126/scisignal.2003212

[68] Kudoh A, Takahama S, Sawasaki T, Ode H, Yokoyama M, Okayama A, Ishikawa A, Miyakawa K, Matsunaga S, Kimura H, Sugiura W, Sato H, Hirano H, Ohno S, Yamamoto N, Ryo A. The phosphorylation of HIV-1 Gag by atypical protein kinase C facilitates viral infectivity by promoting Vpr incorporation into virions. Retrovirology. 2014;**11**:9. doi:10.1186/1742-4690-11-9

[69] Tan BH, Suzuki Y, Takahashi H, Ying PH, Takahashi C, Han Q, Chin WX, Chao SH, Sawasaki T, Yamamoto N, Suzuki Y. Identification of RFPL3 protein as a novel E3 ubiquitin ligase modulating the integration activity of human immunodeficiency virus, type 1 preintegration complex using a microtiter plate-based assay. Journal of Biological Chemistry. 2014;**289**:26368-26382. doi:10.1074/jbc.M114.561662

[70] Matsuoka K, Komori H, Nose M, Endo Y, Sawasaki T. Simple screening method for autoantigen proteins using the N-terminal biotinylated protein library produced by wheat cell-free synthesis. Journal of Proteome Research. 2010;**9**:4264-4273. doi:10.1021/pr9010553

[71] Ullman EF, Kirakossian H, Singh S, Wu ZP, Irvin BR, Pease JS, Switchenko AC, Irvine JD, Dafforn A, Skold CN, et al. Luminescent oxygen channeling immunoassay: measurement of particle binding kinetics by chemiluminescence. Proceedings of the National Academy of Sciences of the United States of America. 1994;**91**:5426-5430.

[72] Matsunaga S, Sawasaki T, Ode H, Morishita R, Furukawa A, Sakuma R, Sugiura W, Sato H, Katahira M, Takaori-Kondo A, Yamamoto N, Ryo A. Molecular and enzymatic characterization of XMRV protease by a cell-free proteolytic analysis. Journal of Proteomics. 2012;**75**:4863-4873. doi:10.1016/j.jprot.2012.05.047

[73] Hershko A, Ciechanover A. The ubiquitin system for protein degradation. Annual Review of Biochemistry. 1992;**61**:761-807. doi:10.1146/annurev.bi.61.070192.003553

[74] Loo YM, Fornek J, Crochet N, Bajwa G, Perwitasari O, Martinez-Sobrido L, Akira S, Gill MA, Garcia-Sastre A, Katze MG, Gale M, Jr. Distinct RIG-I and MDA5 signaling by RNA viruses in innate immunity. Journal of Virology. 2008;**82**:335-345. doi:10.1128/JVI.01080-07

[75] Nasirudeen AM, Wong HH, Thien P, Xu S, Lam KP, Liu DX. RIG-I, MDA5 and TLR3 synergistically play an important role in restriction of dengue virus infection. PLoS Neglected Tropical Diseases. 2011;**5**:e926. doi:10.1371/journal.pntd.0000926

[76] Tsai YT, Chang SY, Lee CN, Kao CL. Human TLR3 recognizes dengue virus and modulates viral replication *in vitro*. Cellular Microbiology. 2009;**11**:604-615. doi:10.1111/j.1462-5822.2008.01277.x

[77] Liang Z, Wu S, Li Y, He L, Wu M, Jiang L, Feng L, Zhang P, Huang X. Activation of toll-like receptor 3 impairs the dengue virus serotype 2 replication through induction of IFN-beta in cultured hepatoma cells. PLoS One. 2011;**6**:e23346. doi:10.1371/journal.pone.0023346

[78] Takeuchi O, Akira S. Pattern recognition receptors and inflammation. Cell. 2010;**140**:805-820. doi:10.1016/j.cell.2010.01.022

[79] Honda K, Takaoka A, Taniguchi T. Type I interferon [corrected] gene induction by the interferon regulatory factor family of transcription factors. Immunity. 2006;**25**:349-360. doi:10.1016/j.immuni.2006.08.009

[80] Schneider WM, Chevillotte MD, Rice CM. Interferon-stimulated genes: a complex web of host defenses. Annual Review of Immunology. 2014;**32**:513-545. doi:10.1146/annurev-immunol-032713-120231

[81] Sen GC. Viruses and interferons. Annual Review of Microbiology. 2001;**55**:255-281. doi:10.1146/annurev.micro.55.1.255

[82] Kane M, Zang TM, Rihn SJ, Zhang F, Kueck T, Alim M, Schoggins J, Rice CM, Wilson SJ, Bieniasz PD. Identification of interferon-stimulated genes with antiretroviral activity. Cell Host Microbe. 2016;**20**:392-405. doi:10.1016/j.chom.2016.08.005

[83] Schoggins JW, Wilson SJ, Panis M, Murphy MY, Jones CT, Bieniasz P, Rice CM. A diverse range of gene products are effectors of the type I interferon antiviral response. Nature. 2011;**472**:481-485. doi:10.1038/nature09907

[84] Brass AL, Huang IC, Benita Y, John SP, Krishnan MN, Feeley EM, Ryan BJ, Weyer JL, van der Weyden L, Fikrig E, Adams DJ, Xavier RJ, Farzan M, Elledge SJ. The IFITM proteins mediate cellular resistance to influenza A H1N1 virus, West Nile virus, and dengue virus. Cell. 2009;**139**:1243-1254. doi:10.1016/j.cell.2009.12.017

[85] Chan YK, Huang IC, Farzan M. IFITM proteins restrict antibody-dependent enhancement of dengue virus infection. PLoS One. 2012;**7**:e34508. doi:10.1371/journal.pone.0034508

[86] Shu Q, Lennemann NJ, Sarkar SN, Sadovsky Y, Coyne CB. ADAP2 is an interferon stimulated gene that restricts RNA virus entry. PLoS Pathogens. 2015;**11**:e1005150. doi:10.1371/journal.ppat.1005150

[87] Jiang D, Weidner JM, Qing M, Pan XB, Guo H, Xu C, Zhang X, Birk A, Chang J, Shi PY, Block TM, Guo JT. Identification of five interferon-induced cellular proteins that inhibit West Nile virus and dengue virus infections. Journal of Virology. 2010;**84**:8332-8341. doi:10.1128/JVI.02199-09

[88] Helbig KJ, Carr JM, Calvert JK, Wati S, Clarke JN, Eyre NS, Narayana SK, Fiches GN, McCartney EM, Beard MR. Viperin is induced following dengue virus type-2 (DENV-2) infection and has anti-viral actions requiring the C-terminal end of viperin. PLoS Neglected Tropical Diseases. 2013;**7**:e2178. doi:10.1371/journal.pntd.0002178

[89] Fink J, Gu F, Ling L, Tolfvenstam T, Olfat F, Chin KC, Aw P, George J, Kuznetsov VA, Schreiber M, Vasudevan SG, Hibberd ML. Host gene expression profiling of dengue virus infection in cell lines and patients. PLoS Neglected Tropical Diseases. 2007;**1**:e86. doi:10.1371/journal.pntd.0000086

[90] Pan XB, Han JC, Cong X, Wei L. BST2/tetherin inhibits dengue virus release from human hepatoma cells. PLoS One. 2012;**7**:e51033. doi:10.1371/journal.pone.0051033

[91] Hishiki T, Han Q, Arimoto K, Shimotohno K, Igarashi T, Vasudevan SG, Suzuki Y, Yamamoto N. Interferon-mediated ISG15 conjugation restricts dengue virus 2 replication. Biochemical and Biophysical Research Communications. 2014;**448**:95-100. doi:10.1016/j.bbrc.2014.04.081

[92] Dai J, Pan W, Wang P. ISG15 facilitates cellular antiviral response to dengue and West Nile virus infection *in vitro*. Virology Journal. 2011;8:468. doi:10.1186/1743-422X-8-468

[93] Schoggins JW, Dorner M, Feulner M, Imanaka N, Murphy MY, Ploss A, Rice CM. Dengue reporter viruses reveal viral dynamics in interferon receptor-deficient mice and sensitivity to interferon effectors *in vitro*. Proceedings of the National Academy of Sciences of the United States of America. 2012;109:14610-14615. doi:10.1073/pnas.1212379109

[94] Yi Z, Sperzel L, Nurnberger C, Bredenbeek PJ, Lubick KJ, Best SM, Stoyanov CT, Law LM, Yuan Z, Rice CM, MacDonald MR. Identification and characterization of the host protein DNAJC14 as a broadly active flavivirus replication modulator. PLoS Pathogens. 2011;7:e1001255. doi:10.1371/journal.ppat.1001255

[95] Suzuki Y, Chin WX, Han Q, Ichiyama K, Lee CH, Eyo ZW, Ebina H, Takahashi H, Takahashi C, Tan BH, Hishiki T, Ohba K, Matsuyama T, Koyanagi Y, Tan YJ, Sawasaki T, Chu JJ, Vasudevan SG, Sano K, Yamamoto N. Characterization of RyDEN (C19orf66) as an interferon-stimulated cellular inhibitor against dengue virus replication. PLoS Pathogens. 2016;12:e1005357. doi:10.1371/journal.ppat.1005357

[96] Diamond MS, Roberts TG, Edgil D, Lu B, Ernst J, Harris E. Modulation of dengue virus infection in human cells by alpha, beta, and gamma interferons. Journal of Virology. 2000;74:4957-4966.

[97] Mangus DA, Evans MC, Jacobson A. Poly(A)-binding proteins: multifunctional scaffolds for the post-transcriptional control of gene expression. Genome Biology. 2003;4:223. doi:10.1186/gb-2003-4-7-223

[98] Wolin SL, Cedervall T. The La protein. Annual Review of Biochemistry. 2002;**71**:375-403. doi:10.1146/annurev.biochem.71.090501.150003

[99] Merret R, Descombin J, Juan YT, Favory JJ, Carpentier MC, Chaparro C, Charng YY, Deragon JM, Bousquet-Antonelli C. XRN4 and LARP1 are required for a heat-triggered mRNA decay pathway involved in plant acclimation and survival during thermal stress. Cell Reports. 2013;**5**:1279-1293. doi:10.1016/j.celrep.2013.11.019

[100] Tcherkezian J, Cargnello M, Romeo Y, Huttlin EL, Lavoie G, Gygi SP, Roux PP. Proteomic analysis of cap-dependent translation identifies LARP1 as a key regulator of 5'TOP mRNA translation. Genes and Development. 2014;**28**:357-371. doi:10.1101/gad.231407.113

[101] Kozlov G, Safaee N, Rosenauer A, Gehring K. Structural basis of binding of P-body-associated proteins GW182 and ataxin-2 by the Mlle domain of poly(A)-binding protein. Journal of Biological Chemistry. 2010;285:13599-13606. doi:10.1074/jbc.M109.089540

[102] Balinsky CA, Schmeisser H, Wells AI, Ganesan S, Jin T, Singh K, Zoon KC. IRAV (FLJ11286), an interferon stimulated gene with antiviral activity against dengue virus, interacts with MOV10. Journal of Virology. 2016. doi:10.1128/JVI.01606-16

[103] Kurane I, Innis BL, Nimmannitya S, Nisalak A, Meager A, Ennis FA. High levels of interferon alpha in the sera of children with dengue virus infection. American Journal of Tropical Medicine and Hygiene. 1993;48:222-229.

[104] Ajariyakhajorn C, Mammen MP, Jr., Endy TP, Gettayacamin M, Nisalak A, Nimmannitya S, Libraty DH. Randomized, placebo-controlled trial of non-pegylated and pegylated forms of recombinant human alpha interferon 2a for suppression of dengue virus viremia in rhesus monkeys. Antimicrobial Agents and Chemotherapy. 2005;49:4508-4514. doi:10.1128/AAC.49.11.4508-4514.2005

[105] Green AM, Beatty PR, Hadjilaou A, Harris E. Innate immunity to dengue virus infection and subversion of antiviral responses. Journal of Molecular Biology. 2014;426:1148-1160. doi:10.1016/j.jmb.2013.11.023

[106] Manokaran G, Finol E, Wang C, Gunaratne J, Bahl J, Ong EZ, Tan HC, Sessions OM, Ward AM, Gubler DJ, Harris E, Garcia-Blanco MA, Ooi EE. Dengue subgenomic RNA binds TRIM25 to inhibit interferon expression for epidemiological fitness. Science. 2015;350:217-221. doi:10.1126/science.aab3369

[107] Bidet K, Dadlani D, Garcia-Blanco MA. G3BP1, G3BP2 and CAPRIN1 are required for translation of interferon stimulated mRNAs and are targeted by a dengue virus non-coding RNA. PLoS Pathogens. 2014;**10**:e1004242. doi:10.1371/journal.ppat.1004242

2

Optical Diagnostic of Dengue Virus Infected Human Blood using Raman, Polarimetric and Fluorescence Spectroscopy

Shamaraz Firdous and Shahzad Anwar

Abstract

In this chapter, we present the optical diagnosis of normal and dengue viral-infected human blood using Raman, Polarimetric, Transmission, and Fluorescence Spectroscopic techniques. The possibility of using light in diagnosis and treating illness has been known for thousands of years. The properties of light and lasers provided many modern applications at home, in industry, and in the field of medicine. Laser use in the field of medicine is large and steadily growing. This growth is based on the versatility of laser light. Efficient and accurate diagnosis of dengue is of primary importance for clinical care. A range of laboratory diagnostic methods has been developed to support patient management and disease control. The choice of diagnostic method depends on the purpose for which the testing is done, the type of laboratory facilities and technical expertise available, costs, and the time of sample collection. The dengue viral infection is mostly diagnosed through laboratory tests; these tests include detection of the virus, virus antigen, anti-dengue virus antibody, complement fixation test, neutralization tests, and detection of virus nucleic acid. As dengue infection most rapidly increases in different regions, early diagnostic confirmation of dengue infection in patients allows for timely clinical intervention, etiological investigation, and disease control. Hence, diagnosis of dengue disease during the acute phase should be a priority and is a public health concern. Lasers and optics have many applications in medical sciences; diagnosis and treatment of diseases with lasers and light are latest and noninvasive techniques. Development of light-based apparatus has evolved into tools for improved diagnosis and treatment modalities in medical sciences. The methods of the laser spectroscopy make it possible to obtain direct information regarding the structure and dynamics of the functional groups of biomolecules. Development of new light sources, optics, and diode laser of different wavelengths makes them attractive for spectroscopy of biological molecules. In our study, more than 600 dengue viral-infected blood or blood sera samples and 25 non-dengue healthy blood samples were analyzed using four different optical methodologies. In the first study, Raman spectrum peaks for normal samples observed at 1527, 1170, and 1021 cm^{-1} show the presence of different biological materials, including lipids, carbohydrates, skeletal C–C stretch of acyl chains, and guanine. Raman peaks at 1467, 1316, 1083, and 860 cm^{-1} were observed in dengue-infected patients, representing CH2/CH3 deformation of lipids and collagen, guanine, lipids, and protein peaks using 532 nm laser sources. In our second study, an optical diagnosis of dengue virus infection in the whole blood is presented utilizing Mueller matrix polarimetry. Mueller matrices were extracted using light source from 500 to 700 nm with scanning step of 10 nm. Polar decomposition of the Mueller matrices for all the blood samples was performed that yielded polarization properties including depolarization, diattenuation, degree of polarization, retardance and optical activity, out of which, depolarization index clusters up the diseased and healthy into different groups. The average depolarized light in the case of dengue infection in the whole blood decreases, whereas for the healthy blood samples it increased. This suggests that the depolarization index of the polarized light was at wavelengths 500–700 nm; in this case, we find that depolarization index values are higher for dengue viral infection when compared to normal samples. This technique can effectively be used for the characterization of the dengue virus infected at an early stage of the disease. In the third experiment, the transmission absorption spectra of dengue-infected whole blood samples were observed in ultraviolet to near infrared range (400–800 nm) of about 30 conformed infected patients and were compared to normal blood samples. Transmitted spectra of dengue-infected blood showed two strong spectrum peaks at 540 and 580 nm wavelength of illuminating light, whereas in case of normal blood below 600 nm total attenuation was observed. The two strong absorption peaks from 500 to 600 nm are characteristic of cell damage and dengue virus antibodies IgG and IgM produced against dengue antigen. In the last study, we report an optical diagnosis of dengue-infected whole blood and controlled samples with Laser Scanning Confocal Microscopy (LSCM) over a laser excitation of 488, 543, and 633 nm wavelength. Based on our findings, the system has potential applications in the detection and quantification of dengue virus-infected cells, antigen, and antibodies in blood in vitro.

Keywords: optical diagnosis, dengue viral infection, transmission Raman spectroscopy, polarimetry, confocal laser scanning microscopy (CLSM)

---

1. Introduction

Dengue is an endemic viral disease affecting tropical and subtropical regions around the world and is a viral infection transmitted by the bite of an infected female Aedes mosquito. There are four distinct serotypes of the dengue virus (DEN 1, DEN 2, DEN 3, and DEN 4). Symptoms appear in the first 15 days after the infection. Dengue virus affects humans from newborn baby to aged persons, mostly children and young ones. Dengue fever has no treatment yet, but precautions, early diagnoses, and proper care can protect patients from severity [1–4]. Recently, most of dengue viral infection cases are from Asia, Europe, Africa, and even America. Last year, majority of cases were from Asia and Africa. In 2013, indigenous transmission of dengue was also reported in America and Europe. Dengue spread in America and Europe is mostly by the movement of infected persons and goods; the lack of healthy environment and preventive arrangements also contribute to the global increase of dengue [5–7].

The World Health Organization estimates that worldwide each year, there may be approximately 100 million cases of dengue virus infections [8, 9]. Dengue spread is mostly related with special kind of mosquito bites; however, some normal mosquitoes are infected through dengue virus and then become the source of infection. Dengue virus spreads from person to person but not directly. In fact, it can never transfer from one person to another directly [10, 11].

An evaluation of commercial capture immunosorbent assay for detection of immunoglobulin M and G antibodies produced during dengue infection and Pan Bio kit was evaluated with paired serum specimens from patients. They proved that ELISA should be useful in the clinical diagnosis of dengue infection. Similarly, an evaluation of a commercial ELISA kit for the detection of IgM during dengue infection revealed that primary dengue infection was detected positive for anti-dengue antibodies. Study of Pan Bio duo ELISA and MRL dengue fever IgM capture ELISA for the diagnosis of dengue virus infection in Southeast Asia was done, and comparing the specificity and sensitivity of the tests at different cutoff values revealed that similarly in distinguishing dengue virus from non-flaviviruses showed significantly better distinction between dengue virus and other viruses [12]. Dengue-infected person generates antibodies against dengue virus, which cannot be observed in normal blood or blood sera. The optical changes observed are reflection of biochemical changes in blood. This is the basic principle of dengue fever diagnosis based on optical spectroscopic techniques [13].

Medical tools and sensors based on lasers and optics are used in many applications. Optical diagnostic apparatus are very effective as compared to conventional disease detection methods. Optical techniques are noninvasive, direct, cost-effective, and easy to use with high specificity, sensitivity, and small size. Optical diseases diagnostic research and development has been useful to healthcare, environmental applications, biotechnology industry, and medical sciences [14, 15]. For the development of new optical equipment to be used in medical sciences and devices for practical applications, all the experimental findings and practical aspects, such as robustness, reproducibility, simplicity, and shelf life, should be carefully considered. In these experimental results and optical detection of different diseases using light allows construction of sensitive, simple, and cheap analytical devices with a wide variety of possible applications in screening and monitoring of diseases for use in personalized medicine, remote areas or in developing countries where the availability of inexpensive diagnostic tools are not accessible [16, 17].

2. Raman spectroscopy

Raman spectroscopy was carried out using high-resolution Raman spectroscopy system. The main elements of setup are laser sources 532nm, samples slides, and chamber light collection optics detection system. The target material, blood serum of normal, and dengue samples on glass substrate at room temperature (300±2 K) are used as optimized parameters. The sample was excited by He-Cd laser of 532 nm wavelength and 80 mw power, and output intensity signal detected with objective lens and air-cooled charge-coupled device (CCD) detector. The Raman spectra collected in Raman shift of 600–1800 cm^{-1}. We used the accumulate acquisition mode to reduce noise and thermal fluctuation and improve signal to noise ratio [18–20].

For normal blood sera, the Raman shifts are observed at 1527, 1170, and 1023 cm^{-1} with intensity level of 7200–9500 pixels, showing a compound that occurs in guano and fish scales and is one of the four constituent bases of nucleic acids. A pure derivative, it is paired with cytosine in double-stranded DNA (guanine). Adenine is used in forming nucleotides of the nucleic acids. Adenine can be found in DNA and RNA, in first with two hydrogen bonds for the nucleic acid structures stabilization and in second for protein synthesis. Tryptophan is α-amino acid that is used in the biosynthesis of proteins TRP (protein) carbohydrates peak for solids. Carbon skeletons are the backbones of organic molecules. They are composed of carbon-carbon atoms that form chains to make an organic compound. Length, shape, location, and amount of double bonds are characteristics of carbon skeletons (skeletal C-C), and Cardiolipins are a subclass of glycerophospholipids containing four acyl chains and three glycerol groups that are particularly abundant in the inner mitochondrial membrane. They are believed to activate enzymes involved with oxidative phosphorylation (stretch of lipids acyl chains) as shown in **Figure 1A**. The Raman shifts observed in Raman spectrum of a dengue-infected blood serum are at 1467, 1316, 1083, and 860 cm^{-1} with intensity level of 6000–7500 pixels attributed to the bands of stretching and deformation vibrations of CH_2, C-CH_3, and OCH_3 groups in the infrared and Raman spectra (CH_2/CH_3) deformation of lipids and collagen, guanine, lipids, and protein bands as shown in **Figure 1B**.

The main dengue viral infection sera peaks appear at 1467 and 860 cm^{-1}. The intensity of these peaks, as well as those at 1316 and 1081 cm^{-1}, is plotted against the intensity level in **Figure 1B**. In our previous chapter [6], we reported transmission spectra of dengue-infected whole blood samples irradiated with light of 400–800 nm wavelength. We collected data of 30 conformed infected patients and compared them to normal blood samples. Transmission spectra of dengue-infected blood show strong and prominent peaks at 540 and 580 nm. In case of normal blood, total absorption has been observed from 400 to 600 nm of wavelength. In case of dengue, the peaks indicate damage and dengue virus antibodies immunoglobulin G (IgG) and immunoglobulin M (IgM) produced against dengue antigen. In another chapter, we determined that normal whole blood and serum characteristic peaks were excited at 442 and 532 nm. In dengue-infected whole blood and serum, two peaks at 1614 and 1750 cm^{-1} are observed, which are due to the presence of immunoglobulin antibodies IgG and IgM.

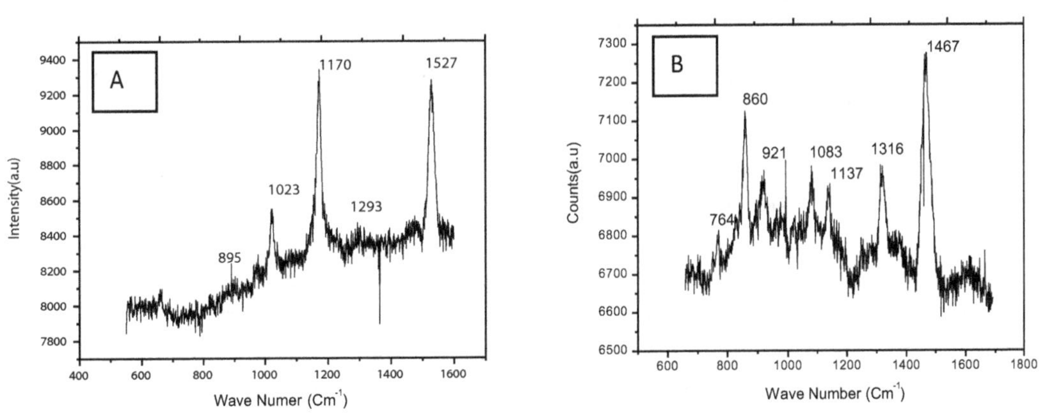

Figure 1. Raman spectrum of (A) normal blood and (B) dengue blood at 532nm wavelength of light.

Raman spectroscopy has proven to be an effective analytical approach in geology, semiconductor, materials, and polymer science fields. The application of Raman spectroscopy and microscopy within biology is rapidly increasing because it can provide chemical and compositional information. Raman spectroscopic technique based on protein and lipid changes due to antibodies and antigen reactions, while the Protein and lipids concentration totally changes in dengue viral sample as compared to normal ones [21].

3. Mueller matrix polarimetry

Polarimeters are optical instruments used for determining the polarization properties of light beams and samples. To perform accurate polarimetry, all the issues necessary for careful and accurate radiometry must be considered together with many additional polarization issues. Mueller matrix polarimetry yields four optical parameters, namely depolarization coefficient, linear retardance, optical activity, and diattenuation, which can be used to characterize the tissues or turbid media [22–34]. We represented very interesting results from the dengue-infected whole blood by exploiting the depolarization nature of polarized light in whole blood; this can be used for the discrimination between the healthy and viral infection diseased blood samples [5].

Mueller matrices from all the 30 ultra-thin smeared blood slides were acquired using Mueller Matrix Polarimeter AxoScan™ (Axometrics, USA). AxoScan™ system employs dual rotating retarder as discussed in our previous study [5]. A tunable light source ranging from 400 to 800 nm, coupled with 200 nm multimode fiber optic probe, is used to shine the sample through Polarization State Generator (PSG). Light source consists of a low-noise 150 W Xenon arc lamp and a scanning diffraction-grating monochromatic light. PSG consists of a fixed linear polarizer along with a rotating linear retarder. As the retarder rotates, a wide variety of polarization states, including linear (horizontal, vertical), elliptical (−45°/+45°), and circular (left/right),is generated. These six polarization states are steered to pass through the smeared blood slides. The rotating retarder in PSG is rotated five times faster than the retarder in the generator for different combinations of the rotation angles of retarders in PSG and Polarization State Analyzer (PSA); light coming out from PSA is collected by a very sensitive detector. The resulting combination of polarization states at different rotation angles of retarders in PSG and PSA is adequate for determining the Mueller matrix of the sample.

In the present study, Mueller matrices from all the blood samples were measured from 500 to 800 nm, and their polar decomposition yields the polarization parameters for each wavelength, out of which depolarization coefficients showed distinct differentiation. **Figures 2** and **3** displayed the diattenuation and retardance of the dengue-infected and non-dengue healthy blood samples as a function of wavelength. We find that in the case of dengue viral infection, diattenuation and retardance values are lower when compared to normal samples. The diattenuation and retardance of both types of samples can be used for the characterization of the early stage detection of dengue infection in the human blood. The Mueller matrix is generally a diagonal matrix having m_{00}= 1 and m_{11}= m_{22}. The m_{11}= m_{22} is due to axial symmetry of the material.

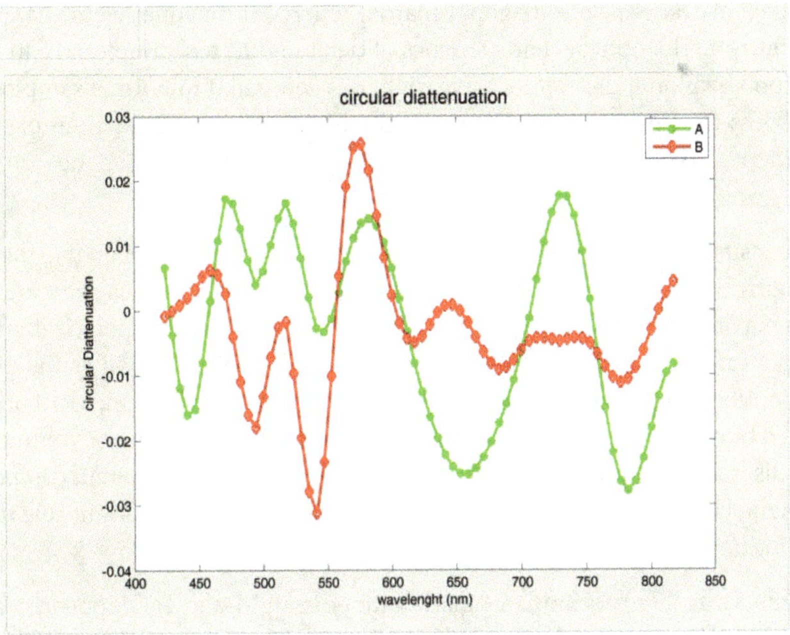

Figure 2. Polarization properties in terms of Mueller matrix, diattenuation of normal (—●—), and of dengue-infected blood (—◆—) at 400–800nm wavelength.

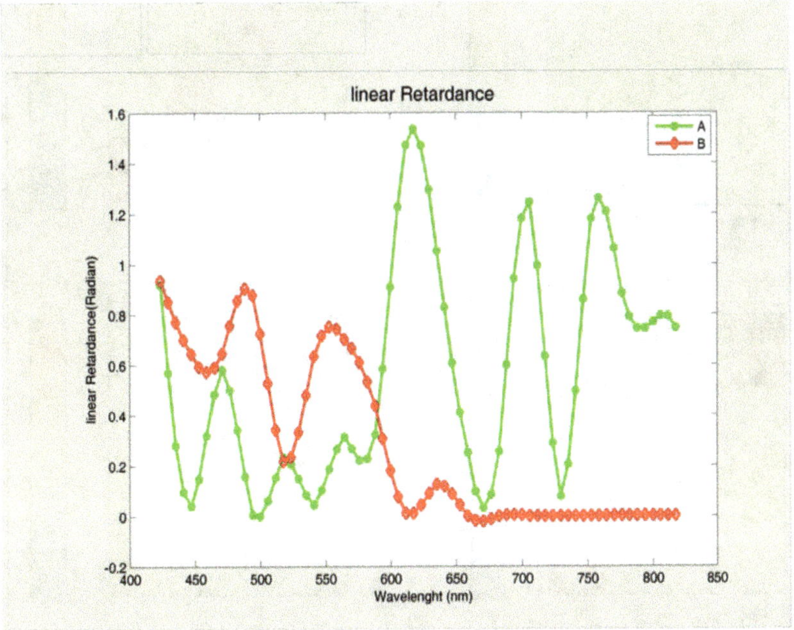

Figure 3. Polarization properties in terms of Mueller matrix, retardance of normal (—●—), and of dengue-infected blood (—◆—) at 400–800nm wavelength.

The retardance matrix is also a diagonal matrix, where all diagonal elements are equal as shown in **Figure 4**. The optical characteristics of dengue-infected samples at 540 nm of light showing depolarization index values were higher as compared to normal samples. The diattenuation is less than polarization as seen in the first row and first column of the Mueller matrix. In the retardance matrix, image m_{11} and m_{22} are same. m_{33} depends on the size of scatterers.

The color intensity of the elements m_{11}, m_{22}, and m_{33} increases when compared to the retardance image of **Figure 4** of dengue-infected ones. The depolarization image is showing a diagonal matrix with maximum intensity at diagonal elements. It is clear that depolarization coefficient decreases as a function of wavelength for both types of samples, as well as the difference of depolarization coefficients reduces for both types of the samples. The hematocrit of the dengue virus-infected blood increases due to decreasing platelets; this increasing of volume fraction of red blood cells may be responsible for the more depolarization coefficient in comparison with the non-dengue healthy blood samples as red blood cells play an important role in scattering that causes the depolarization of polarized light.

In the dengue virus-infected human blood, antibodies IgM and IgG appeared against the infection by the defensive system. These antibodies are like protein structures that must also be responsible for producing more depolarization effects in the dengue-infected blood samples.

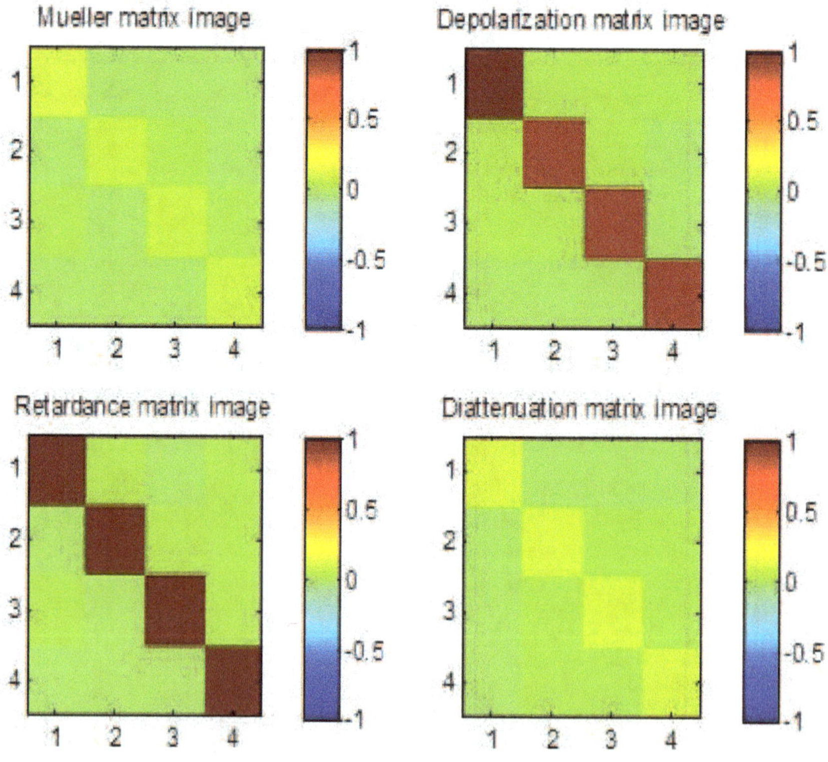

Figure 4. Polarization properties in terms of Mueller matrix, depolarization, retardance, and diattenuation matrix of dengue-infected blood at 540 nm of light.

Mueller matrix polarimetry has been exploited successfully for the optical diagnosis of dengue virus infection in human blood. Depolarization coefficient of the dengue-infected and non-dengue human blood samples is clearly distinct in light spectra for the characterization of both types of samples. In addition, diattenuation, retardance, and depolarization coefficients may be helpful for monitoring the disease from time to time and to monitor very minute structural changes in the tissue of blood chemistry.

4. Transmission spectroscopy

In this study, we provide transmission spectroscopy of dengue viral infection analysis. The cell culture method is still considered the standard for viral diagnosis as it has the advantages of detecting infectious viral particles and the ability to achieve low detection limits. This new method has the potential to be extended for the detection of other viruses and adapted into a portable, automated system for detection of viruses from environmental samples. The presented results are very effective for initial screening of dengue-infected patients and to minimize the diagnostic cost [6].

We used Avaspec. Spectrometer (Avantes Inc, Netherlands) of wavelength range 400–1000 nm and Avaspec.software to record data. About 50 μl drop of whole blood excited with light as shown in **Figure 5**. Two prominent absorption peaks at 540 and 580 nm of blood spectrum, as measured within a set of about 30 essentially conformed dengue-infected individuals, are observed as shown in **Figure 6**. The change represented by these peaks in the protein and blood cells within the human body is a manifestation of significant biochemical changes due to the antibodies IgG activated after 2–3 days of dengue virus infection and IgM produced after one week. We have recorded transmission spectra of other viral-infected blood samples, like hepatitis and malaria, besides dengue infection, but there is no transmission in the range of 400–600 nm. The spectrum peaks at 540 and 580 nm are only in dengue-infected samples.

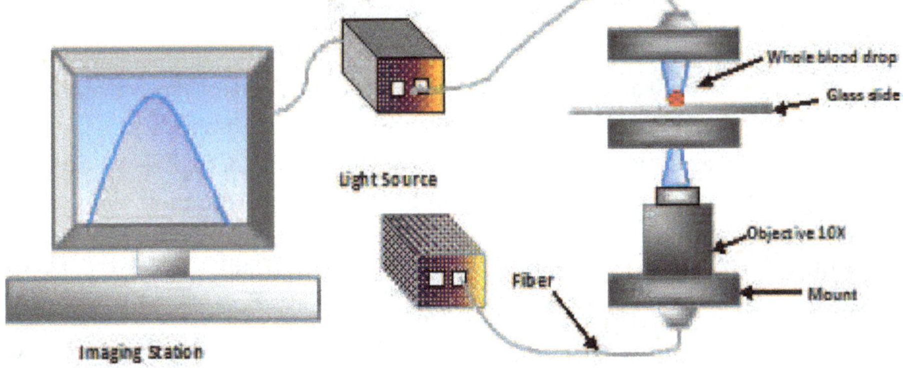

Figure 5. Experimental setup for the whole blood dengue infection diagnosis with light spectroscopy.

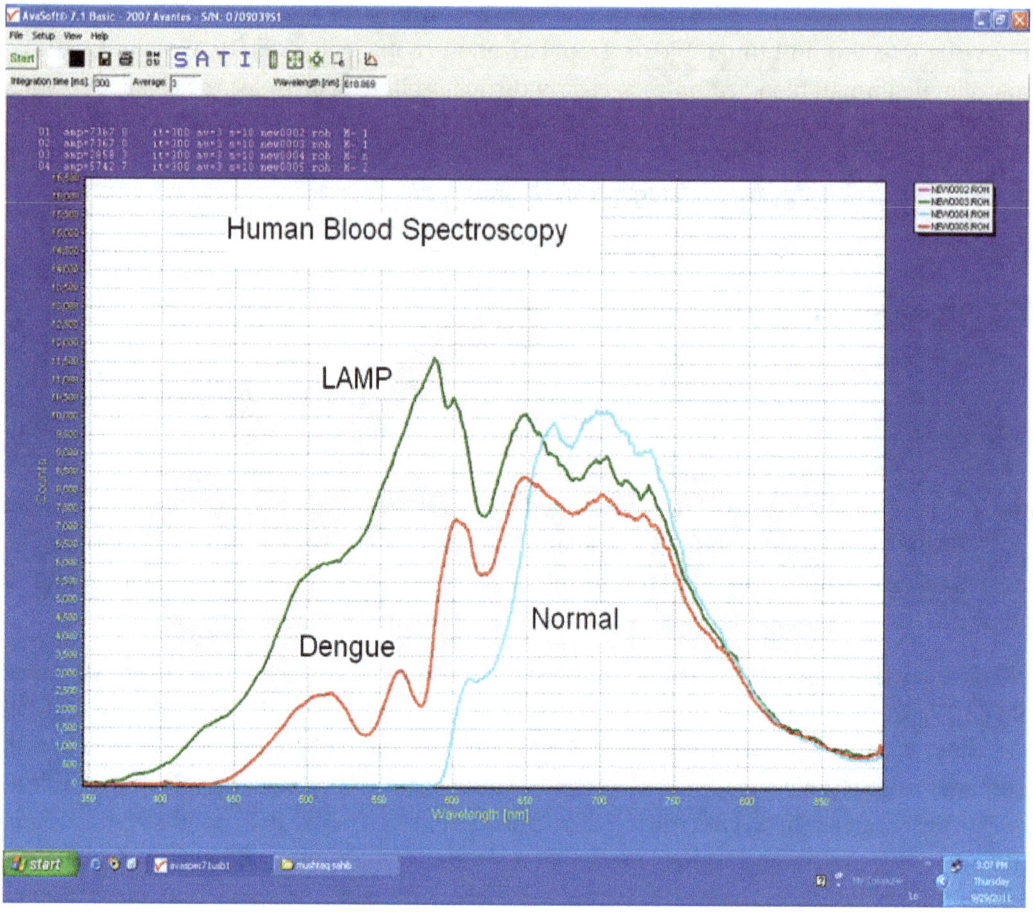

Figure 6. The transmission spectroscopy of normal and dengue-infected whole blood spectrum at 400–1000 nm wavelength.

5. Confocal microscopic analysis

We have used light spectroscopy, Raman and absorption spectroscopy, and Laser scanning confocal microscopy (LSCM) techniques for repaid screening of dengue infection. LSCM has become an invaluable tool for a wide range of investigations in the biological and medical sciences for imaging thin optical sections in living and fixed specimens. To image the dengue-infected blood, a drop of 50μl whole blood was placed on quartz glass slide and seen through (63X, 100X) water and oil emulsions objectives of LSCM (LSM-510, Carl Zeiss, Micro Imaging Inc., Germany) equipped with 451, 471, 488, and 517nm line of Argon ion, 553 and 633 nm He-Ne lasers, 10 to 100X water and oil emulsions objectives and three Photo Multiplier Tubes (PMTs). Fluorescence light from the sample was collected by the objective, directed to an analyzer, and spatially filtered by the confocal pinhole in the detection path. Reflected light that passed through the pinhole was spectrally separated by dichroic filters and directed to three PMTs to detect light at each wavelength. Images were acquired as 8-bit TIFF files (512 × 512 pixel frame) and processed using Zen software (Carl Zeiss, Micro Imaging Inc., Germany).

We demonstrated the dengue-infected human blood in in vitro using LSCM. The confocal images of normal and dengue-infected whole blood samples are analyzed with LSCM and fluorescence is detected. The dengue cells are different in looks compared to the normal ones, and the fluorescence from dengue infected is prominent than normal as shown in **Figure** 7. The whole blood analyzed on day 10 and day 13 shows antibodies IgG and IgM structure over blood cells. We suggest that as platelets decrease, fluorescence increase due to complex interactions between the virus and host cells, leading to the activation of transcription factors, cytokines, and enzymatic factors. The simple blood images taken at day 3 of infection are shown in **Figure** 7 and fluorescence of cells at day 10 is shown in **Figure** 8. These interactions may induce not only pathologic prion flammatory responses that influence the severity and progression of the disease but also virus clearance and apoptotic pathways that could be controlling infection by anti-viral mechanisms. The present study may, therefore, contribute to a better understanding of the cell activation mechanisms triggered during dengue infections occurring in human target cells. The viral infection images at day 10 and 13 after infection are shown in **Figure** 8.

Blood sample analysis with LSCM provides a way for diagnosis of infection. The results obtained can be used in the development of new methods and optimization of existing ones for dengue-infected patients. The presented techniques can be used for new light-based diagnostic apparatus for the quantities analysis of dengue patients. In our previous research findings,

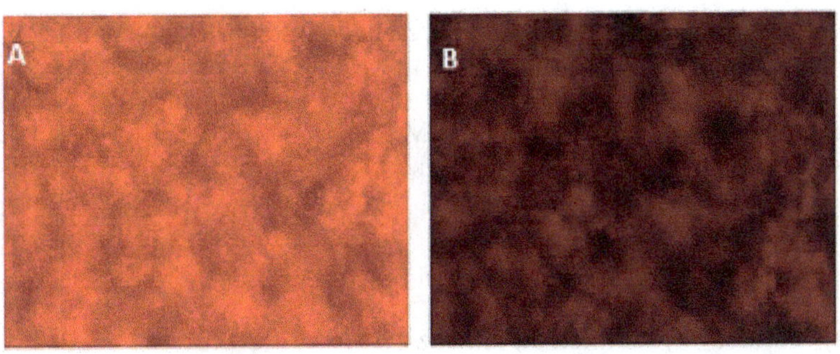

Figure 7. An early comparison of dengue-infected blood samples with a confocal microscope (63×). (A) normal blood drop on glass slide and (B) dengue-infected blood at day 4 after infection.

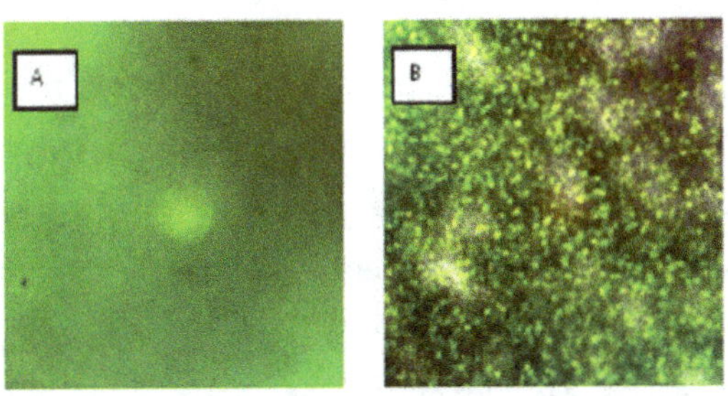

Figure 8. An early comparison of dengue-infected blood samples with a confocal microscope (63×). (A) normal blood drop on glass slide and (B) dengue-infected blood at day 10 after infection.

we have characterized tissues and biomaterials for optical imaging to diagnose diseases and develop optical detection equipments [35–53].

Author details

Shamaraz Firdous* and Shahzad Anwar

*Address all correspondence to: shamaraz@gmail.com

Biophotonics Laboratories, National Institute of Lasers and Optronics (NILOP), Islamabad, Pakistan

References

[1] Meinke GM, Helfmann J,Friebel M (2007) Optical properties of platelets and blood plasma and their influence on the optical behavior of whole blood in the visible to near infrared wavelength range. J Biomedical Optics 12(1):14024-14032

[2] Shu PY, Huang HJ (2004) Current advances in dengue diagnosis. Clin Diagn Lab Immunol 11:642-650

[3] Monath TP (1994) Dengue: the risk to developed and developing countries. Proceedings of the National Academy of Sciences of United States of America. 91:395-400

[4] Rehman A, Anwar S, Firdous S, Ahmed M, Rasheed R, Nawaz M (2012) Dengue blood analysis by Raman spectroscopy. Laser Physics 22(6):1085-1089

[5] Shahzad Anwar, Shamaraz Firdous (2016) Optical diagnosis of dengue virus infected human blood using Mueller matrix polarimetry. Opt Spectrosc 121(2):322-325

[6] Firdous S, Ahmed M, Rehman A, Nawaz M, Anwar S, Murtaza S (2012) Transmission spectroscopy of dengue viral infection. Laser Phys Lett 9(4):317-321

[7] Firdous S, Anwar S (2017) Confocal microscopic analysis of dengue infected blood.

[8] Verma SP (1986) Low levels of irradiation modify lipid domains in model membranes: a laser Raman study. Radiation Research 107(2):183-193

[9] World Health Organization (1986) Dengue haemorrhagic fever: diagnosis, treatment and control. Geneva: WHO, pp. 1-58

[10] Chakravarti A, Matlani M, Kashyap B, Kumar A (2012) Awareness of changing trends in epidemiology of dengue fever is essential for epidemiological surveillance. Indian Journal of Medical Microbiology 30:222-226.

[11] Subedi D., Taylor-Robinson AW (2014) Laboratory diagnosis of dengue infection: current techniques and future strategies. Open Journal of Clinical Diagnostics 2014.doi:10.4236/ojcd.2014.41012

[12] Pei-Yun Shu, Jyh-Hsiung Huang (2004) Current advances in dengue diagnosis. Clinical and Laboratory Immunology 11(4) 642-650

[13] Puppels GJ, Garritsen HS, Segers-Nolten GM, de Mul FF, Greve J (1991) Raman micro-spectroscopic approach to the study of human granulocytes. Biophysical Journal 60(5): 1046-1056

[14] Narayahan S, Galloway L, Nonoyama A, Leparc GF, Garcia LH, Potter RL (2002)UV-visible spectrophotometric approach to blood typing II: phenotyping of subtype A2 and weak D and whole blood analysis.Transfusion42(5):619-626

[15] Lagali NS, Burns NK, Zimmerman D, Munger R (2007) Spectroscopic whole-blood indicators of end-stage renal disease and the hemodialysis treatment. Photochemistry and Photobiology 83(5):1186-1192

[16] O'Faolain E, Hunter MB, Byrne JM, Kelehan P, McNamara M, Byrne HJ, et al (2005) A study examining the effects of tissue processing on human tissue sections using vibrational spectroscopy. Vibrational Spectroscopy 38(1-2):121-127

[17] Krishna CM, Sockalingum GD, Kurien J, Rao L, Venteo L, Pluot M et al (2004) Micro-Raman spectroscopy for optical pathology of oral squamous cell carcinoma. Applied Spectroscopy 58(9):1128-1135

[18] Cafferata ML, Bardach A, Rey-Ares L, Alcaraz A, Cormick G, Gibbons L, Romano M, Cesaroni S, Ruvinsky S (2013) Dengue epidemiology and burden of disease in Latin America and the Caribbean: asystematic review of the literature and meta-analysis. Value in Health Regional Issues 2:347-356

[19] Firdous S, Anwar S, Waheed A, Maraj M (2016) Optical characterization of pure vegetable oils and their biodiesels using Raman spectroscopy. Laser Physics 26(4):045601

[20] S. Anwar, S. Firdous, A. Rehman, and M. Nawaz, Raman Optical Diagnostic of Breast Cancer using Raman, Polarimetric Fluorescence Spectroscopy, Laser phy. Letter 12(4) 045601 (2015).

[21] Shamaraz Firdous, Shahzad Anwar (2015)Dengue viral infection monitoring from diagnostic to recovery using Raman spectroscopy. Laser Physics Letters 12(8):085601

[22] Firdous S, Atif M, Nawaz M(2011) Stokes vector determination of polarized light propagation in turbid medium. Optics and Spectroscopy 110(3):438-441

[23] Firdous S, Hassan K, Ikram M (2005)Formulation of Mueller matrix and modeling of depolarizing and scattering of nitrobenzene in a Kerr Cell. Applied Optics 44(7):1171-1177

[24] Firdous S, Ikram M (2005) Polarized Mueller matrix analytical model for glucose measurement in vitro. Turkish Journal of Medical Science 35:145-159

[25] Firdous S, Atif M, Nawaz M (2010)The optical polarimetric study of blood malignancy in vitro for diagnostic and treatment of blood diseases. Lasers in Engineering 19(5-6):291-305

[26] Firdous S, Fuzail M, Atif M, Nawaz M (2011) Polarimetric characterization of ultra-high molecular weight polyethylene (UHMWPE) for bone substitute biomaterials. Optik 122(2):99-104

[27] Firdous S, Ahmed A, Nawaz M, Ikram M (2013) Optical characterization of chitosan for application as an engineered biomaterial. Optik: International Journal for Light and Electron Optics 124(12):1297-1302

[28] Firdous S, Waqas W, Idrees M, Nawaz M, Ikram M (2013) Polarization sensitive optical imaging of biomaterials using Mueller matrix polarimetric algorithm. Lasers in Engineering 26(3/4):157-180

[29] Ahmed M, Ali S, Mehmood S, Khurshid A, Firdous S, Ikram M (2013) Ex-vivo assessment of carbon tetrachloride(CCL_4) induced chronic injury using polarized light spectroscopy. Applied Spectroscopy 67(12):1382-1389

[30] Aziz T, Firdous S, Rehman T, Khan MA (2013) Polarimetric study of leukemia human peripheral blood smears in 400-800nm spectral range. Optik: International Journal for Light and Electron Optics124(1):2936-2942

[31] Rehman A, Ahmad I, Rehman K, Anwar S, Firdous S, Nawaz M (2015) Optical properties measurement of highly diffusive tissue phantoms for biomedical applications. Laser Physics 25(2):025605

[32] Anwar S, Mubarik M, Waheed A, Firdous S (2015)Polarization imaging and characterization of Chitosan for applications in tissue engineering. Optik:International Journal for Light and Electron Optics 126:871-876

[33] Kamal A, Bashir M, Firdous S, Yasin T, Tariq M, Ikram M, Mehmood MS (2016) Optical properties of ultra-high molecular weight polyethylene (UHMWPE): a material of choice for total joint applications. Radiation Physics and Chemistry118:102-106

[34] Firdous Shamaraz, Anwar Shahzad (2016) Noninvasive optical diagnostic of breast cancer using depolarization of light. Optik 127(5):3035-3038

[35] Rice William, Firdous Shamaraz, Gupta Sharad, Hunter Martin, Foo Cheryl WP, Wang Yongzhong, Kim Hyeon Joo, Kaplan David L, Georgaukodi Irene (2008) Non-invasive characterization of structure and morphology of silk fibroin biomaterials using nonlinear microscopy. Biomaterials 29:2014-2021

[36] Atif M, Firdous S, Khurshid A, Noreen L, Zaidi S, Ikram M (2009) In vitro study of 5 aminolevulinic acid (5-ALA) based photodynamic therapy for apoptosis in human cervical HeLa cell line. Laser Physics Letters 6(12):886-891

[37] Khan Y, Mehmood M, Ahmad J, Riaz Khan M, Firdous S (2010) Low temperature synthesis of fluorescent ZnO nanoparticles. Applied Surface Science 257:1756-1761

[38] Ullah H, Atif M, Firdous S, Mehmood S, Ikram M, Kurachi C, Grecco C, Nicolodelli G, Bagnato VS (2010) Femtosecond light distribution at skin and liver of rats: analysis for use in optical diagnostics. Laser Physics Letters 7-12:889-898

[39] Atif M, Firdous S, Nawaz M (2010) Laser induced effects in different biological samples. Lasers in Medical Sciences 25(4):545-550

[40] Khursid A, Atif M, Firdous S, Zaidi S, Suleman R, Ikram M (2010)Study of the efficacy of 5 ALA_mediated photodynamic therapy of human larynx squamous cell carcinoma (Hep2c) using 5-aminolevulanic acid in vitro. Laser Physics 20(7):1673-1678

[41] Alam F, Roohi S, Atif M, Firdous S, Amir N, Zahoor R (2010) Labelling and optimization of photofrin with ^{99m}Tc. Radiochimica Acta 98:1-6

[42] Atif M, Alam F, Firdous S, Zaidi S, Suleman R, Ikram M. (2010) Study of the efficacy of 5-ALA mediated photodynamic therapy on human rhabdomyosarcoma cell line (RD). Laser Physics Letters 7:757-764

[43] Ullah H, Atif M, Firdous S, Mehmood S, Hamza Y, Imran M, Hussan G, Ikram M. (2011) Optical properties of normal and thermally coagulated chicken liver tissue measured ex vivo with diffuse reflectance. Optics and Spectroscopy 11(2):311-317

[44] Ikram M, Khan R, Firdous S, Atif M, Nawaz M (2011) Photodynamic therapy of non-melanoma skin cancers. Laser Physics 21(2):427-433

[45] Atif M, Firdous S, Mahmood R, Fakhar_e_Alam M, Zaidi SSZ, Suleman R, Ikram M, Nawaz M. Cytotoxic and photocytotoxic effect of photofrin® on human laryngeal carcinoma (Hep2c) cell line. Laser Physics 21(7):1235-1242

[46] Khan RU, Khurshid N, Ikram M, Firdous S, Atif M (2011)Pain during topical photodynamic therapy in Pakistani and Afghani patients. Photodiagnosis and Photodynamic Therapy 8(2):145-146

[47] Fakhar_e_Alam M, Firdous S, Atif M, Khan Y, Zaidi SSZ, Suleman R, Rehman A, Khan RU, Nawaz M, Ikram M (2011) The potential applications of ZnO nanoparticles conjugated with ALA and photofrin as a biomarker in HepG2 cells. Laser Physics 21(11):2156-2154

[48] Fakhar-e-Alam M, Atif M, Rehman T, Sadia H, Firdous S (2011) The role of sensitivity of ALA (PpIX)-based PDT on human embryonic kidney cell line (HEK293T).Laser Physics 21(8):1428-1437

[49] KhurshidA, Firdous S, Ahmat L, Ferraria J, Vollet-Filho JD, Kurachi C, Bagneto VS, Nawaz M, Ikram M, Ahmad M (2012) In vivo study of laser irradiation of fractionated drug administration based mechanism for effective photodynamic therapy in rat liver. Laser Physics 22(1):317-321

[50] Rehman A, Firdous S, Nawaz M, Ahmad M (2012) Optical parameters measurement for diagnostic and photodynamic therapy of human cervical adenocarcinoma (HeLa) cell line. Laser Physics 22(1):322-326

[51] Firdous S, Nawaz M, Ikram M, Ahmed M (2012) In vitro study of cell death with 5-Aminolevulinic acid based photodynamic therapy to improve the efficiency of cancer treatment. Laser Physics 22(3):626-633

[52] Firdous S, Nawaz M, Ahmed M, Anwar S, Rehman A, Rashid R, Mahmood A (2012) Measurement of diabetic sugar concentration in human blood using Raman spectroscopy. Laser Physics 22(6):1-5

[53] Anwar S, Firdous S (2015) Optical diagnostic of Hepatitis B(HBV) and C (HCV) from human blood serum using Raman spectroscopy. Laser Physics Letters 12(7):076001

3

Ecology of *Aedes* Mosquitoes, the Major Vectors of Arboviruses in Human Population

Eliningaya J. Kweka, Vito Baraka, Leah Mathias, Beda Mwang'onde, Germana Baraka, Lucile Lyaruu and Aneth M. Mahande

Abstract

Aedes aegypti (Stegomyia) has been human vectors for many human diseases globally. In recent years, dengue virus has been diagnosed in different regions such as Asia and Latin America vectored by *Aedes* spp. mosquitoes. Dengue cases have been reported again in the several parts of African and other continental hospital. The different types of breeding sites have been found to be abundant in both urban and rural areas. The abundance of adult *Ae. aegypti* and habitat productivity in different settings escalates the risk of dengue transmission if viruses are found in asymptomatic population. The insecticide resistance has been found to occur in the wild population of *Aedes aegypti* to insecticides commonly used for indoor residual spray and long-lasting insecticidal net treatments. The control of human vector population is still a challenge as the vector has a diurnal feeding and outdoor resting behavior. Environmental management is still the best practice to be adopted in many countries for *Aedes aegypti* control. The currently discovered dengue vaccine might be an immediate arsenal for the community immunization.

Keywords: *Aedes aegypti*, ecology, insecticide resistance, control, arboviruses

1. Introduction

Mosquitoes are small, midge-like flies that constitute the family Culicidae. Females of most species are ectoparasites feeding on vertebrates' blood through piercing the hosts' skin to suck the blood. To-date, approximately 3500 species of the Culicidae have been described. The family Culicidae is a large and abundant group which occurs throughout temperate and tropical regions of the world and well beyond the Arctic Circle [1]. There are two subfamilies of Culicidae, that is, the Anophelinae (3 genera) and the Culicinae (110 genera). The subfamily Culicidae, *Aedes* is the largest tribe of mosquitoes with 1256 species classified into 10 genera: Aedes sensu (931), Armigeres (58), Eretmapodites (48), Haemagogus (28), Heizmannia (38), Opifex (2), Psorophora (49), Udaya (3), Verrallina (95), and Zeugnomyia (4) [2].

The public health concern of *Aedes* mosquitoes particularly *Ae. aegypti* and *Ae. albopictus* in the transmission of arboviruses such as dengue virus, chikungunya virus, ZIKV virus, and yellow fever virus is kept on increasing globally. Over half of the world's population is at risk of dengue and chikungunya infections [3]. The Caribbean, South America, and Europe are no longer spared from chikungunya infection, a disease which was previously limited to Africa and Asia [3]. According to the World Health Organization, about 2.5 billion people globally live in dengue endemic regions [4]. Dengue is the most worldwide important mosquito-transmitted viral infection [4]. Over 100 countries in Africa, North and South America, Southeast Asia, Europe, and the Pacific are reported to have had severe dengue outbreaks [5]. The annual occurrence of dengue fever infections ranges from 50 to 100 million with which around 500,000 facing severe morbidity causing to over 20,000 mortalities, pediatrics beings the most cases [5]. The chikungunya virus infections (CHIKV) have been documented in over 60 countries in Asia, Africa, Europe, and the Americas [6]. The estimated number of chikungunya cases in Americas in 2016 was 693,000, and Zika virus (ZIKV) disease was 500,000 [6, 7]. Yellow fever cases in Africa were 130,000 with an estimated 31,000 annual disability adjusted life years and 500 deaths [8, 9].

About 80% of the world's population is at risk for at least of exposure to one vector-borne disease; these diseases account for about 17% of the estimated global burden of communicable diseases and cause over 700,000 deaths annually, affecting disproportionately poorer populations [6, 9]. They hamper economic development through direct medical costs and indirect costs such as the loss of productivity and tourism. The social, demographic, and environmental factors strongly influence transmission patterns of vector-borne pathogens. Vector control is an important component for decision science in the prevention and control of vector-borne disease approaches. Consequently, the global distribution and ecology of these vectors and the geographical determinants of their ranges are essential in order to be effective. Therefore, it is important to work out where these mosquito species are found around the globe to identify the areas at risk. It is also important to predict where these species could become established if they were introduced, in order to identify areas that could become at risk in the future.

1.1. *Aedes* distribution

Ae. aegypti and *Ae. albopictus* are worldwide distributed between 35° N and 35° S, latitudes that roughly correspond to a 10°C winter isotherm which appears to be the limiting temperatures that the species can tolerate while overwintering [5]. The species are highly adapted to urban environments, breeding in stagnant water found in manufactured containers, garbage heaps, and tyres. However, the distribution of *Ae. albopictus* has been highly biased to temperate climates [10] though the vector is now widely distributed throughout the Americas (excluding Canada), Europe, Asia, Africa, Australia, and the Pacific [11].

The geographic distribution of *Ae. aegypti* based on the order of higher levels of occurrence for each continent reveals that in the Americas, the Brazil ranks the highest (**Table 1**). In Africa, occurrence of the vectors have been recorded in Senegal, Cameroon, Kenya, Tanzania, Ivory Coast, Nigeria, Madagascar, Gabon, and Sierra Leone (**Table 1**). In Asia/Oceania, occurrence of *Ae. aegypti* has been reported and documented (**Table 1**) [3, 12].

1.2. Ecology of *Aedes* mosquitoes

1.2.1. Aedes aegypti

Ae. aegypti is an arthropod closely associated with humans and their habitats. They are mostly anthropophilic [13] with high preference to the urban environment [14]. They get blood meals from human, and human creates conducive environment for their population growth through up haphazardly disposal of water-holding containers/obsoletes around our homes. The mosquito lays her eggs on the sides of containers with water, and eggs hatch into larvae after a rain or flooding. A larva changes into a pupa in about a week and into a mosquito in 2 days. The *Aedes* main habitat is aquatic, and they can thrive better from tree cavities to toilets. People also furnish shelter as *Ae. aegypti* preferentially rests in darker cool areas, such as closets leading to their ability to bite indoors.

Ae. aegypti has adaptations to the environment that makes them highly resilient, or with the ability to rapidly bounce back to initial numbers after disturbances resulting from natural phenomena (e.g., droughts) or human interventions (e.g., control measures). One such adaptation is the ability of the eggs to withstand desiccation (drying) and to survive without water for several months on the inner walls of containers. For example, if we were to eliminate all larvae, pupae, and adult *Ae. aegypti* at once from a site, its population could recover 2 weeks later as a result of egg hatching following rainfall or the addition of water to containers harboring eggs.

It is likely that *Ae. aegypti* is continually responding or adapting to environmental change. For example, it was recently found that *Ae. aegypti* is able to undergo immature development in broken or open septic tanks resulting in the production of hundreds or thousands of *Ae. aegypti* adults per day. In general, it is expected that control interventions will change the spatial and temporal dispersal of *Ae. aegypti* and perhaps the pattern of habitat utilization.

1.2.2. Aedes albopictus

Aedes albopictus (*Stegomyia albopicta*), from the mosquito (Culicidae) family, also known as (Asian) tiger mosquito or forest mosquito, is a mosquito native to the tropical and subtropical areas of Southeast Asia; however, in the past few decades, this species has spread to many countries through the transport of goods and international travel [15]. The eggs of *Ae. albopictus* are desiccation resistant, which enhance survival in inhospitable environments [16]. *Ae. albopictus* is among the aggressive outdoor species of mosquito, and they are day biter that has a very broad host range and attacks humans, livestock, amphibians, reptiles, and birds [17]. Their biting rate level can be as high as 30 to 48 bites per hour [18]. *Ae. albopictus* survives at a large range of temperatures [19].

	Country	Occurrences		Country	Occurrences		Country	Occurrences
Ae. aegypti								
Americas	Brazil	5044	Europe/ Africa	Senegal	112	Asia/ Oceania	Taiwan	9490
	USA	436		Cameroon	55		Indonesia	603
	Mexico	411		Kenya	52		Thailand	495
	Cuba	177		United Republic of Tanzania	44		India	423
	Argentina	170		Côte d'Ivoire	40		Australia	282
	Trinidad and Tobago	152		Nigeria	35		Viet Nam	223
	Venezuela	130		Madagascar	28		Malaysia	112
	Colombia	128		Gabon	27		Singapore	44
	Puerto Rico	120		Mayotte	20		Philippines	36
	Peru	89		Sierra Leone	20		Cambodia	29
Ae. albopictus								
Americas	Brazil	3441	Europe/ Africa	Italy	203	Asia/ Oceania	Taiwan	15,339
	USA	1594		Madagascar	58		Malaysia	186
	Mexico	50		Cameroon	42		Indonesia	161
	Cayman Islands	15		France	37		India	150
	Haiti	13		Gabon	27		Japan	97
	Guatemala	12		Albania	22		Thailand	82
	Venezuela	7		Mayotte	21		Singapore	44
	Colombia	3		Greece	18		Lao People's Democratic Republic	26
	Cuba	3		Israel	17		Philippines	22
	Puerto Rico	3		Lebanon	15		Viet Nam	18

Note: This table was contributed by Kramer a leading author of the paper published in E-life journal (https://doi.org/10.7554/eLife.08347.003).

Table 1. The ***Aedes aegypti*** and ***Ae. albopictus*** distribution globally.

Ae. albopictus is a treehole mosquito, and so its breeding places in nature are small, restricted, shaded bodies of water surrounded by vegetation. It inhabits densely vegetated rural areas. However, its ecological flexibility allows it to colonize many types of man-made sites and urban regions. It may reproduce in cemetery flowerpots, birdbaths, soda cans and abandoned containers, and water recipients. Tyres are particularly useful for mosquito reproduction as they are often stored outdoors and effectively collect and retain rainwater for a long time. The addition of decaying leaves from the neighboring trees produces chemical conditions similar to tree holes, which provides an excellent substrate for breeding. *Ae. albopictus* can also establish and survive throughout nonurbanized areas lacking any artificial containers, raising additional public health concerns for rural areas [17].

1.2.3. Aedes mosquitoes life cycle

Aedes mosquito species, *Ae. aegypti,* and *Ae. albopictus* are major public health concern due to their role in transmission of diseases [3]. *Ae. aegypti* mosquito is widespread in (sub-)tropical regions and is largely responsible for vector-borne arboviral infections, yellow fever virus (YFV), ZIKV, dengue virus (DENV), West Nile virus (WNV), CHIKV and transmission, and outbreaks in various regions [3, 7]. The *Ae. aegypti* is known to have high vectorial capacity due to its anthropophilic behavior, well domesticated, and adapted to survive in different geographical regions including Africa, Americas, Asia, and Europe [1, 3].

The *Aedes* spp. mosquitoes are known to have a complex life cycle involving aquatic and terrestrial life [2]. Mosquitoes acquire the infection after a blood-meal form the host in order for the eggs to develop. The vector needs water to lay their eggs in the preferred breeding container, including tyres, water storage containers, disposed tyres, coconut shells, and flowerpots [20]. *Aedes* spp. prefers to lay their eggs on the inner wet walls of containers with water, hence the name "container breeder". The development of the eggs occurs between 2 and 7 days in the aquatic phase (**Figure 1**) where the larvae hatch from the eggs. The larva survival depends on the microorganisms found in the aquatic environment. Larvae go through developmental stages (stage 1–4) in which they molt or shed their skin; these larval stages are called the first to fourth instars [20]. When a larva is a fully grown fourth instar, it undergoes metamorphosis into a new form called a pupa in approximately 4 days, the "cocoon" stage for the mosquito. This developmental stage of the mosquitoes also occurs in the aquatic environment. After 1–2 days, the fully developed adult mosquito forms and breaks through the skin of the pupa and a fully grown adult emerges. The adult mosquito is able to fly and has a terrestrial habitat inhabiting inside and outside households [20].

Interestingly, *Aedes* has developed a survival mechanism during the dry seasons; the eggs can enter a dormancy (quiescence) for up to 8 months at the end of embryogenesis [21]. If the habitat is dry, the eggs remain dormant but after rainfall, the eggs hatch and development continues [20]. In addition to being desiccation resistant, *Aedes* spp. is well adapted to produce, eggs can withstand months of dormancy, so-called "extended quiescence" in the unfavorable abiotic environment [21]. The male *Aedes* spp. mosquitoes feed on flowers' nectar or plant juices, unlike the female that needs a blood meal [22]. The vector becomes infected

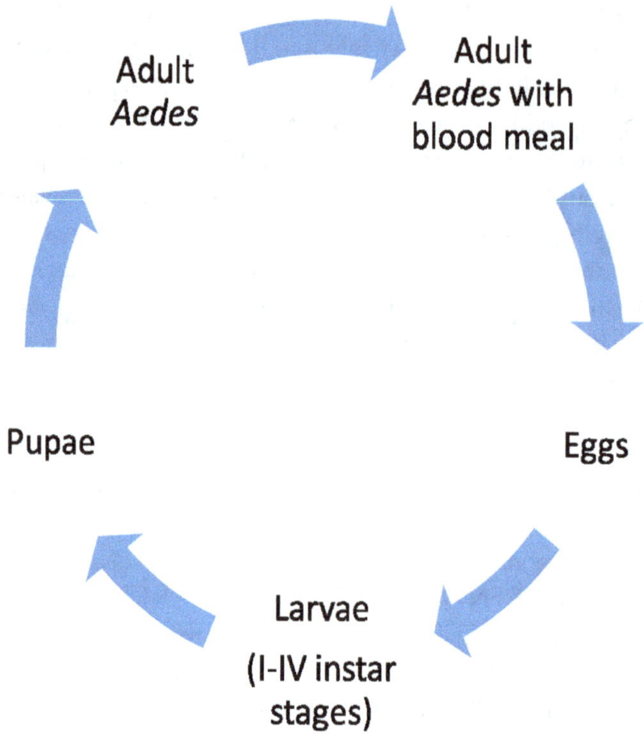

Figure 1. *Aedes* mosquito life cycle in aquatic and terrestrial phases.

when they feed on infected humans, and transmission may occur when the vector bites the host, which is believed to be promoted by mosquito salivary protein.

Historically, *Ae. aegypti* is believed to have originated from zoophilic subspecies *Ae. Aegypti formosus* inhabiting forests in sub-Saharan Africa [12]. This subspecies is found in the forests, breed in the tree holes and feeding on other mammals. The evolution of the ancestral *Ae. aegypti* resulted in the domesticated *Ae. aegypti* subspecies with a strong preference for biting humans and breed in man-made containers [20]. This evolved as the dominant vector of several diseases including yellow fever and DENV, ZIKV infections worldwide. The domestication of the vector was associated with the human migrations, trade, transportation, and urbanization [20, 23]. The domestic *Ae. aegypti* thrive in (sub-)tropical and temperate regions and can inhabit either terrestrial or aquatic depending on the stages of the growth. *Ae. aegypti* is primarily a container breeding vector and is known to predominate in urban areas where there is the vast composition of favorable man-made breeding container environment [20]. The breeding sites range from natural to artificial including vegetation, discarded tyres, discarded containers, bottle tops, water storage containers (especially in places with erratic tap water supply), flowerpots and vases, metal drums, and coconut shells [9, 24]. Other breeding sites include the open or unsealed septic tanks, water wells, and water meters. The ecological factors determine the crucial characteristics of different stages of the life and eventually its success. The *Ae. aegypti* larvae feed on nutritious materials available in the aqueous phase in the breeding containers including the plant particles, animal debris, and phytoplankton such as microalgae found in the water-filled containers [25]. The ecological characteristics are important in the life cycle of the adult vector including the longevity, fecundity body mass, and vectorial competence [26]. For instance, some algae species, *Cladophora sp.*, *Chlorella ellipsoidea*, and *Rhizoclonium hieroglyphicum*, were shown to exhibit larvicidal properties that affect the development of the immature stages [25]. Evidence suggests that the developmental stage from first instar larval stage to adult mosquito is faster when the organic matters are abundant in the breeding container, in addition, the survival rate of the immature stage is enhanced [27]. In contrast, low concentration or exhaustion of the nutrients is required to trigger pupation presumably in response to the increasing level of ecdysteroid hormone [3, 28, 29]. Temperature is important for the survival larva density and competence of the *Ae. aegypti*. In areas where the temperature is warmer, the development of the aquatic stage temperature was associated with shorter development time from hatch to the emergence of the adult mosquito [4]. Similarly, longer light exposure was also shown to shorten the development time [30]. The evidence explains the widespread distribution and pattern of *Ae. aegypti* in (sub-)tropical regions. Furthermore, evidence suggests increasing *Ae. aegypti* abundance in urban areas leading to outbreaks [31]. It is evident that developing countries are becoming more urbanized; however, poor city planning and sanitation have increased mosquito breeding sites [7]. The "ecological plasticity" exhibited by the vector is arguably among the reasons for reason that explain it its worldwide widespread and success as a human vector.

1.3. Insecticide resistance in *Aedes* spp.

The emergence of insecticide resistance to multiple classes of insecticides has been widely reported in *Ae. aegypti* in different regions [24, 32–34]. WHO defines resistance as the ability of mosquitoes to survive exposure to a standard dose of insecticide; this ability may be the result of physiological or behavioral adaptation [35]. The emergence and spread of resistance to the main insecticides could compromise the effectiveness of the preventive measures, operational implementation of control programs, and outbreak management.

1.4. Mechanisms of insecticide resistance

There are three major categories of insecticide resistance that have been described, namely, physiological resistance (target-site resistance and metabolic resistance) and behavioral avoidance. First, physiological resistance may develop due to the target-site resistance. Target site mutations are known to cause amino acid substitutions, which could affect the influx of insecticides into the target site. This may compromise the action of the insecticide rendering the vector tolerant or fully resistant to the insecticide. Another form of physiological resistance is due to metabolic resistance due to detoxification of insecticides by cytochrome P450 monooxygenases which allow the resistant vector to metabolize insecticides [36]. Glutathione S-transferases (GSTs) and carboxylesterases (ESTs) are also described in this process. Over expression of P450s was associated with insecticide resistance in diverse vector species including *Ae. aegypti* [37]. The resistant vectors accumulate high levels of efficient enzymes that detoxify the toxins. The second mechanism of resistance is known as behavioral adaptation or avoidance of the vector, this is well characterized in *Anopheles* mosquitoes. Therefore, monitoring insecticide resistance is crucial in the implementation of vector control strategies.

1.4.1. Physiological resistance in Aedes spp.

In Tanzania, like many other African settings, there is limited information on the *Ae. aegypti* resistance, most of the resistance data were collected mainly in the Americas and Asia. Our recent study in Dar es Salaam [24] demonstrated that the majority of *Ae. aegypti* strains were resistant to pyrethroid class of insecticide; mortality ranging from 83 to 92% in Dar es Salaam City. Data on molecular markers of resistance are scarce; however, studies elsewhere have correlated the occurrence of the knockdown resistance (kdr) mutations and resistance to pyrethroid and DDT [29, 34, 37, 38].

The mechanism of action of the pyrethroid compounds is through their toxic effect and subsequent disruption of the VGS channels in the insect nervous system [32]. The evidence suggests that *Ae. aegypti* resistance to pyrethroids is conferred by the *kdr* mutations in the VGS channel [29, 39]. Nonsynonymous mutations in *kdr* gene are associated with insecticide resistance to DDT and pyrethroids on codon V1016I and F1534C in domains II and III of the VSG channel in *Aedes* spp. [40]. Other studies demonstrated the role of *kdr* gene mutation I1011M/V and F1269C in association with *Ae. aegypti* resistance [33, 34, 41]. In African settings, the occurrence of F1534C in concurrence with the V1016I mutation was also observed in Ghanaian *Ae. aegypti* population [42]. The more recent study demonstrated the significant role of *kdr* mutation V410L alone or in combination with the F1534C in reducing the sensitivity of *Ae. aegypti* to both type I (e.g., permethrin) and type II (e.g., deltamethrin) pyrethroids [32].

In addition to the *kdr* mutations, metabolic resistance is also know to lead to a physiological resistance due to the increase in the synthesis of detoxifying enzymes or in their specificity to metabolize the insecticide, both resulting in an enhancement of the insect detoxifying capacity of the vector [43, 44]. The P450 monooxygenases were shown to play a significant role in modulating resistance as revealed by high-throughput assays, by comparing the overall profile at genomic and transcriptome levels between resistant and susceptible populations [37]. A study that characterized several P450s, four CYP's, 9 J32, 9 J24, 9 J26, and 9 J28, conferring insecticide resistance in *Ae. aegypti* [37]. The CYPs were shown to be capable of metabolizing deltamethrin and permethrin; two common pyrethroid-based insecticides are widely used in vector interventions. Furthermore, there is evidence on the role of glutathione transferase (GST) enzymes in conferring resistance to several classes of insecticides [45]. In *Ae. aegypti*, the GST occurs as a cluster of genes in chromosome 2 and is shown to play a significant role in the metabolism of DDT [46]. Over expression of the GST enzyme is associated with DDT and pyrethroid resistant in *Ae. aegypti* populations. We, therefore, characterized additional members of this class in *Ae. aegypti* and provide evidence for a role of two additional GSTs in conferring resistance to insecticides.

1.4.2. Behavioral resistance in Aedes spp.

Thus is defined as the ability of a vector to detect and escape from an insecticide-treated area and avoid the toxin. This type of resistance has been shown in different classes of insecticides, including organochlorines, organophosphates, carbamates, and pyrethroids [47]. It has been shown that vectors are capable of avoiding feeding if they come across certain insecticides or escape the area sprayed with the insecticides. There are currently limited studies exploring this mechanism of resistance in *Ae. aegypti*. This paucity of information could hamper control programs since insecticide resistance could spread and render the insecticides ineffective. Therefore, more studies to assess the current susceptibility status of insecticides used for vector control are needed to describe the status to support control strategies.

2. Disease transmission by *Aedes aegypti*

Ae. aegypti mosquito is a major vector of dengue virus represented by four closely related serotypes called dengue 1, 2, 3, and 4 cause different illness including dengue fever, dengue shock syndrome, and dengue haemorrhagic fever. Dengue virus (DENV) belonging to the family Flaviviridae and genus *Flavivirus* [48].

Transmission of dengue fever (DF) occurs when a female *Aedes* spp. mosquito obtains its blood meal from an infected person during the period of viraemia. Mosquito-borne viruses multiply in both invertebrate and vertebrate cells where they cause cytopathic effects and cell destruction. Vector mosquitoes become infected when they feed on blood of a viremic vertebrate host in which there are sufficient circulating viral particles to provide an infectious dose to the mosquito.

A mosquito with salivary gland infection may transmit infectious virions during salivation as it probes the tissues of another vertebrate host. Transovarial transmission of virions occurs from the female mosquito to her progeny, and females of the next generation can transmit the virus orally without having been infected through blood feeding. There is also a venereal transmission of some arboviruses from male to female mosquito as observed and reported by Amarasinghe and others [49] (**Figure 2**).

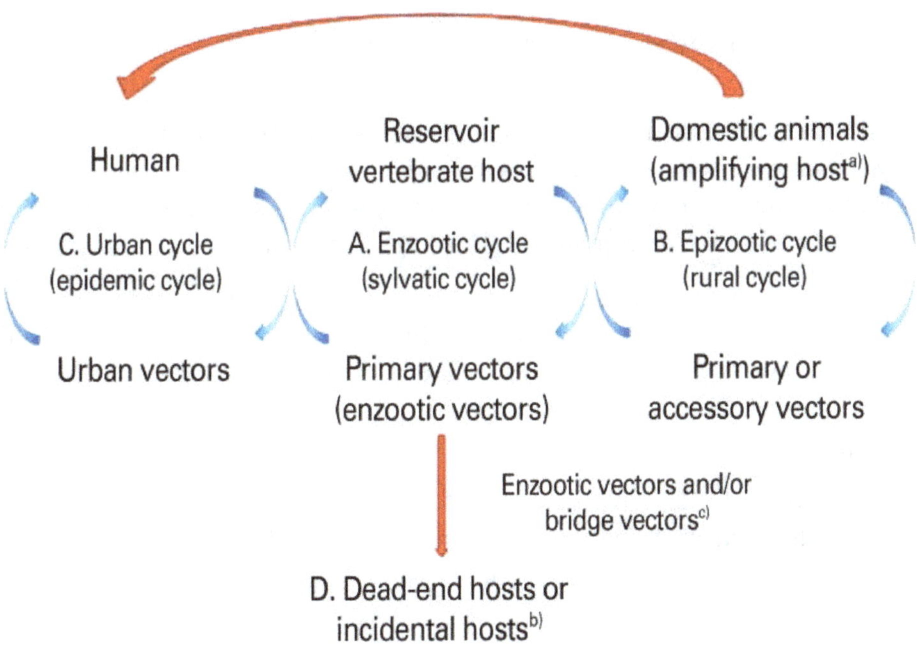

Figure 2. Arboviral transmission cycle vectored by *Aedes* mosquitoes.

Transmission of dengue virus occurs in 3 cycle, namely, enzootic cycle, epizootic cycle, and epidemic cycle. The enzootic cycle involves monkey-Aedes-monkey cycle, and this cycle is primitive and has been reported in South Asia and Africa [50]. The second is epizootic cycle, which involves the transmission of dengue virus from nonhuman primates to the next human in epidemic cycles by Aedes mosquito. Lastly, the epidemic cycle where the transmission cycle is through human *Ae. aegypti* contact, human cycle with periodic, or cyclical epidemic (**Figure 2**).

In this life cycle (human-to-*Ae. aegypti* mosquito-to-human cycle), the main dengue virus transmission is through mosquito that usually acquires the virus after feeding on the blood of an infected person. Replication of the virus occurs in the epithelial lining of the mosquito's midgut and then the virus move to haemocoele to infect the salivary glands. The virus can be transmitted though saliva during probing or blood feeding. The extrinsic incubation period may take 8–12 days, and this mosquito remains infected in all her life [50].

Infected humans are the major carriers of the virus where mosquito can acquire the virus through biting. The incubation time varies from virus to virus, but generally, arboviruses exhibit between 2–15 days from inoculation to development of clinical symptoms. During this period, *Aedes* mosquito can acquire the virus after feeding this person.

The reemergence of dengue disease in other places may be associated with the transovarial (via the eggs) transmission of dengue virus by *Ae. aegypti.* Dengue fever cannot spread directly from one person to another. Usually, *Ae. aegypti* prefers to feed mammalian hosts and will like to feed on humans, and even in the presence of other hosts (anthropophilic behavior), this behavior together with multiple feeding habit and highly domesticated behavior can make it an efficient vector.

3. Seasonality and intensity of transmission

Usually, dengue transmission occurs in rainy seasons with appropriate temperature and humidity for surviving of adult and larva mosquito. On the other hand, in arid areas, the rainfall is scant, and therefore, during the dry season, the man-made containers become the main breeding sites for the *Aedes* mosquito. Therefore, this can increase disease transmission.

In the ambient temperature, the life cycle of *Aedes* is shortening; also, there is production of small size mosquitoes, which may lead to the reduction of extrinsic incubation period. This small size mosquito may take more blood meal for egg production, which may lead to the increase in the number of infected mosquito and speedup the disease epidemic in the next dry season [50–52].

Several entomological factors have been associated with the initiation and maintenance of the epidemic including behavior, density, and vectorial capacity of mosquito vector population and introduction of the virus into a community.

4. Control and surveillance

4.1. Community education

This can be done by professionals by giving the public awareness, which can help to empower people to take control of mosquito breedings around their surroundings and adult control. The public can be provided with the tools needed to reduce mosquito annoyance. This is when the community, families, and individuals involved in planning and implementation of local vector control activities in order to ensure that the program meets priorities and the needs of the people in the community.

4.2. Larval mosquito control

Frequent larval breeding sites should be searched and treated as frequent as possible by trained field technicians and trained community members. Mosquito elimination in larval stages before emerging to adults will reduce the adult mosquito population. Reduction of mosquito breeding sites such as jars, barrels, pots, vases, bottles, tins, water coolers, and tyres can be done by environmental management, removing of solid waste and managing artificial man-made habitats. All domestic water storage containers should be cleaned and covered daily.

4.3. Adult control of *Aedes aegypti*

This should aim to control *Ae. aegypti* population. The use of insecticides such as lambda cyhalothrin- or deltamethrin-treated material by hanging them on windows and used as water jar covers may reduce *Ae. aegypti* population [53]. The use of insecticide space spraying, coils, and vaporizers in the community may reduce the mosquito population.

4.4. Use of repellents

Application of repellents such as DEET, DIMP, and of like is of paramount importance in reducing or controlling human to vector contact. The application should be done during active hours of the day.

4.5. Surveillance

Surveillance is important detect mosquito species in a certain area and changes in populations. By having valuable data, we are capable of more successfully time larvicide applications and more correctly target the adulticide activities. The WHO recommends of regular household surveys of *Aedes* spp. collecting evidence on the ecological and epidemiological indices to guide prevention and control strategies. This involves determining the habitat productivity, preference of the breeding sites, containers for the presence of egg, larvae and pupae as well as the collection of adult mosquitoes for further identification. Larval surveys involve identifying the presence of immature mosquitoes in breeding sites such as discarded tyres, containers, and water storage vases in the defined targeted area. Through this assessment, it is possible to identify most containers that are positive for *Aedes* spp. and parameters such Container Index (CI) and Breteau Index (BI) [6]. On the other hand, pupal survey is performed in houses and other breeding sites to identify the productivity in the breeding habitat [7]. In addition, surveys to determine the prevalence and circulating serotypes of DENV, ZIKV, CHIKV, and YFV as a part of regular surveillance are required to inform strategies to prevent transmission and provide early warning signal of outbreaks of clinical infections.

5. Discussion

Ae. aegypti remains a serious public health threat due to its importance in arboviral transmission, DENV, CHIKV, and ZIKV transmission. Globally, the incidence of DENV infections is on the rise, and recently, reemergence of CHIKV and ZIKV has been observed. Vaccine, prophylaxis, and therapeutics for most arboviral infections are still in development pipeline; hence, integrated vector management remains the cornerstone to stop outbreak transmission and sustainable control. Therefore, understanding of the ecology is important for outbreak prediction and effective planning of strategies to control transmission of arboviral infections.

Studies on the ecology of *Ae. aegypti* are important to better understand the preference of the vector in terms of the oviposition and colonization of mosquitoes [8]. The ecological factors play a role on influencing the population dynamics of larvae and pupae. The evidence is clear that both abiotic and biotic factors are important determinants of adulthood characteristics of life cycle such as longevity, fecundity, and body size [8, 9]. The factors are important to explain the vectorial capacity of *Ae. aegypti* on disease transmission. Furthermore, there is compelling evidence that *Ae. aegypti* is most productive in containers, which varies among regions, geographical settings, and seasonality [10]. In addition, it undoubtedly clears that water storage containers and discarded containers influence the vector density and risk of arboviral transmission particularly in poorly planned cities in (sub-)tropical regions [11]. Unless appropriate actions are taken, increasing urbanization, poor environmental management will continue to influence the stability of the *Ae. aegypti* populations. In addition, the vector density is influenced significantly by environment factors and urbanization [9, 11, 13]. *Ae. aegypti* feed exclusively on human and is increasingly a threat particularly in unplanned (peri-)urban areas. The recent data highlight the increasing *Aedes* spp. abundance and urbanization that could potentially escalate the risk of arboviral outbreaks [31]. Furthermore, the environment contributes to the breeding and ecological colonization of the vector. The presence of organic nutrients and microorganisms such as cyanobacteria seems to have influence on the productivity and development of *Ae. aegypti* [11, 15]. The presence of microalgae in the larval habitats, therefore, represents high adequacy of nutrients for immature stages of *Ae. aegypti* [11, 15]. Microalgae are associated with the presence and abundance of the vectors being the source of food for the larvae in breeding habitats. The evidence suggests that better understanding of these factors may be a useful indicator for mosquito population control. Measures to control microalgae to deprive nutrients to the vector could be explored for additional measures of the vector control. Importantly, approaches targeting immature stages of *Ae. aegypti* are highly recommended for effective and sustainable vector control. *Ae. aegypti* vector lays eggs in containers, buckets, care tyres and water storage vases; thus, the appropriate intervention such as proper disposal and management of containers and discarded tyres for source reduction could prove effective in reducing the vector population and mitigate the risk of arboviral transmission. Therefore, implementation of strategies to address the challenge of reemergence and expansion of arboviral infections will require a strong multisector commitment and integration for effective surveillance and control at regional, national, and program levels.

There is widespread resistance to the commonly widely used insecticide, pyrethroids and organophosphates in *Aedes* spp. control. Insecticide resistance is likely to impact disease outbreak and transmission measures and cost of the interventions [16, 17]. This is currently a major concern in South America where organophosphates, pyrethroids, and DDT have been widely used in vector control. However, there is also evidence on decreased susceptibility to pyrethroids in Sub-Saharan Africa and Asia [10, 13]. The origin and evolution of *Aedes* spp. resistance to insecticides remain unclear; however, it is assumed that the use of the insecticide in other vector interventions such as malaria control and agricultural may have exerted selective pressure on the *Aedes* spp. The mechanism of *Ae. aegypti* resistance to insecticides seems to be mediated by the nonsynonymous mutations *kdr* gene [18, 19]. Other studies suggest the role of enhanced enzymatic biodegradation or sequestration [20, 21]. Studies suggest the potential role of the metabolic enzymes including cytochrome P450s and GSTs in conferring resistance to pyrethroids and organophosphates in *Aedes* spp. Evidence on the possible behavioral resistance or avoidance is patchy, and more investigation is needed to understand how it may affect the current interventions. Despite the worsening *Ae. aegypti* resistance to pyrethroids and organophosphates, studies on susceptibility profile of *Bti* are reassuring that *Aedes* spp. retains considerable susceptibility to the biolarvicides [17]. Therefore, *Bti* remains a suitable alternative for prevention and control tool in regions where resistance to pyrethroids is widespread. To mitigate the risk of resistance and its public health consequences, it is crucial to strengthen monitoring and surveillance at all levels. Susceptibility testing of the commonly used insecticides and biolarvicides using the standardized WHO bioassay protocol should be integrated as part of the surveillance program and profiling of molecular markers of resistance may be considered as appropriate.

6. Conclusion

Aedes aegypti is the most important vector in outbreak and transmission of arboviral infections. The environmental factors favor mosquitoes and risk of disease transmission. The diseases are expanding particularly in (sub-)urban settings with frequent water shortage, high human population, poor planning, and poor waste disposal systems. Primary prevention and control measures are to reduce the vector exposure, but current vector control tools are unsustainable and there is increasing threat due to insecticide resistance. Integration of *Aedes* spp. vector control with other ongoing program and coordination of insecticide resistance monitoring and management is crucial to increase the impact of interventions. Future interventions will require deployment of effective vaccines against arboviral infections combined with integrated vector management.

Author details

Eliningaya J. Kweka[1,2*], Vito Baraka[3], Leah Mathias[4], Beda Mwang'onde[5], Germana Baraka[6], Lucile Lyaruu[2] and Aneth M. Mahande[7]

*Address all correspondence to: eliningaya.kweka@tpri.go.tz

1 School of Medicine, Department of Parasitology and Entomology, Catholic University of Health and Allied Health Sciences, Mwanza, Tanzania

2 Tropical Pesticides Research Institute, Arusha, Tanzania

3 National Institute for Medical Research, Tanga Centre, Tanzania

4 Ministry of Education Science and Technology, Mzumbe High School, Morogoro, Tanzania

5 Sokoine University of Agriculture, Morogoro, Tanzania

6 College of Natural Sciences, University of Dar es Salaam, Dar es Salaam, Tanzania

7 Tropical Pesticides Research Institute, Mabogini Field Station, Moshi, Tanzania

References

[1] Harbach R. Mosquito Taxonomic Inventory. 2013. p. 2015

[2] Wilkerson RC, Linton Y-M, Fonseca DM, Schultz TR, Price DC, Strickman DA. Making mosquito taxonomy useful: A stable classification of tribe Aedini that balances utility with current knowledge of evolutionary relationships. PLoS One. 2015;**10**:e0133602

[3] Kraemer MU, Sinka ME, Duda KA, Mylne AQ, Shearer FM, Barker CM, et al. The global distribution of the arbovirus vectors *Aedes aegypti* and *Ae. albopictus*. eLife. 2015;**4**:e08347

[4] WHO. Global Strategy for Dengue Prevention and Control 2012-2020. Geneva, Switzerland: WHO; 2012. p. 43, 43

[5] Fredericks AC, Fernandez-Sesma A. The burden of dengue and chikungunya worldwide: Implications for the southern United States and California. Annals of Global Health. 2014;**80**:466-475

[6] WHO, UNICEF. Global vector control response 2017-2030. Geneva: WHO and UNICEF; 2017

[7] Schaffner F, Mathis A. Dengue and dengue vectors in the WHO European region: Past, present, and scenarios for the future. The Lancet Infectious Diseases. 2014;**14**:1271-1280

[8] Sang RC. Dengue in Africa. In: Report of the Scientific Working Group Meeting on Dengue. Geneva: WHO Special Programme for Research and Training in Tropical Diseases. 2007. pp. 50-52

[9] Mboera LEG, Mweya CN, Rumisha SF, Tungu PK, Stanley G, Makange MR, et al. The risk of dengue virus transmission in Dar es Salaam, Tanzania during an epidemic period of 2014. PLoS Neglected Tropical Diseases. 2016;**10**:e0004313

[10] Capinha C, Rocha J, Sousa CA. Macroclimate determines the global range limit of *Aedes aegypti*. EcoHealth. 2014;**11**:420-428

[11] Brady OJ, Golding N, Pigott DM, Kraemer MUG, Messina JP, Reiner RC Jr, et al. Global temperature constraints on *Aedes aegypti* and *Ae. albopictus* persistence and competence for dengue virus transmission. Parasites & Vectors. 2014;**7**:338

[12] Weetman D, Kamgang B, Badolo A, Moyes CL, Shearer FM, Coulibaly M, et al. Aedes mosquitoes and aedes-borne arboviruses in Africa: Current and future threats. International Journal of Environmental Research and Public Health. 2018;**15**:220

[13] Ponlawat A, Harrington LC. Blood feeding patterns of *Aedes aegypti* and *Aedes albopictus* in Thailand. Journal of Medical Entomology. 2005;**42**:844-849

[14] Zahouli JB, Utzinger J, Adja MA, Müller P, Malone D, Tano Y, et al. Oviposition ecology and species composition of Aedes spp. and *Aedes aegypti* dynamics in variously urbanized settings in arbovirus foci in southeastern Côte d'Ivoire. Parasites & Vectors. 2016;**9**:523

[15] Scholte E-J, Schaffner F. Waiting for the tiger: Establishment and spread of the *Aedes albopictus* mosquito in Europe. In: Takken W, Knols BG, editors. Emerging Pests and Vector-Borne Diseases in Europe. Vol. 1. Wageningen: Wageningen Academic Publisher; 2007. p. 241

[16] Juliano SA, Philip Lounibos L. Ecology of invasive mosquitoes: Effects on resident species and on human health. Ecology Letters. 2005;**8**:558-574

[17] Eritja R, Escosa R, Lucientes J, Marques E, Roiz D, Ruiz S. Worldwide invasion of vector mosquitoes: Present European distribution and challenges for Spain. Biological Invasions. 2005;**7**:87

[18] Cancrini G, Romi R, Gabrielli S, Toma L, Di Paolo M, Scaramozzino P. First finding of Dirofilaria repens in a natural population of *Aedes albopictus*. Medical and Veterinary Entomology. 2003;**17**:448-451

[19] Delatte H, Gimonneau G, Triboire A, Fontenille D. Influence of temperature on immature development, survival, longevity, fecundity, and gonotrophic cycles of *Aedes albopictus*, vector of chikungunya and dengue in the Indian Ocean. Journal of Medical Entomology. 2009;**46**:33-41

[20] Powell JR, Tabachnick WJ. History of domestication and spread of *Aedes aegypti*-a review. Memórias do Instituto Oswaldo Cruz. 2013;**108**:11-17

[21] Diniz DFA, Albuquerque CMR, Oliva LO, Melo-Santos MAV, Ayres CFJ. Diapause and quiescence: Dormancy mechanisms that contribute to the geographical expansion of mosquitoes and their evolutionary success. Parasites & Vectors. 2017;**10**:310

[22] Whitehead SS, Blaney JE, Durbin AP, Murphy BR. Prospects for a dengue virus vaccine. Nature Reviews Microbiology. 2007;**5**:518

[23] McBride CS, Baier F, Omondi AB, Spitzer SA, Lutomiah J, Sang R, et al. Evolution of mosquito preference for humans linked to an odorant receptor. Nature. 2014;**515**:222

[24] Mathias L, Baraka V, Philbert A, Innocent E, Francis F, Nkwengulila G, et al. Habitat productivity and pyrethroid susceptibility status of *Aedes aegypti* mosquitoes in Dar es Salaam, Tanzania. Infectious Diseases of Poverty. 2017;**6**:102

[25] Ahmad R, Chu W-L, Lee H-L, Phang S-M. Effect of four chlorophytes on larval survival, development and adult body size of the mosquito *Aedes aegypti*. Journal of Applied Phycology. 2001;**13**:369-374

[26] Barrera R, Amador M, Clark GG. Ecological factors influencing *Aedes aegypti* (Diptera: Culicidae) productivity in artificial containers in Salinas, Puerto Rico. Journal of Medical Entomology. 2006;**43**:484-492

[27] Tun-Lin W, Burkot T, Kay B. Effects of temperature and larval diet on development rates and survival of the dengue vector *Aedes aegypti* in North Queensland, Australia. Medical and Veterinary Entomology. 2000;**14**:31-37

[28] Levi T, Ben-Dov E, Shahi P, Borovsky D, Zaritsky A. Growth and development of *Aedes aegypti* larvae at limiting food concentrations. Acta Tropica. 2014;**133**:42-44

[29] Brito LP, Linss JG, Lima-Camara TN, Belinato TA, Peixoto AA, Lima JBP, et al. Assessing the effects of *Aedes aegypti* kdr mutations on pyrethroid resistance and its fitness cost. PLoS One. 2013;**8**:e60878

[30] Couret J, Dotson E, Benedict MQ. Temperature, larval diet, and density effects on development rate and survival of *Aedes aegypti* (Diptera: Culicidae). PLoS One. 2014;**9**:e87468

[31] Zahouli JB, Koudou BG, Müller P, Malone D, Tano Y, Utzinger J. Urbanization is a main driver for the larval ecology of Aedes mosquitoes in arbovirus-endemic settings in South-Eastern Côte d'Ivoire. PLoS Neglected Tropical Diseases. 2017;**11**:e0005751

[32] Haddi K, Tomé HV, Du Y, Valbon WR, Nomura Y, Martins GF, et al. Detection of a new pyrethroid resistance mutation (V410L) in the sodium channel of *Aedes aegypti*: A potential challenge for mosquito control. Scientific Reports. 2017;**7**:46549

[33] Harris AF, Rajatileka S, Ranson H. Pyrethroid resistance in *Aedes aegypti* from grand Cayman. The American Journal of Tropical Medicine and Hygiene. 2010;**83**:277-284

[34] Brengues C, Hawkes NJ, Chandre F, McCarroll L, Duchon S, Guillet P, et al. Pyrethroid and DDT cross-resistance in *Aedes aegypti* is correlated with novel mutations in the voltage-gated sodium channel gene. Medical and Veterinary Entomology. 2003;**17**:87-94

[35] WHO. Test Procedures for Insecticide Resistance Monitoring in Malaria Vector Mosquitoes. Geneva, Swirtzeland: WHO; 2016

[36] Feyereisen R. Insect CYP genes and P450 enzymes. In: Insect Molecular Biology and Biochemistry. London: Elsevier, Academic Press; 2012. pp. 236-316

[37] Stevenson BJ, Pignatelli P, Nikou D, Paine MJ. Pinpointing P450s associated with pyrethroid metabolism in the dengue vector, *Aedes aegypti*: Developing new tools to combat insecticide resistance. PLoS Neglected Tropical Diseases. 2012;**6**:e1595

[38] de Lourdes Macoris M, Martins AJ, Andrighetti MTM, Lima JBP, Valle D. Pyrethroid resistance persists after ten years without usage against *Aedes aegypti* in governmental campaigns: Lessons from São Paulo state, Brazil. PLoS Neglected Tropical Diseases. 2018; **12**:e0006390

[39] Smith LB, Kasai S, Scott JG. Pyrethroid resistance in *Aedes aegypti* and *Aedes albopictus*: Important mosquito vectors of human diseases. Pesticide Biochemistry and Physiology. 2016;**133**:1-12

[40] Kasai S, Ng LC, Lam-Phua SG, Tang CS, Itokawa K, Komagata O, et al. First detection of a putative knockdown resistance gene in major mosquito vector, *Aedes albopictus*. Japanese Journal of Infectious Diseases. 2011;**64**:217-221

[41] Saavedra-Rodriguez K, Urdaneta-Marquez L, Rajatileka S, Moulton M, Flores A, Fernandez-Salas I, et al. A mutation in the voltage-gated sodium channel gene associated with pyrethroid resistance in Latin American *Aedes aegypti*. Insect Molecular Biology. 2007;**16**:785-798

[42] Kawada H, Higa Y, Komagata O, Kasai S, Tomita T, Yen NT, et al. Widespread distribution of a newly found point mutation in voltage-gated sodium channel in pyrethroid-resistant *Aedes aegypti* populations in Vietnam. PLoS Neglected Tropical Diseases. 2009;**3**:e527

[43] David J-P, Ismail HM, Chandor-Proust A, Paine MJI. Role of cytochrome P450s in insecticide resistance: Impact on the control of mosquito-borne diseases and use of insecticides on earth. Philosophical Transactions of the Royal Society, B: Biological Sciences. 2013;**368**

[44] Faucon F, Gaude T, Dusfour I, Navratil V, Corbel V, Juntarajumnong W, et al. In the hunt for genomic markers of metabolic resistance to pyrethroids in the mosquito *Aedes aegypti*: An integrated next-generation sequencing approach. PLoS Neglected Tropical Diseases. 2017;**11**:e0005526

[45] Hemingway J, Hawkes NJ, McCarroll L, Ranson H. The molecular basis of insecticide resistance in mosquitoes. Insect Biochemistry and Molecular Biology. 2004;**34**:653-665

[46] Lumjuan N, Rajatileka S, Changsom D, Wicheer J, Leelapat P, Prapanthadara L-A, et al. The role of the *Aedes aegypti* Epsilon glutathione transferases in conferring resistance to DDT and pyrethroid insecticides. Insect Biochemistry and Molecular Biology. 2011;**41**:203-209

[47] Hemingway J, Ranson H. Insecticide resistance in insect vectors of human disease. Annual Review of Entomology. 2000;**45**:371-391

[48] Malik A, Earhart K, Mohareb E, Saad M, Saeed M, Ageep A, et al. Dengue hemorrhagic fever outbreak in children in Port Sudan. Journal of Infection and Public Health. 2011; **4**:1-6

[49] Amarasinghe A, Kuritsky JN, Letson GW, Margolis HS. Dengue virus infection in Africa. Emerging Infectious Diseases. 2011;**17**:1349

[50] Gubler DJ. Dengue and dengue hemorrhagic fever. Clinical Microbiology Reviews. 1998; **11**:480-496

[51] Gubler DJ, Clark GG. Community-based integrated control of *Aedes aegypti*: A brief overview of current programs. The American Journal of Tropical Medicine and Hygiene. 1994;**50**:50-60

[52] Thongcharoen P, Jatanasen S. Epidemiology of dengue and dengue haemorrhagic fever. Monograph on Dengue/Dengue Haemorrhagic Fever. 1999:1-8

[53] Kroeger ALA, Ochoa M, Villegas E, Levy M, Alexander N. Effective control of dengue vectors with curtains and water container covers treated with insecticide in Mexico and Venezuela: Cluster randomised trials. BMJ. 2006;**332**:1247

4

RNA Association, RNA Interference, and microRNA Pathways in Dengue Fever Virus-Host Interaction

Imran Shahid

Abstract

Dengue fever is a fatal vector transmitted disease and is one of the most significant health problems which have magnified its impact globally by afflicting 390 million people across 110 countries. The causative agent of this life-threatening disease is a positive single-stranded RNA arbovirus known as dengue virus (DENV), which uses *Aedes aegypti* mosquito as an intermediate host. It has been well demonstrated that virus evades mosquito's RNA interference (RNAi)-mediated antiviral defense and manipulates host microRNA (miRNA) profile to its own benefit. However, the exact mechanisms are still not exclusively elucidated. The molecular mechanisms which characterize the role of novel DENV-encoded small RNAs and other viral proteins in host miRNA modulation and evasion of RNA interference are still elusive. Furthermore, the possibility of small activating RNAs-(RNAa)-mediated activation in mosquitoes in conjunction with dengue virus genes is not fully explored. This book chapter pragmatically overviews intricate interplay between virus-host interactions, how virus invades host antivirus defense mechanisms, and possibly the potential emerging therapeutic role of RNA activation (RNAa) and RNAi for the infections, which can be cured by specific gene activation and gene silencing, respectively.

Keywords: dengue fever, dengue fever virus, *Aedes aegypti*, RNA interference, microRNAs, RNA association, host-virus interaction, DENV therapy

1. Introduction

Dengue virus (DENV) is a major arbovirus that uses *Aedes aegypti* mosquitoes as an intermediate host to be transmitted to human and is the causative agent of most serious mosquito-borne viral disease (i.e., dengue fever) afflicting around more than 390 million people worldwide [1]. Despite substantial efforts to control dengue virus vector, it is still emerging rapidly [2]. Therapeutic options are limited as the available treatments are just supportive, and there is no specific therapy or approved vaccine available. DENV belongs to *Flaviviridae* family, which comprises lipid-enveloped, positive-sense single-stranded RNA viruses [3]. DENV is classified into four closely related serotypes based on antigen distinction and represented as DENV-1 to DENV-4. The length of DENV genome is 10.7 kilobases comprising a single open reading frame (ORF) flanked by highly conserved 5′ and 3′ nontranslated regions. Single ORF encodes a polyprotein of approximately 3391 amino acids, which is further processed by host (furin and signalase) and viral proteases (NS2B/NS3 protease complex) to generate three structural (C, prM, and E) and seven nonstructural genes (NS1, NS2A, NS2B, NS3, NS4A, NS4B, and NS5) [4, 5].

RNA interference (RNAi) is evolutionarily conserved phenomenon, constituting a major component of mosquito innate immune response to virus infections [6]. It has been demonstrated that dengue virus elicits RNAi response in *Ae. aegypti* but is unable to completely repress viral replication instead it may just modulate virus replication to maintain persistent viral infection to ensure long-term survival of infected mosquitoes [7]. It has been explored that DENV employs two different mechanisms to inhibit RNAi pathway, involving RNAi suppression protein NS4B and subgenomic flavivirus RNA (sfRNA). Dengue virus encoded nonstructural protein, NS4B, has been reported to suppress RNAi pathway in both human Huh-7 cells by the mechanism still not fully understood [8]. Furthermore, dengue virus infection produces 3′ NTR degradation product sfRNA that is thought to incapacitate RNAi pathway by inhibiting dicer-mediated cleavage of dsRNA [9]. Recently, it has been ferreted out that in Culex mosquitoes, West Nile virus (WNV) replication is repressed by cytokine-like secreted antiviral protein "vago" in a dicer-2-dependent manner [10]. However, the possible effect of vago protein against dengue virus replication in *Ae. aegypti* research area is not explored yet. Such evidence clearly indicates that dengue virus opts variety of mechanisms to evade mosquito immune response to successfully replicate in the mosquitoes.

Apart from small interference RNAs (siRNA) reputation to inhibit gene expression through a phenomenon called RNAi, the target gene can also be induced by a mechanism called RNA activation (RNAa). The term RNAa was first coined by Li, who named them after he surprisingly found up regulation of human E-cadherin, p21, and VEGF genes by synthetic dsRNAs designed to target promoters of these genes [11]. He further named those promoters targeting small RNAs as short activating RNAs (saRNAs). Recent studies in which authors evaluated RNAa of above-said genes in monkey, rat, and mouse found that RNAa is highly conserved among all mammals [12]. However, the term RNA activation is not necessarily limited to transcriptional activation by saRNA, targeting promoter region only, rather it should be used to describe all small RNA-mediated gene and epigenome activation mechanisms, including transcriptional activation by targeting 3′ terminal regions of genes with saRNAs [13], piwi-interacting RNA (piRNAs)-mediated epigenetic activation [14], and microRNA (miRNA)-mediated translation activation [15]. One of the key differences between RNAi and RNAa is their kinetics. RNAi effect is known to occur within a couple of hours and disappears 5–7 days following siRNA transfection, while RNAa effect does not appear until about 48 h posttransfection and lasts much longer (at least 2 weeks) [16]. This delay may be due to the more complex mechanism of RNAa involving nuclear access and chromatin restructuring as compared to RNAi [17].

microRNAs (miRNAs) represent one of the shortest functional classes of noncoding RNAs, depicting hottest spot of gene regulation research. They were first reported in 1993 in small round worms *Caenorhabditis elegans* [18]. Since then, miRNAs have been implicated in regulating all cellular pathways in eukaryotes ranging from development to oncogenesis. These 20–24 nucleotide-long noncoding RNAs have been demonstrated to be encoded by a diverse range of organisms including plants, humans, insects, and even viruses [19]. The miRNA shows a very high degree of evolutionary sequence conservation among species [20] proved by the presence of miRNA biogenesis complex in archaea and eubacteria [21]. Historically, these microRNAs were thought to regulate different gene expressions either by degradation of particular mRNA or inhibition of translation [22, 23]. However, recent studies have revealed that these small noncoding RNAs can also activate the target gene expression through mRNA stabilization [15, 24]. As the molecular biology, bioinformatics approaches and protocols of small RNA sequencing continue to grow and sophisticate, so is the number of miRNAs discovered in different species. It is becoming more and more apparent that miRNAs not only constitute a fundamental part of regulatory machinery but also may act as molecular decoys to interfere with the function of regulatory RNA-binding proteins [25]. miRNA is involved in fundamental physiological and pathological processes like cancer development and host-pathogen interactions [26–29]. The pathogens have evolved to use to host machinery by altering the expression level of host miRNAs for their benefit [30]. Furthermore, microorganism-encoded miRNAs have also been reported to vary the host gene expression to their advantage [30]. Despite recent advances, there are still significant gaps in our understanding of miRNAs role in host-pathogen interactions, which is probably due to lack of miRNA characterization.

This pragmatic book chapter overviews the possibility of RNAi suppressor activity of DENV in the context of different viral genes. By characterizing the role of different DENV genes in RNAi suppression, we will review to gather valuable lead into the mechanism that governs DENV RNAi evasion in mosquitoes and the viral genes that are responsible for it. We will also explicit the possibility of RNA activation (RNAa) in insect, especially mosquitos. It is interesting to characterize whether RNAa has any role in host pathogen interaction because, despite the difference in their mode of action, RNAa use same RNAi machinery to induce gene activation. Although very few virus-encoded miRNAs have been fully characterized, it is understandable that they can target both viral and host genes. The information will produce a better understanding of microRNAs role in DENV replication and further deeper insight into characterization of DENV-mediated differential expression of *Ae. aegypti* miRNAs.

2. Dengue virus genome organization

The dengue virus (DENV) genome comprises a single open reading frame (ORF) of approximately 10.7 kilobases flanked by 5′ and 3′ nontranslated regions (NTRs) [30]. The nontranslated regions contain highly conserved secondary structures and coding regions in ORF, which play integral roles in viral life cycle. The composition of secondary structures is based on the sequencing of DENV-2 (a southeast Asian strain) strain, which is similar to other

Structural proteins	Protein functions
C	Viral RNA packaging
prM	Prevention of premature fusion
E	Envelope glycoprotein, receptor binding and fusion
Non-structural proteins	**Protein functions**
NS1	Signal transduction
NS2B	Co-factor for NS3 serine protease
NS3	Serine protease/helicase; NTPase
NS4B	Inhibition of interferon signal transduction
NS5	RNA-dependent RNA polymerase (RdRP); methyltransferase
RNA elements	**Functions**
5' UTR	Viral RNA synthesis and non-canonical translation
3' UTR	Cap-dependent and non-canonical translation; viral RNA synthesis

Table 1. Functions of DENV genome structural and nonstructural proteins.

different viral strains and serotypes. Although most of the DENV proteins are with known functions but some remains to be explored (**Table 1**) [31].

3. Viral entry

DENV is mostly introduced in human by infected *Ae. aegypti* mosquitoes. After the introduction, DENV particularly targets mononuclear phagocyte lineage cells including the skin resistant Langerhans cells [31, 32]. However, in mosquitoes, DENV is thought to initially target midgut and then extends and replicate in other peripheral tissues [33]. DENV can infect a very diverse range of cell lines including human, mosquito, monkey, hamster, and murine cell linages. This suggests that either DENV uses a ubiquitous receptor or it uses multiple receptors for its entry [33]. In mosquito cells, different independent groups have reported many potential DENV receptors like heat shock protein 70 (HSP), R80, R60, and 45 kDa protein [33]. In human beings, heparan sulfate [34], Hsp90 [35], CD14 [36], GRP78/BiP [37], and a 37/67-kDa high-affinity laminin receptor have been reported [38]. DENV particles interact with human myeloid cells by C-type lectin receptors (CLR) including DC-specific intracellular adhesion molecule 3 (ICAM-3)-grabbing no integrin (DC-SIGN, CD209) [39, 40], mannose receptor (MR), and C-type lectin domain family 5, member A (CLEC5, MDL-1) [41].

4. Viral replication

DENV like other flaviviruses, after adsorption to receptors, is endocytosed by cells in clathrin-dependent manner and then is further transported to endosomes [42]. However, according to one study, DENV can adopt clathrin-independent pathways as well to gain entry into mammalian cells in particular [43]. DENV nucleocapsid is released into cytosol after acidic pH triggered rearrangements of envelope protein in late endosomes leading to fusion of viral envelope and cellular endosome membrane [44, 45]. The nucleocapsid disassembles, and viral genome is translated by endoplasmic reticulum (ER)-located ribosomes generating numerous copies of viral proteins. NS5 and other viral nonstructural proteins along with various host proteins establish replication complexes [46]. At replication complex, the viral polymerase (NS5) transcribes negative viral RNA, which serves as a template for synthesis of subsequent positive viral RNA copies. Viral replication is regulated by 5′-3′ UTR sequences (upstream of AUG region) present in 5′-3′ UTRs, which are actively involved in the circularization of DENV RNA [47]. These newly synthesized positive DENV RNAs interact with core proteins to assemble into nucleocapsids [48]. The nucleocapsid buds into ER lumen, thereby getting enveloped in a membrane bilayer carrying the viral prM and E proteins [46]. From ER lumen, immature viral particles are transported through cellular secretary pathways, furin protease cleaves prM, and results in the formation of mature viral particles capable of infecting naïve cells [49].

5. Virus-host interactions

In nature, almost every organism engages in ecological or molecular interactions whether antagonistic or mutualistic with other organisms of different species to thrive and excel. These interactions are major drivers of diversification and adaptive evolution. Among these interactions, most fascinating examples are those involved in invertebrate susceptibility to pathogens [50]. According to a recent study, the susceptibility of *Ae. aegypti* to dengue virus has a genetic basis for genotype-by-genotype interactions [51]. It is evident by the fact that despite pathogenic nature of dengue virus in human, its interaction with *Ae. aegypti* mosquito is somehow mutualistic. DENV has somehow improvised to overcome mosquito defenses and manipulate its cellular machinery in a way still not well known that emancipates its replication without interfering too much with normal growth of mosquitos.

6. RNA interference (RNAi)

RNA interference (RNAi) is a major component of innate defense of invertebrates against pathogens. Most arboviruses cause persistent infections within their arthropod vectors. However, how viruses maintain persistent infection in the face of a robust RNAi response is still not fully understood. Many plants and animal viruses have evolved molecular mechanisms for subverting the host RNAi response. For example, Flock house virus (FHV) encodes B2 protein, which directly binds to dsRNA to inhibit DCR2 activity, to inert siRNA pathway [52]. In another study, researchers have found that plasmid-expressed La Crosse virus (LACV) NSs protein successfully inhibits interferon (IFN) and RNAi pathway in mammalian cells and mice, while fails to show any RNAi-suppressive effect in transfected U4.4 cells and C6/36 cells infected with LACV [53]. A recent publication has revealed that DENV NS4b functions as an RNAi suppressor in human Huh-7 cells via inhibition of dsRNA processing by Dicer [8]. However, whether NS4b behaves similarly in mosquitoes has not been investigated, and to date, no RNAi suppressor activity has been described for an arbovirus protein during mosquito infection. Given that DENV successfully develops persistent infection in mosquitoes despite their RNAi response, the precise mechanism of RNAi evasion is definitely a significant point of interest.

7. RNA activation (RNAa)

RNA activation (RNAa) is one of the nascent phenomena around the scientific field. RNAa is considered to be a potent emerging therapeutic strategy for the disease that can be cured by particular gene activation [54]. However, most of the studies relating to RNAa research have been carried out in human cell line. Till date, proper mechanism of RNAa is still not clear. However, it has been demonstrated that it is mostly a nuclear event that leads to chromatin restructuring [17]. RNA activation is still in its infancy, so its exact mechanism is still elusive. Recently, Portnoy et al. has proposed a model for the promoter-directed-small-activating-RNA (saRNAs)-mediated RNA activation. In this model, authors proposed that an exogenously introduced saRNA or endogenously produced small noncoding RNA, (e.g., miRNA) is loaded into an Ago protein in the cytoplasm. The Ago protein processes the saRNA by discarding its passenger strand to form an active Ago-RNA complex. Ago-RNA complex enters the nucleus through active transport/passive diffusion cell division. Guide strand directs Ago-RNA complex to complementary genomic DNA sequences usually in promoter region or to noncoding RNA (ncRNA) sequences, which tethers to the DNA. After that, the Ago-RNA complex initiates a process that differs from RNAi, which alter chromatin structure and epigenetic states of target gene via two different potential mechanistic models. In model A, the saRNA guide strand leads the Ago protein to its DNA target by constituting an RNA–DNA duplex or triplex structure, while Ago protein then serves as a docking platform to attract histone-modifying activities, like opening of chromatin structure and active transcription. On the other hand, in model B, the RNA guide strand binds to cognate promoter transcripts making saRNA-RNA complex and then Ago protein recruits histone modifiers to introduce active chromatin marks on local chromosome, resulting in activation of transcription [17].

8. MicroRNAs (miRNAs)

As the molecular biology, bioinformatics approaches and protocols of small RNA sequencing continue to grow and sophisticate, so is the number of miRNAs discovered in different species. Virus-encoded miRNAs have been known to be crucial for the viral replication. miRNAs encoded by DNA viruses have been well studied in comparison with those by RNA viruses because RNA viruses lack nuclear access [55]. However, recent discovery of noncanonical miRNA biogenesis pathways that utilize Argonaute (Ago) 2 for processing of pre-miRNA to mature miRNA has highlighted the fact that RNA viruses may opt similar pathway to generate functional miRNAs. Similar noncanonical pathways might be used to generate functional miRNAs derived from RNA viruses that replicate in the cytoplasm. Several examples up to now have been accumulated like cellular miRNAs, miR-124, is expressed from a cytoplasmic RNA virus, Sindbis virus (SINV) [56]. Several miRNAs were found to be produced by a retrovirus, Bovine leukemia virus (BLV), based on DNA polymerase III transcription *in vivo* as well as *in vitro* [57]. Recently, Hussain et al. have identified six DENV-encoded miRNA like small RNAs in which one of miRNAs directly targets DENV NS1 gene during late infection to autoregulate its replication. Functional analysis has revealed that viral miRNAs can target both cellular and viral mRNAs to regulate viral replication leading to a successful infection [58]. Although, very few virus-encoded miRNAs have been fully characterized, it is understandable that they can target both viral and host genes.

Flaviviruses are well reported to manipulate host miRNA machinery to facilitate their replication. It has been well reported that DENV induce differential expression of miRNAs in human peripheral blood mononuclear cells (PBMCs) [59]. It has been previously reported that miR-124a, -128a, -218, and -let-7c may be important for neurological symptoms caused by a chimeric tickborne encephalitis/dengue virus [60]. Additional studies have shown that miR-122 and miR-142 of the host cells are involved in restricting dengue virus [61, 62]. However, most of the above work has been done in human. Very little is known about the differential miRNA expression of *Ae. aegypti* influenced by DENV infection, leaving a significant gap in our understanding of DENV-*Aedes aegypti* interaction. Although a recent study has shown aberrant host small RNA (sRNA) profiles in *Ae. aegypti* during DENV infection, it mainly focused on piRNAs [63] leaving a significant gap in understanding the differential expression of *Ae. aegypti* miRNAs during DENV replication.

9. miRNA biogenesis

9.1. miRNAs genomic arrangement and transcription

miRNAs are usually encoded by different regions of genome ranging from coding as well as noncoding [64]. Seventy percent of mammalian miRNAs are the intron products of protein coding genes, while rest comes from the noncoding transcription units. miRNAs have been found to be originated from both senses and antisense strands of DNA [65]. Studies have shown that about 30% of *C. elegans* miRNA genes are on the antisense strand overlapping protein coding region [66]. In Drosophila too, many miRNAs are originated from antisense strand overlapping protein coding region [67]. Multiple miRNAs can be transcribed as one long transcript named clusters [18].

Majority of miRNAs are transcribed by RNA polymerase II; however, some miRNAs usually located near Alu repeats are transcribed by RNA polymerase III, from independent genes having their own promoter or represent introns of protein-coding genes [18]. Nearly, all the independent miRNA promoters have particular features of Pol II promoters, including initiator elements and TATA boxes [18].

9.1.1. Canonical pathway of miRNA biogenesis

So far, a vast majority of reported miRNAs are produced through an RNase III enzyme-controlled canonical pathway. Transcription of primary transcript (i.e., pri-miRNA) harboring one or several stem loop structures by RNA polymerase II or otherwise RNA polymerase III kick start the biogenesis process in nucleus [68, 69]. pri-miRNAs are then further processed at stem loop sites by two RNase III proteins Drosha and DGCR8/Pasha (DiGeorge critical region 8) to produce about 70 nucleotide pre-miRNA [70]. This pre-miRNA is then exported to cytoplasm with the help of exportin-5 and RanGTP proteins [71]. Once in cytoplasm, pre-miRNA is chopped down into 22 nucleotide miRNA duplexes. Apart from above-mentioned proteins, many other proteins also work as cofactors to influence the outcome of miRNA biogenesis [65, 72].

9.1.2. Noncanonical pathway of miRNA biogenesis

Although, it was thought earlier that there is only one universal mechanism of all mature miRNAs biogenesis; however, multiple recent discoveries have led us to the conclusion that there may be several other miRNA biogenesis pathways as well. Biogenesis of quite a few miRNAs has been demonstrated to be not only Drosha independent, but also Dicer dependent [73]. It has been reported that in Drosophila and C. *elegans* along with some other vertebrates, mature miRNAs called "mirtrons" can be produced after splicing from intron hairpins independently of Drosha processing [74–76]. Recent studies have revealed that mature functional miRNAs can arise from highly conserved small nucleolar RNA (snoRNAs) in human and *Giardia lamblia* [77, 78] as well as DicerII-processed endogenous siRNAs mostly derived from transposable elements and load into AgoI in Drosophila [76]. Furthermore, researchers have identified miRNAs derived from transfer RNA (tRNA) in mouse embryonic stem cells [79].

Recent studies have led to the discovery of other types of miRNA noncanonical biogenesis pathway that is Dicer independent. One prime example of this is miR-451 biogenesis, which is Dicer independent as pre miR-451 has ~18 nucleotide stem duplex that is too short for Dicer activity. However, pre miR-451 requires AgoII for its maturation [80]. A few examples of other types of noncanonical biogenesis come from virus-encoded miRNAs. For example, several miRNAs are produced by a retrovirus, Bovine leukemia virus (BLV), based on DNA polymerase III transcription *in vivo* as well as *in vitro* [57]. The products of these transcripts were too small to be recognized by Drosha; therefore, these were directly processed by Dicer-1 to mature miRNAs.

10. Mode of action of miRNAs

After the production of mature miRNA by either canonical or noncanonical pathway, the resulting mature miRNA duplex is loaded into miRNA inducing silencing complex (miRISC) having Ago as core component [81]. After degradation of one strand, other strands of duplex, representing mature miRNA, then guide miRISC complex to target mRNA to determine its fate [82]. The stability of the base pairs at the ends of the strands of miRNA duplex usually determines which strand will be degraded. Usually, less stable strand avoids degradation [82]. There are different modes of action of miRNAs that influence the expression of target gene ranging from mRNA degradation, translational repression to activation of transcription [16, 83, 84]. Whatever the outcome is, the general way of miRNA-mRNA interaction relies on the sufficient sequence complementarity between mRNA and 5′ seed region (usually 2–8 nucleotides) of miRNA [85]. Perfect complementarity between mRNA and miRNA is likely to downregulate the expression of target gene through its mRNA degradation by endonuclease activity of miRISC complex. This type of miRNA-mediated gene regulation is mostly evident in plants [86]. However, in animals, there is mostly imperfect complementarity between mRNA and miRNA, which usually leads to translational repression of target gene [86]. Interestingly, there are solid experimental evidences that miRNAs are also involved in upregulation of target genes as well. One of its well-characterized examples is host miR-122-mediated upregulation of HCV RNA replication by stabilizing HCV RNA and preventing its decay [87].

11. Virus-encoded miRNAs

As most viruses need host genes to facilitate their replication, one cannot rule out the possibility of viruses encoding miRNAs in order to manipulate host gene expression or keep viral copy number under check to ensure persistent infection. Possible benefits of virus-encoded miRNAs are that they usually do not elicit immune response, require less coding ability, and they have ability to constantly evolve to target new transcripts. Till date, more than 200 viral miRNAs have been identified. Most of the well-characterized viral-encoded miRNA comes from DNA viruses as compared to RNA viruses, with herpes viruses as a major contributor having average copy number of more than 10/genome [58]. Different recent studies have identified novel microRNAs from different RNA viruses. Bovine leukemia virus (BLV), a retrovirus, also encodes microRNAs [57]. Hussain et al. has reported microRNA like small RNAs in both West Nile virus and Dengue virus [88]. These viral-encoded miRNAs are produced through canonical as well as noncanonical biogenesis pathways. Based on their function, viral encoded miRNAs can be classified into two broad classes:

i. Virus-encoded miRNA regulating host genes

ii. Virus-encoded miRNAs regulating virus copy number

Important functions of viral miRNAs, which target host genes, include promoting cell survival through downregulation of apoptotic factors, thus promoting infected cells survival and proliferation, as well as modulating the immune response of the host cell [89]. It is becoming increasingly evident that one mechanism the viruses have evolved to facilitate regulatory control over their hosts is by generating transcripts, which outmatch cellular miRNAs. Interestingly, Human Kaposi's sarcoma-associated herpes virus (KSHV) and chicken oncogenic Marek's disease virus (MDV) transcribe miR-K12-11 and miR-M4, respectively; these miRNAs appear to be an ortholog of miR-155 to identical seed region [90, 91]. miR-155 has been reported to be involved in many malignancies [92], so exploitation of its targets by viruses may contribute to viral oncogenesis. Recently, it has been reported that a flavivirus named West Nile virus encode an miRNA KUN-miR-1 that specifically induces the expression of GATA4 in *Ae. albopictus* that in turn facilitates the WNV replication [88].

Interestingly, virus-encoded miRNAs can regulate their own replication as well their own benefit. For example, simian virus 40 (SV40)-encoded miRNA miR-S1, expressed during late infection, has been shown to downregulate viral T-antigen, which is crucial to evade cytotoxic T cell response [93]. Another example is HvAV-miR-1 encoded by *Heliothis virescens* ascovirus (HvAV), an insect with dsDNA virus that downregulate viral replication by targeting viral DNA polymerase I [94]. Recently, it has been reported that Dengue virus (DENV)-encoded miRNA like viral small RNA DENV-vsRNA-5 plays an important role in the autoregulation of DENV replication by directly targeting dengue virus NS1 protein during late infection [30].

12. miRNA role in host-viral interactions

Regulative control of miRNAs over gene expression in every organism is the core reason why pathogens try to hijack them. This takeover may include disruption of miRNA biogenesis pathway, inhibiting a specific host miRNA that hinders pathogen propagation or differential miRNA expression. In case of human, it has been well documented that miR-146 and miR-155 are involved in upregulating immune function in response to various bacterial infections including *H. pylori* [95] and *Salmonella enterica* [96]. Many viruses encode miRNAs, having the potential to not only the viral genomes, which encode them, but also to target host transcripts, which facilitate their replication [97, 98]. Functions of viral miRNA targeting host genes include cell survival through downregulation of apoptotic factors as well as modulation of host immune response [89]. One example is upregulation of GATA4 by WNV-encoded miRNA, which has been found to be very important in virus replication in mosquito cells [88]. Recently, it has been demonstrated that viruses have evolved to encode miRNAs that mimic host miRNAs. Kaposi's sarcoma-associated herpes virus (KSHV) encoded miR-K12-11 that is an ortholog of human miR-155 sharing same seed region homology that will likely be able to regulate all targets of miR-155 [90].

12.1. miRNA role in *Aedes aegypti* with an insect-specific flavivirus

Previous studies demonstrated that mosquito miRNAs could be affected by different viral infections. However, those studies were restricted to pathogenic viruses, mainly restricted to the role of differently expressed miRNAs with limited characterization. Limited knowledge is available about the modulation of host miRNAs with respect to insect-specific flaviviruses (ISFs, e.g., Palm Creek virus (PCV)). ISFs share the similar genome organization with other flaviviruses; however, their rate of vertical transmission between insect hosts is higher than other vertebrate-infecting flaviviruses. Although it is still unclear that why ISFs fail to replicate in mammalian cells, it is assumed that ISFs potentially lack to antagonize the host interferon system. Similarly, ISFs express a high adaptation level in insect hosts, which may further limit their replication in vertebrate hosts. Recently, Lee et al. explicated the potential role of miRNAs in Palm Creek virus (PCV) infection using the *Ae. aegypti* mosquito model [99]. They proposed differently expressed miRNAs after combining small-RNA sequencing and bioinformatics tools although the results hardly predicted the potential involvement of PCV infection to alter host miRNAs. They revealed that only one miRNA (i.e., aae-miR-2940-5p) out of 101 reported miRNAs of *Ae. aegypti* that had significantly altered expression over the course of PCV infection. The level of aae-miR-2940-5p was induced within 2 days p.i. and suppressed at 12 days p.i.; however, a different pattern of miRNA screening was demonstrated in *Ae. aegypti* Aa20 cell line without displaying any significant change upon PCV infection. Further *in vitro* miRNA inhibition experiments while using aae-miR-2940-5p inhibitors demonstrated that this miRNA did not directly impact on PCV replication and has no significant role in PCV-*Ae. aegypti* interaction. This variable response to virus infection in cell lines and host mosquito might be due to tissue tropism of the virus. At mRNA target level, the study reported the inconsistent expression level of MetP with miR-2940-5p expression although previously it was reported a potential target of aae-miR-2940-5p with positive interaction. It means that there was no correlation of MetP expression to PCV infection because silencing the gene did not significantly affect the virus replication. The pair MetP--aae-miR-2940-5p also positively regulate West Nile virus (WNV) virion production where aae-miR-2940-5p was selectively downregulated upon WNV infection in infected cells. The MetP human ortholog like M41 ftsh, YME1L, plays an important role as an antiapoptotic factor. It is assumed that the induction of aae-miR-2940-5p in PCV-infected cells during infection boosts MetP transcript levels and thus protects infected cells undergoing apoptosis under stress responses. However, the MetP physiological role is still uncertain in insects and requires further investigation [99].

13. RNA interference in *Aedes aegypti* with an insect-specific flavivirus

RNA interference is considered a vital antiviral defense response in mosquitoes as lot of studies reported the production of viral-specific small RNAs for different viruses. However, several reports also confirm the establishment of persistent viral infection only in mosquitoes either infected by pathogenic mosquito-borne viruses or insect-specific viruses that produce these small RNAs. While doing so, viral-derived DNA (vDNA) is produced by reverse transcription during persistent infection and may survive in extrachromosomal or integrated forms. Such vDNAs increase RNAi-mediated antiviral response in mosquitoes to boost mosquito tolerance to arbovirus infection while establishing persistent infection. In one study, Lee et al. detected PCV-specific 21 nucleotide small-RNAs in mosquitoes at different time points of infection (2, 6, and 12 days p.i.) as a potential indicator of active viral replication in the mosquitoes [99]. These findings complied with other studies where the researchers demonstrated the similar phenomenon for other pathogenic mosquito-borne flaviviruses (e.g., DENV) and insect-specific flaviviruses (e.g., cell fusing agent viruses). Their presence as hot spots suggests that either those are the potential targets of Dicer-2, or are more stable or can be reverse-transcribed into vDNA. All these might be the potential cause to enhance RNAi antiviral response. However, the authors are also afraid of bias, which could be due to technical issues such as library preparation. In addition to RNAi, piRNAs (piwi RNAs) have been reported in mosquitoes and knockdown of piRNAs-related specific proteins indicates their endogenous antiviral activity instead of well-established exogenous RNAi activities in mosquitoes. Similarly, virus-specific piRNAs with typical A_{10} bias in sense RNA and U_1 bias in antisense RNA have been reported to be produce by Bunya viruses and alphaviruses. However, the piRNAs expressed by dengue virus and cell fusing agent virus have only A_{10} bias in sense RNA. Interestingly, the PCV-specific small RNAs do not show either A10 or U1 bias features. In this scenario, it is uncertain that either they are piRNAs or just viral degradation products. This situation is very similar seen in other flavivirus-specific piRNAs, which map to very small number of sequences in the genome where the presence of one copy of genome indicates more specific targeting than random RNA degradation. The production of virus small RNAs and piRNAs through vDNA synthesis is also documented in mosquitoes or in their derived cell lines. It is worth mentioning to note the contribution of vDNA in the production of small RNAs of virus and piRNAs in mosquitoes, although insect-specific viruses like PCV establish persistent infection in their hosts [99].

14. Long intergenic noncoding RNAs (lincRNAs) and their association with DENV-host interaction

Considering as another important class of regulatory RNAs, lincRNAs (sometimes known as dark matter) have various biological functions including genomic imprinting and cell differentiation specifically in host-pathogen interaction [100]. A growing number of evidences also reflect their possible role in gene regulation either epigenetics or nonepigenetics. However, their role in immune cell differentiation and activation is poorly understood, but the recent discoveries show their potential role in defense system as well as rapid responses to various stimuli and stress factors. Some studies also predict their active role to enhance viral replication or decrease antiviral immunity. It was also depicted that some lincRNAs also interact with other noncoding RNAs like miRNAs. The *Ae. aegypti*-linked lincRNAs are shorter in length (approximately 3000 nucleotide bases) than their protein-coding genes. Similarly, their GC content was also lower (mean:40.1%) than their protein-coding gene sequences (mean:47.8%). However, the AT enrichment or lower GC content is a typical characteristic of lincRNAs and congruent with other lincRNAs in other species [100].

Etebari et al. identified lincRNAs in dengue fever vector *Ae. aegypti* and demonstrated their potential role in host antiviral defense [100]. They evaluated lincRNA's expression in DENV serotype 2 (DENV-2) and *Wolbachia*-infected and noninfected adult mosquitoes as well as in Aa20 cells. The findings revealed the increased number of host lincRNAs under the circumstances of DENV-2 infection, some of which inhibit viral replication in mosquito cells. Furthermore, the silencing of only one lincRNA_1317 by RNA interference enhanced the viral replication in host cells, which clearly indicates their possible role in host antiviral defense. The lincRNA_1317 suppression was confirmed by reverse transcription quantitative polymerase chain reaction (RT-qPCR). It was found that the lincRNA_1317 expression was increased substantially upon the progression of infection, indicating the possible role of this lincRNA in antiviral defense. The findings might be consistent as the highly overexpressed lincRNA_1317 expression (2.33 fold) was reported in *Wolbachia*-infected mosquitoes as compared to noninfected [100].

The authors also described lincRNAs potential involvement in mosquito-pathogen interaction by determining its association with host-endogenous small RNAs and its direct interaction with DENV-2 infection. lincRNA_1317 was not found to be located in any of the known piRNA clusters; however, no differences were found in the mapping pattern and mapped read length distribution when reads from DENV-infected and noninfected small RNA libraries were mapped to lincRNA_1317. Gene silencing like role of piRNAs on lincRNA_1317 transcriptome was also speculated. However, a little information is available about piRNA-mediated lincRNA although some recent studies predict piRNA-mediated degradation of lincRNAs in mouse's late spermatocytes [100].

The researchers also tested the hypothesis that *Ae. aegypti* lincRNA_1317 response to microbial challenge could be due to cross regulation between miRNAs and the lincRNAs. For this purpose, the normalized minimum free energy (mfe) of hybridization for each *Ae. aegypti* miRNA and lincRNA_1317 was calculated by using RNAhybrid core script. The basic objective was to identify *Ae. aegypti* miRNA recognition elements on lincRNA_1317. The results were quite interesting as binding sites enrichment for a few miRNAs with more than two recognition elements were detected on lincRNA_1317 (e.g., more than four recognition sites for miR-278-5p and miR-252-3p were predicted on lincRNA_1317). Furthermore, some hot spots for miRNA recognition sites on lincRNA_1317 were also identified, which may facilitate multiple miRNAs to bind the same regions. microRNAs contain the capability to shake lincRNA stability by targeting their transcripts similar to targeted mRNAs. Similarly, lincRNAs possessing multiple recognition sites might act as a competitive inhibitor of miRNA by eliminating them to bind their genuine targets by sequestration. The mfe values of hybridization for miRNA-lincRNA recognition sites could be a strong predictor of a binding event between two; however, further investigations and trials are still needed to validate this interface [100].

15. IsomiRs and their impact on miRNAs in dengue fever vector *Ae. aegypti*

microRNAs may exist in various lengths and sequence variations, which are known as isomiRs [101]. Earlier, those were considered as sequencing errors; however, some studies predicted to be physiologically relevant and posttranscriptionally modified miRNA variants. IsomiRs may express affinities for different targets than their canonical miRNA counterparts. Furthermore, nucleotide heterogeneity could be found at both ends of miRNA sequence in the form of nucleotide substitutions despite the variations are more frequent at 3′ end. The molecular biology, genome structure, and epigenetics of isomiRs are still poorly understood, and the mechanisms of their biogenesis are also considered very complex and even cell-type specific. Some variations in miRNA sequences are supposed to be the product of template variations, which might be brought by the exonuclease activity of Drosha and Dicer [101].

It is a well-documented fact that miRNAs may play a vital role to modulate the capability of vectors to propagate the infection for widely damaging arboviruses (e.g., dengue virus) [101]. It has been demonstrated that miRNA could be modified in mosquitoes upon the induction of DENV infection. As genetic variations in isomiR prevalence have significant impact on gene regulation, a clear understanding of the role of isomiR profile of mosquitoes in DENV and other arboviruses infection propagation is urgently needed. Etebari et al. in one study found this altered posttranscriptional modification role of miRNAs in *Ae. aegypti* mosquitoes after DENV infection in comparison with uninfected mosquitoes. For this purpose, they utilized already published RNA-seq data from 2-, 4-, and 9-day DENV-infected and uninfected mosquitoes. The findings showed significant variations in miRNA prevalence in response to dengue virus infection although the effects were not ubiquitous, and no remarkable alteration in overall pattern of isomiR expression was noted upon DENV infection. They calculated the exact/all read count ratio as an index for isomiR production rate for all known *Ae. aegypti* miRNAs. DENV-infected mosquitoes increased the isomiR production of 3 miRNAs (miR-2c, miR-210, and miR-34) with notable impact on two miRNAs (miR-276 and miR-10) with less read count by DENV infection. The data also demonstrated that 3 isomiRs of miR-34-5p were also significantly altered by dengue virus infection. Collectively, those alterations might have net benefit to determine the mosquito's role upon DENV infection propagation; however, potential biological significances of these modifications are still unclear except to infer that some evolutionary function of miRNAs. Similarly, it is also ambiguous that why some specific isomiRs potentially modify more in response to DENV infection in *Ae. aegypti*. Furthermore, it was also noted that one particular miRNA with significant increase in one specific isomiR variants upon DENV infection also contained a common variant in at least one other isomiR as well. The authors speculated that establishment and persistence of DENV infection might cause significant changes in activity levels of some enzymes involved in the production of isomiRs, which ultimately modify the isomiR production frequencies of some specific miRNAs. The isomiR production power against different *Ae. aegypti* miRNAs was also demonstrated differently as observed by the read count. The "true" miRNAs were considered as those which had an exact match to the canonical sequence (already reported and available in miRbase), while the "false" ones were classified as those which significantly differed to that reported in miRbase. The authors explicated that in *Ae. aegypti*, most abundant miRNA sequences matched to true miRNAs were just 45%, while 55% miRNAs produced by *Ae. aegypti* miRNAs were false miRNAs, and interestingly, this overall trend was not altered by DENV infection. Although the findings are striking and indicate that little variations in miRNA sequences may significantly impact target affinities in DENV-host interaction as well as in infection propagation, still extensive studies are required in the field to validate such hypothesis [101].

16. Conclusions

An over-growing number of reports and continuous publication of journals and books illustrate an intricate interplay between virus-host interactions in dengue fever virus infection. Similarly, an increase in morbidity and mortality rate with DENV infection and still unavailability of standard care to treat the infection have diverted the DENV-research to explore new paradigms in treatment and to map/identify cellular/molecular pathways to better understanding of disease progression in infected vectors, either mosquitoes or humans. Small interference

RNA and microRNA as anti-mRNA-based treatment strategies with strong evidences are evolutionary, but unfortunately still not a successful and reliable treatment line in viral infections with certain issues of drug delivery and long-term therapeutic effects. The involvement of lincRNAs and variations in miRNA epigenetic profile in disease-specific arboviruses (e.g., dengue virus) during infection also indicate complex genome interactions between virus and hosts. RNA association as a novel therapeutic approach to treat infection by gene activation, to find out some specific modulators of gene regulation in viral replication as well as in disease progression is still in an explanatory phase specifically for disease-specific or insect-specific flaviviruses. In conjunction, the molecular approaches to find out disease progression pathways in disease-specific arboviruses are still investigative and antiviral treatment approaches in the form of siRNAs, microRNAs as well as RNA association still need to be explored fully before their practical implementations in diagnostics and as some antiviral therapeutics.

Author details

Imran Shahid[1,2*]

*Address all correspondence to: iyshahid@uqu.edu.sa

1 Department of Pharmacology and Toxicology, College of Pharmacy, Umm-Al-Qura University, Makkah, Saudi Arabia

2 Applied and Functional Genomics Laboratory, Center of Excellence in Molecular Biology (CEMB), University of the Punjab, Lahore, Pakistan

References

[1] Gubler DJ. Dengue/dengue hemorrhagic fever: History and current status. Novartis Foundation Symposium. 2006;**277**:3-16. discussion 16-22, 71-13, 251-253

[2] Tatmen AJ, Hay SI, Rogers DJ. Global traffic and disease vector dispersal. Proceedings of the National Academy of Sciences of the United States of America. 2006;**103**:6242-6247

[3] Clyde K, Kyle JL, Harris E. Recent advances in deciphering viral and host determinants of dengue virus replication and pathogenesis. Journal of Virology. 2006;**80**:11418-11431

[4] Lindenbach BD, Pragai BM, Montserret R, Beren RKF, Pyle AM, Penin F, et al. The C terminus of hepatitis C virus NS4A encodes an electrostatic switch that regulates NS5A hyperphospholylation and viral replication. Journal of Virology. 2007;**81**:8905-8918

[5] Sampath A, Padmanabhan R. Molecular targets for flavivirus drug discovery. Antiviral Research. 2009;**81**:6-15

[6] Blair CD. Mosquito RNAi is the major innate immune pathway controlling arbovirus infection and transmission. Future Microbiology. 2011;**6**:265-277

[7] Sanchez-Vargas I, Scott JC, Poole-Smith BK, Franz AWE, Barbosa-Solomieu V, Wilusz J, et al. Dengue virus type 2 infections of italic *Aedes aegypti* are modulated by the mosquito's RNA interference pathway. PLoS Pathogens. 2009;**5**:e1000299

[8] Kakumani PK, Ponia SS, S RK, Sood V, Chinnappan M, Banerjea AC, et al. Role of RNA interference (RNAi) in dengue virus replication and identification of NS4B as an RNAi suppressor. Journal of Virology. 2013;**87**:8870-8883

[9] Pijlman GP, Funk A, Kondratieva N, Leung J, Torres S, van der Aa L, et al. A highly structured, nuclease-resistant, noncoding RNA produced by flaviviruses is required for pathogenicity. Cell Host & Microbe. 2008;**4**:579-591

[10] Paradkar PN, Trinidad L, Voysey R, Duchemin J-B, Walker PJ. Secreted Vago restricts West Nile virus infection in Culex mosquito cells by activating the Jak-STAT pathway. Proceedings of the National Academy of Sciences. 2012;**109**:18915-18920

[11] Li LC, okino ST, Zhao H, Pookot D, Place RF, Urakami S, et al. Small dsRNAs induce transcriptional activation in human cells. Proceedings of the National Academy of Sciences of the United States of America. 2006;**103**:17337-17342

[12] Huang V, Qin Y, Wang J, Wang X, Place RF, Lin G, et al. RNAa is conserved in mammalian cells. PLoS One. 2010;**5**:e8848

[13] Yue X, Schwartz JC, Chu Y, Younger ST, Gagnon KT, Elbashir S, et al. Transcriptional regulation by small RNAs at sequences downstream from 3′ gene termini. Nature Chemical Biology. 2010;**6**:621-629

[14] Yin H, Lin H. An epigenetic activation role of piwi and a piwi-associated piRNA in Drosophila melanogastor. Nature. 2007;**450**:304-308

[15] Vasudevan S, Tong Y, Steitz JA. Switching from repression to activation: MicroRNAs can up-regulate translation. Science. 2007;**318**:1931-1934

[16] Place RF, Li LC, Pookot D, Noonan eJ, Dahiya R. MicroRNA-373 induces expression of genes with complementary promoter sequences. Proceedings of the National Academy of Sciences of the United States of America. 2008;**105**:1608-1613

[17] Portnoy V, Huang V, Place RF, Li LC. Small RNA and transcriptional upregulation. Wiley Interdisciplinary Reviews. RNA. 2011;**2**:748-760

[18] Lee Y, Jeon K, Lee JT, Kim S, Kim VN. MicroRNA maturation: Stepwise processing and subcellular localization. The EMBO Journal. 2002;**21**:4663-4670

[19] Almeida MI, Reis RM, Calin GA. MicroRNA history: Discovery, recent applications, and next frontiers. Mutation Research, Fundamental and Molecular Mechanisms of Mutagenesis. 2011;**717**:1-8

[20] Bartel DP. MicroRNAs: Genomics, biogenesis, mechanism, and function. Cell. 2004;**116**: 281-297

[21] Pillai RS, Bhattacharyya SN, Filipowicz W. Repression of protein synthesis by miRNAs: How many mechanisms? Trends in Cell Biology. 2007;**17**:118-126

[22] Baek D, Villen J, Shin C, Camargo FD, Gygi SP, Bartel DP. The impact of microRNAs on protein output. Nature. 2008;**455**:64-71

[23] Guo H, Ingolia NT, Weissman JS, Bartel DP. Mammalian microRNAs predominantly act to decrease target mRNA levels. Nature. 2010;**466**:835-840

[24] Fabian MR, Sonenberg N, Filipowicz W. Regulation of mRNA translation and stability by microRNAs. Annual Review of Biochemistry. 2010;**79**:351-379

[25] Eiring AM, Harb JG, Neviani P, Garton C, Oaks JJ, Spizzo R, et al. miR-328 functions as an RNA decoy to modulate hnRNP E2 regulation of mRNA translation in leukemic blasts. Cell. 2010;**140**:652-665

[26] Asgari S. Role of MicroRNAs in insect host-microorganism interaction. Frontiers in Physiology. 2011;**2**:48

[27] Cui Q, Yu Z, Purisima EO, Wang E. Principles of microRNA regulation of a human cellular signaling network. Molecular Systems Biology. 2006;**2**:46

[28] Lau NC, Lim LP, Weinstein EG, Bartel DP. An abundant class of tiny RNAs with probable regulatory roles in *Caenorhabditis elegans*. Science. 2001;**294**:858-862

[29] Lim LP, Glasner ME, Yekta S, Burge CB, Bartel DP. Vertebrate microRNA genes. Science. 2003;**299**:1540

[30] Hussain M, Frentiu FD, Moreira LA, O'Neill SL, Asgari S. Wolbachia uses host microRNAs to manipulate host gene expression and facilitate colonization of the dengue vector *Aedes aegypti*. Proceedings of the National Academy of Sciences of the United States of America. 2011;**108**:9250-9255

[31] Jessie K, Fong MY, Devi S, Lam SK, Wong KT. Localization of dengue virus in naturally infected human tissues, by immunohistochemistry and in situ hybridization. The Journal of Infectious Diseases. 2004;**189**:1411-1418

[32] Wu SJ, Grouard-Vogel G, Sun W, Mascola JR, Brachtel E, Putvatana R, et al. Human skin Langerhans cells are targets of dengue virus infection. Nature Medicine. 2000;**6**:816-820

[33] Rodrigueza A, Griffiths-Jones S, Ashurst JL, Bradley A. Identification of mammalian microRNA host genes and transcription units. Genome Research. 2004;**14**:1902-1910

[34] Germi R, Crance JM, Garin D, Guimet J, Lortat-Jacob H, Ruigrok RW, et al. Heparin sulfate-mediated binding of infectious dengue virus type 2 and yellow fever virus. Virology. 2002;**292**:162-168

[35] Reyes-Del Valle J, Chavez-Salinas S, Medina F, Del Angel RM. Heat shock protein 90 and heat shock protein 70 are components of dengue virus receptor complex in human cells. Journal of Virology. 2005;**79**:4557-4567

[36] Chen YC, Wang SY, King CC. Bacterial lipopolysaccharide inhibits dengue virus infection of primary human monocytes/macrophages by blockade of virus entry via a CD14-dependent mechanism. Journal of Virology. 1999;**73**:2650-2657

[37] Jindadamrongwech S, Thepparit C, Smith DR. Identification of GRP 78 (BiP) as a liver cell expressed receptor element for dengue virus serotype 2. Archives of Virology. 2004;**149**: 915-927

[38] Thepparit C, Smith DR. Serotype-specific entry of dengue virus into liver cells: Identification of the 37-kilodalton/67-kilodalton high-affinity laminin receptor as a dengue virus serotype 1 receptor. Journal of Virology. 2004;**78**:12647-12656

[39] Lozach PY, Burleigh L, Staropli I, Navarro-Sanchez E, Harriague J, Virelizier JL, et al. Dendritic cell-specific intercellular adhesion molecule 3-grabbing non-integrin (DC-SIGN)-mediated enhancement of dengue virus infection is independent of DC-SIGN internalization signals. The Journal of Biological Chemistry. 2005;**280**:23698-23708

[40] Navarro-Sanchez E, Altmeyer R, Amara A, Schwartz O, Fieschi F, Virelizier JL, et al. Dendritic-cell-specific ICAM3-grabbing non-integrin is essential for the productive infection of human dendritic cells by mosquito-cell-derived dengue viruses. EMBO Reports. 2003;**4**:723-728

[41] Miller JL, de Wet BJ, Martinez-Pomares L, Radcliffe CM, Dwek RA, Rudd PM, et al. The mannose receptor mediates dengue virus infection of macrophages. PLoS Pathogens. 2008;**4**:e17

[42] Stiasny K, Fritz R, Pangerl K, Heinz FX. Molecular mechanisms of flaviviruses membrane fusion. Amino Acids. 2011;**41**:1159-1163

[43] Acosta EG, Castilla V, Damonte EB. Alternative infectious entry pathways for dengue virus serotypes into mammalian cells. Cellular Microbiology. 2009;**11**:1533-1549

[44] Harrison SC. Viral membrane fusion. Natural Structural & Molecular Biology. 2008;**15**: 690-698

[45] Modis Y, Ogata S, Clements D, Harrison SC. Structure of the dengue virus envelope protein after membrane fusion. Nature. 2004;**427**:313-319

[46] Welsch S, Miller S, Romero-Brey I, Merz A, Bleck CK, Walther P, et al. Comparison and three-dimensional architecture of the dengue virus replication and assembly sites. Cell Host & Microbe. 2009;**5**:365-375

[47] Villorodo SM, Gamarnik AV. Genome cyclization as strategy for flavivirus RNA replication. Virus Research. 2009;**139**:230-239

[48] Ivanyi-Nagy R, Darlix JL. Intrinsic disorder in the core proteins of flaviviruses. Protein and Peptide Letters. 2010;**17**:1019-1025

[49] Li L, Lok SM, Yu IM, Zhang Y, Kuhn RJ, Chen J, et al. The flavivirus precursor membrane-envelope protein complex: Structure and maturation. Science. 2008;**319**:1830-1834

[50] Schmid-Hempel P, Ebert D. On the evolutionary ecology of specific immune defence. Trends in Ecology & Evolution. 2003;**18**:27-32

[51] Fansiri T, Fontaine A, Diancourt L, Caro V, Thaisomboonsuk B, Richardson JH, et al. Genetic mapping of specific interactions between *Aedes aegypti* mosquitoes and dengue viruses. PLoS Genetics. 2013;**9**:e1003621

[52] Lingel A, Simon B, Izaurralde E, Sattler M. The structure of the flock house virus B2 protein, a viral suppressor of RNA interference, shows a novel mode of double-stranded RNA recognition. EMBO Reports. 2005;**6**:1149-1155

[53] Blakqori G, Delhaye S, Habjan M, Blair CD, Sanchez-Vargas I, Olson KE, et al. La Crosse bunyavirus nonstructural protein NSs serves to suppress the type I interferon system of mammalian hosts. Journal of Virology. 2007;**81**:4991-4999

[54] Janowski BA, Younger ST, Hardy DB, Ram R, Huffman KE, Corey DR. Activating gene expression in mammalian cells with promoter-targeted duplex RNAs. Nature Chemical Biology. 2007;**3**:166-173

[55] Boss IW, Plaisance KB, Renne R. Role of virus-encoded microRNAs in herpesvirus biology. Trends in Microbiology. 2009;**17**:544-553

[56] Rouha H, Thurner C, Mandl CW. Functional microRNA generated from a cytoplasmic RNA virus. Nucleic Acids Research. 2010;**38**:8328-8337

[57] Rosewick N, Momont M, Durkin K, Takeda H, Caiment F, Cleuter Y, et al. Deep sequencing reveals abundant noncanonical retroviral microRNAs in B-cell leukemia/lymphoma. Proceedings of the Natioan Academy of Sciences of the United States of America. 2013;**110**:2306-2311

[58] Kincaid RP, Sullivan CS. Virus-encoded microRNAs: An overview and a look to the future. PLoS Pathogens. 2012;**8**:e1003018

[59] Qi Y, Li Y, Zhang L, Huang J. microRNA expression profilinf and bioinformatic analysis of dengue virus infected peripheral blood mononuclear cells. Molecular Medicine Reports. 2013;**7**:791-798

[60] Heis BL, Maximova OA, Pletnev AG. Insertion of microRNA targets into the flavivirus genome alters its highly neurovirulent phenotype. Journal of Virology. 2011;**85**:1464-1472

[61] Lee TC, Lin YL, Liao JT, Su CM, Lin CC, Lin WP, et al. Utilizing liver-specific microRNA-122 to modulate replication of dengue virus replication. Biochemical and Biophysical Research Communications. 2010;**396**:596-601

[62] Pham AM, Langlois RA, TenOever BR. Replication in cells of hematopoietic origin is necessary for dengue virus dissemination. PLoS Pathogens. 2012;**8**:e10022465

[63] Hess AM, Prasad AN, Ptitsyn A, Ebel GD, Olson KE, Barbacioru C, et al. Small RNA profiling of dengue virus-mosquito interactions implicates the PIWI RNA pathway in anti-viral defense. BMC Microbiology. 2011;**11**:45

[64] Rodrigueza A, Griffiths-Jones S, Ashurst JL, Bradley A. Identification of mammalian micfroRNA host genes and transcription units. Genome Research. 2004;**14**:1902-1910

[65] Finnegan EF, Pasquinelli AE. MicroRNA biogenesis: Regulating the regulators. Critical Reviews in Biochemistry and Molecular Biology. 2013;**48**:51-68

[66] Martinez NJ, Ow MC, Reece-Hoyes JS, Barrasa MI, Ambros VR, Walhout AJ. Genome-scale spatiotemporal analysis of *Caenorhabditis elegans* microRNA promoter activity. Genome Research. 2008;**18**:2005-2015

[67] Berezikov E, Robine N, Samsonova A, Westholm JO, Naqvi A, Hung J-H, et al. Deep annotation of Drosophila melanogaster microRNAs yields insights into their processing, modification, and emergence. Genome Research. 2011;**21**:203-215

[68] Kim VN, Han J, Siomi MC. Biogenesis of small RNAs in animals. Nature Reviews. Molecular Cell Biology. 2009;**10**:126-139

[69] Lee Y, Kim M, Han JJ, Yeom KH, Lee S, Baek SH, et al. MicroRNA genes are transcribed by RNA polymerase II. EMBO Journal. 2004;**23**:4051-4060

[70] Lee Y, Ahn C, Han JJ, Choi H, Kim, Yim J, et al. The nuclear RNase III Drosha initiates microRNA processing. Nature. 2003;**425**:45-419

[71] Ying SY, Lin SL. Intron-derived microRNAs- fine tuning of gene functions. Gene. 2004; **342**:25-28

[72] Ameres SL, Zamore PD. Diversifying microRNA sequence and function. Nature Reviews. Molecular Cell Biology. 2013;**14**:475-488

[73] Ruby JG, Jan CH, Bartel DP. Intronic microRNA precursors that bypass Drosha processing. Nature. 2007;**448**:83-86

[74] Chong MM, Zhang G, Cheloufi S, Neubert TA, Hannon GJ, Litman DR. Canonical and alternate functions of the microRNA biogenesis machinery. Genes & Development. 2010;**24**:1951-1960

[75] Chung WJ, Agius P, Westholm JO, Chen M, Okamura K, Robine N, et al. Computational and experimental identification of mirtrons in Drosophila melanogaster and *Caenorhabditis elegans*. Genome Research. 2011;**21**:286-300

[76] Okamura K, Chung W-J, Ruby JG, Guo H, Bartel DP, Lai EC. The Drosophila hairpin RNA pathway generates endogenous short interfering RNAs. Nature. 2008;**453**:803-806

[77] Ender C, Krek A, Friedlander MR, Beitzinger M, Weinmann L, Chen W, et al. A human snoRNA with microRNA-like functions. Molecular Cell. 2008;**32**:519-528

[78] Saraiya AA, Wang CC. snoRNA, a novel precursor of microRNA in *Giardia lamblia*. PLoS Pathogens. 2008;**4**:e1000224

[79] Babiarz JE, Ruby JG, Wang Y, Bartel DP, Blelloch R. Mouse ES cells express endogenous shRNAs, siRNAs and other microprocessor-independent, dicer-dependent small RNAs. Genes & Development. 2008;**22**:2773-2785

[80] Cifuentes D, Xue H, Taylor DW, Patnode H, Mishima Y, Cheloufi S, et al. A novel miRNA processing pathway independent of dicer requires Argonaute2 catalytic activity. Science. 2010;**328**:1694-1698

[81] Miyoshi K, Okada TN, Siomi H, Siomi MC. Characterization of the miRNA-RISC loading complex and miRNA-RISC formed in the Drosophila miRNA pathway. RNA. 2009;**15**:1282-1291

[82] Winter J, Jung S, Keller S, Gregory RI, Diederichs S. Many roads to maturity: MicroRNA biogenesis pathways and their regulation. Nature Cell Biology. 2009;**11**:228-234

[83] Bartel DP. MicroRNAs: Target recognition and regulatory functions. Cell. 2009;**136**:215-233

[84] Bruno IG, Karam R, Huang L, Bhardwaj A, Lou, Shum EY, et al. Identification of a microRNA that activities gene expression by repressing nonsense-mediated RNA decay. Molecular Cell. 2011;**42**:500-510

[85] Didiano D, Hobert O. Perfect seed pairing is not a generally reliable predictor for miRNA-target interactions. Nature Structural & Molecular Biology. 2006;**13**:849-851

[86] Jackson RJ, Standart N. How do microRNAs regulate gene expression? Science's STKE. 2007;**2**

[87] Conrad KD, Giering F, Erfurth C, Neumann A, Fehr C, Meister G, et al. MicroRNA-122 dependent binding of Ago2 protein to hepatitis C virus RNA is associated with enhanced RNA stability and translation stimulation. PLoS One. 2013;**8**:e56272

[88] Hussain M, Torres S, Schnettler E, Funk A, Grundhoff A, Pijlman GP, et al. West Nile virus encodes a microRNA-like small RNA in the 3′ untranslated region which up regulates GATA4 mRNA and facilitates virus replication in mosquito cells. Nucleic Acids Research. 2012;**40**:2210-2223

[89] Cullen BR. Viral and cellular messenger RNA targets of viral microRNAs. Nature. 2009;**457**:421-425

[90] Skalsky RL, Samols MA, Plaisance KB, Boss IW, Riva A, Lopez MC, et al. Kaposi's sarcoma-associated herpesvirus encodes an ortholog of miR-155. Journal of Virology. 2007;**81**: 12836-12845

[91] Zhao Y, Yao Y, Xu H, Lambeth L, Smith LP, kgosana L, et al. A functional MicroRNA-155 ortholog encoded by the oncogenic Marek's disease virus. Journal of Virology. 2009;**83**: 489-492

[92] Xiao C, Rajewsky K. MicroRNA control in the immune system: Basic principles. Cell. 2009;**136**:26-36

[93] Sullivan CS, Grundhoff AT, Tevethia S, Pipas JM, Ganem D. SV40-encoded microRNAs regulate viral gene expression and reduce susceptibility to cytotoxic T cells. Nature. 2005;**435**:682-686

[94] Hussain M, Taft RJ, Asgari S. An insect virus-encoded microRNA regulates viral replication. Journal of Virology. 2008;**82**:9164-9170

[95] Matsushima K, Isomoto H, Inoue N, Nakayama T, Hayashi T, Nakayama M, et al. MicroRNA signatures in helicobacter pylori-infected gastric mucosa. International Journal of Cancer. 2011;**128**:361-370

[96] Schulte LN, Eulalio A, Mollenkopf HJ, Reinhardt R, Vogel J. Analysis of the host microRNA response to Salmonella uncovers the control of major cytokines by the let-7 family. EMBO Journal. 2011;**30**:1977-1989

[97] Asgari S, Sullivan CS. Role of MicroRNAs as Regulators of Host-Virus Interactions. England: Caister Academic Press; 2010

[98] Skalsky RL, Cullen BR. Viruses, microRNAs, and host interactions. In: Gottesman S, Harwood CS, editors. Annual Review of Microbiology. 2010;**64**:123-141

[99] Lee M, Etebari K, Hall-Mendelin S, van den Hurk AF, Hobson-Peters J, Vatipally S, et al. Understanding the role of microRNAs in the interaction of *Aedes aegypti* mosquitoes with an insect-specific flavivirus. Journal of General Virology. 2017;**98**:1892-1903

[100] Etebari K, Asad S, Zhang G, Asgari S. Identification of *Aedes aegypti* long intergenic non-coding RNAs and their association with Wolbachia and dengue virus infection. PLoS Neglected Tropical Diseases. 2016;**10**(10):e0005069

[101] Etebari K, Osei-Amo S, Blomberg SP, Asgari S. Dengue virus infection alters post-transcriptional modification of mocroRNAs in the mosquito vector *Aedes aegypti*. Scientific Reports. 2015;**30**(5):15968

5

Dengue Fever: A General Perspective

Muhammad Kashif Zahoor, Azhar Rasul, Muhammad Asif Zahoor, Iqra Sarfraz, Muhammad Zulhussnain, Rizwan Rasool, Humara Naz Majeed, Farhat Jabeen and Kanwal Ranian

Abstract

Dengue Fever or commonly known as Dengue, a mosquito-borne arboviral infection has emerged as havoc around the globe. Annually, about 50 million infections are reported, resulting in 22,000 deaths and almost 2.5 billion people are reported living at risk. Dengue infection is caused by Dengue Virus (DENV), which is a member of genus Flavivirus and comprised of ten proteins; three proteins, capsid (C), membrane (M), and envelope (E), play structural role and seven are identified as non-structural that direct DENV replication. Four distinct serotypes: DENV-1, DENV-2, DENV-3 and DENV-4 are transmitted via *Aedes* mosquitoes. Clinically, Dengue patients can be categorized into three groups according to WHO 2009 revised classification. Typical symptoms of dengue include: extreme fatigue; sudden fever (from 3-7 days), headache, joint, muscle, and back pain; vomiting and diarrhea, appetite loss; skin rash along minor bleeding. *Aedes aegypti* is geographically distributed in tropical areas and breeds in artificially filled water containers i.e. drums, tyres, flower vases plastic food containers, tin cans, etc. Due to four viral serotypes and non-availability of the model animal for dengue, producing vaccines is a challenging task. Thus, Dengue can be managed using various vector control strategies through physical, chemical and biological means.

Keywords: dengue fever, dengue hemorrhagic fever, dengue shock syndrome, *Aedes aegypti*, DEN virus

1. Historical background

The word "dengue" is known to be derived from Swahili language "ki denga pepo", which illustrates the meaning as "sudden cramp like seizure". The signs and indications that are suggestive of this viral disease can be tracked back to Chinese Chin Dynasty (265–420 AD) where this infection was believed to be a type of water poison and reported to be linked with insects and water [1]. Some of the historical accounts for dengue fever states that about 500–600 years ago, it appeared from Africa while the first and foremost outbreak of this deadly disease reached other parts of world in 1780s [2]. The detection and isolation of dengue virus date backed to the World War II and it was documented in Japan for the first time in 1942 [3]. Dengue-like symptoms have been reported in early Chinese manuscripts which can be traced back to 992 and to 1600s in the West Indies [4]. In another report, Benjamin Rush observed the first detailed symptoms of dengue shock syndrome (now severe dengue) in 1780 during an outbreak in Philadelphia near Delaware River [5]. Similar disease symptoms were observed in North America along Atlantic coast during eighteenth–nineteenth centuries, on the Caribbean Islands and the Mississippi basin [6]. Bancroft reported for the first time that *Aedes aegypti* mosquito is vector of dengue virus [7]. However, modern research about dengue virus was not started until 1943–1944. For the first time culturing and isolation of this virus was performed from suckling mice brain [8].

2. Geographic distribution

It is scientifically accepted that dengue viruses originated in monkeys and jumped to humans in Africa or Southeast Asia between 100 and 800 years ago. Dengue fever remained geographically

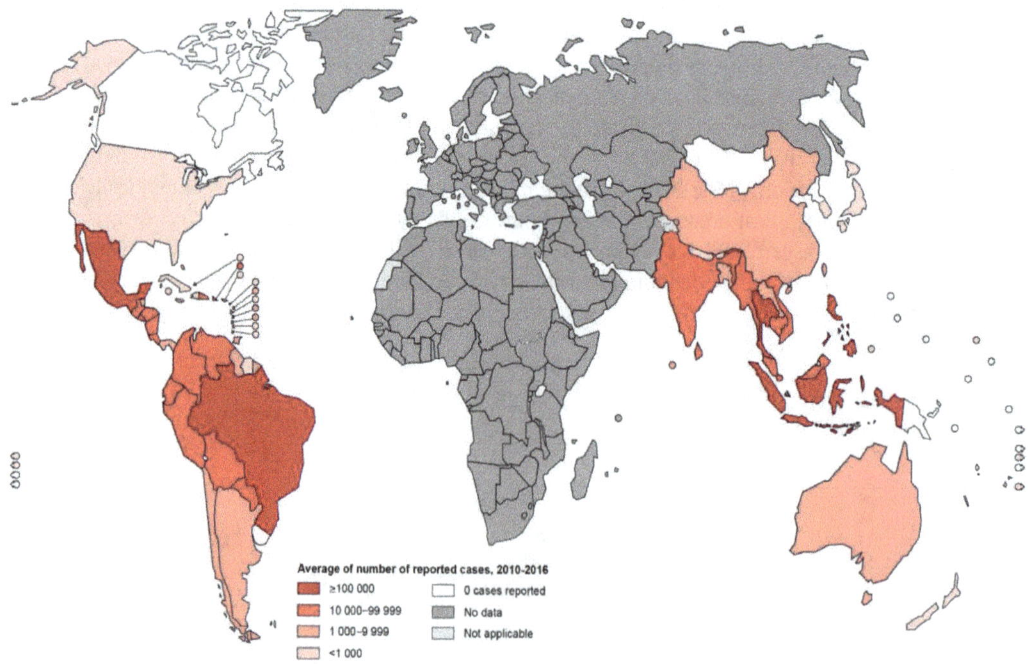

Figure 1. Distribution of dengue worldwide (taken from www.who.int/denguecontrol/ epidemiology/).

restricted till 1950s. But due to the Second World War, transport of *Aedes* mosquitoes happened around the world which played a crucial role in the dissemination of the viruses. Now, approximately 2.5 billion people live in areas where there is a risk of dengue transmission [9–12].

During 1850s, first case of dengue was documented in the Philippines and Thailand. Later, after 1980s large number of cases began to appear in the Caribbean and Latin America. Today, Dengue is endemic in at least 100 countries in Asia, the Pacific, the Americas, Africa, and the Caribbean. Dengue fever is reported to prevail in 26 states [13–15]. DENV-2 was the predominant serotype in dengue outbreaks that occurred before 2000 but DENV-3 was the predominant serotype between 2000 and 2009. After 2010, DENV-1 dominated global dengue outbreaks, and DENV-4 was the least frequently identified serotype [16, 17]. The geographical distribution of dengue with respect to countries has been shown in **Figure 1** which explains the current prevalence of this disease around the world [11].

3. The vector

Dengue virus spreads due to infected females of genus *Aedes*, significantly form *Aedes aegypti* and *Aedes albopictus*. There has been a serious concern amid public health departments. In newly invaded countries, *Aedes albopictus* would cause severe epidemics of arbovirus diseases (it is considered as a competent vector transmitting about 22 arboviruses), especially all four serotypes of dengue; however generally it is transmitted by *Aedes aegypti*. *Aedes albopictus* persists to spread, taking the place of *Aedes aegypti* in some areas. [18] *Aedes albopictus* might serve as a maintenance vector of dengue in non-urban areas of Pacific islands and South-east Asia. *Aedes albopictus* is not considered an imperative urban dengue vector, but in a few countries where *Aedes aegypti* is not present, that is, the Seychelles, parts of China, Japan and Hawaii [18]. The biting females of *Aedes albopictus* were discovered firstly in 1999, in Southern Cameroon; it provoked survey in 2000 and then adults as well as breeding populations were identified in five major cities of the country mainly breeding in old tires imported from Nigeria and USA which were infested with the mosquitoes [19].

Aedes is best known vectors of dengue fever and yellow fever. Some species of *Aedes* are also vectors of viral disease and filariasis [20]. Several serotypes of the dengue virus are carried to human beings via the bites of *Aedes* mosquitoes infected with dengue virus. *Aedes aegypti* is considered one of the most crucial vector whereas *Aedes niveus*, *Aedes albopictus* and *Aedes polynesiensis* have been reported as secondary vectors in most of the regions of the world [9]. *Aedes aegypti* and *Aedes albopictus* are known as the two primary vectors for transmitting the dengue in most parts of South Asia, including India. As the distribution of this affliction is concerned in respect to geographically, it is characteristically parallel to that of the principal vector species, *Aedes aegypti* [21]. Dengue mosquito is a subtropical and tropical species having distribution throughout the world [22]. Dengue virus spreads due to infected females of genus Aedes, specifically through *Aedes aegypti* in urban settings and *Aedes albopictus* in sylvatic areas [18]. *Aedes albopictus* (Diptera: *Culicidae*), is basically endemic to Pacific and Indian Oceanic islands, and from South-east Asia, it spread to America, Europe and Africa in recent decades dormant eggs in the tires. Venereal and possibly vertical transmission of dengue virus takes place by infected female of *Aedes aegypti* to its progeny (transovarian) and also from infected male to the female during the process of copulation, respectively [23].

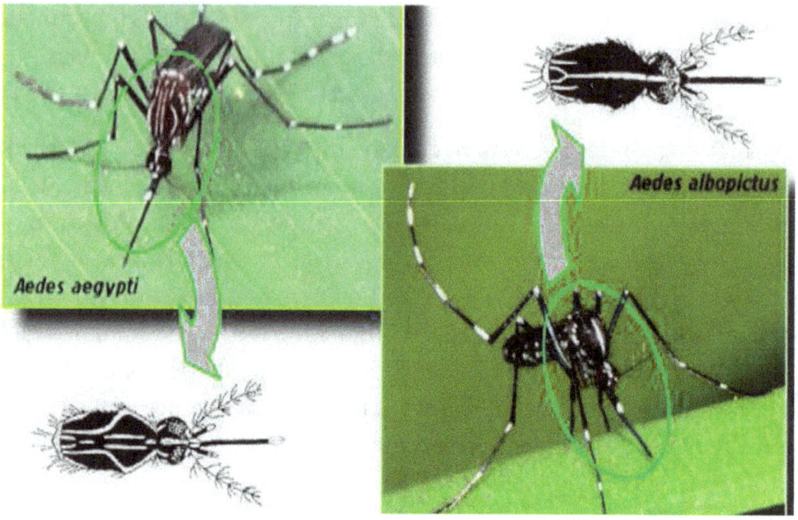

Figure 2. Difference between *Aedes aegypti* and *Aedes albopictus* (Source: http://www.mdsaude.com/wp-content/uploads/2012/04/aedes-aegypti-e-aedes-albopictus.jpg).

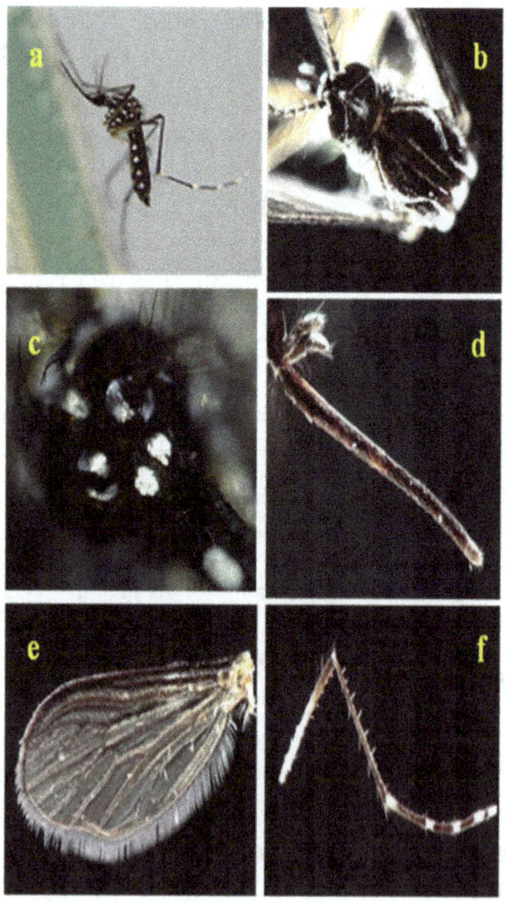

Figure 3. *Aedes aegypti* with its taxonomic characteristics. (a) *Aedes aegypti*; (b) Lyrix at thorax; (c) Clypeus; (d) Proboscis; (e) silvery scales on wing; (f) white stripes on leg.

The adult of yellow fever mosquito have approximately 4–7 mm size and it range from small to medium-sized mosquito. To the human eye, these mosquitoes are similar to the Asian tiger mosquito with a minor dissimilarity in thorax patterns and size. Adults of *Aedes aegypti* have white scales that form the shape of a violin or lyre, on the dorsal side of the thorax while the adults of *Aedes albopictus* is characterized by a white stripe to the middle at the top of the thorax region. Every tarsal portion of the hind legs exhibit white bands, this is what appear to be stripes. Abdomen is usually dark brown to black in color, but also exhibit white scales. Males are smaller than females, and can be discriminated by small palps tipped with white or silver scales. Males are characterized by plumose type of antennae; however, females possess sparse short hairs. Under a microscope, male mouthparts are viewed as modified structure for nectar feeding, and mouthparts of female are modified for feeding f blood. The proboscis from both sexes is darkly colored, and the segment above the proboscis which is known as clypeus has two clusters of white scales. A characteristic feature of all *Aedes* species is the pointed tip of the abdomen (**Figures 2** and **3**) [24].

4. Life cycle of *Aedes aegypti*

Aedes aegypti is geographically distributed in tropical areas and it breeds in artificially filled water containers such as drums, tyres, flower vases such as plastic food containers, tin cans and old motor parts [4]. *Aedes aegypti* is a holometabolous type of insect, going through complete metamorphosis meaning four developmental stages from egg to adult stage. Life span of adult can range from 2 weeks to about 4 weeks but it depends on conditions of environment. A female mosquito lay eggs for about 4–5 times during her entire life span and average number of eggs in single spawn ranges from 10 to 100 eggs. *Aedes aegypti* are found in three different polytypic forms: sylvan, domestic, and peridomestic. The domestic type usually breeds in urban habitats, mostly inside or around houses. The sylvan type is rural form which breeds in tree holes, normally in forests, and the peridomestic form generally lives in environmentally-modified regions as coconut farms and groves (**Figure 4**) [24].

As the spread of mosquitoes is concerned, it occurs by active flight (adult) and passive transportation (immature stages) through international trades. Successive waves of invasion of *Aedes aegypti* and *Culex pipiens* have been aided by commercial passages also from fifteenth century to onward. *Aedes aegypti* substituted *Aedes albopictus* in Asian countries during the twentieth century [25, 26].

5. The virus

Dengue infection is transmitted by dengue virus (DV) which is a member of genus *Flavivirus*. This Arbovirus group of viruses is specifically transmitted via insect vectors. Mature viral particles have diameter of 40–50 nm, spherical shape and 11 kb, having positive single stranded RNA which has a 5′-methyl cap with a single open reading frame. Genus *Flavivirus* has 4 antigenically associated but four distinct serotypes known as DENV-1, DENV-2, DENV-3 and DENV-4 [27, 28]. The serotypes are evolved from a common ancestor and all are considered

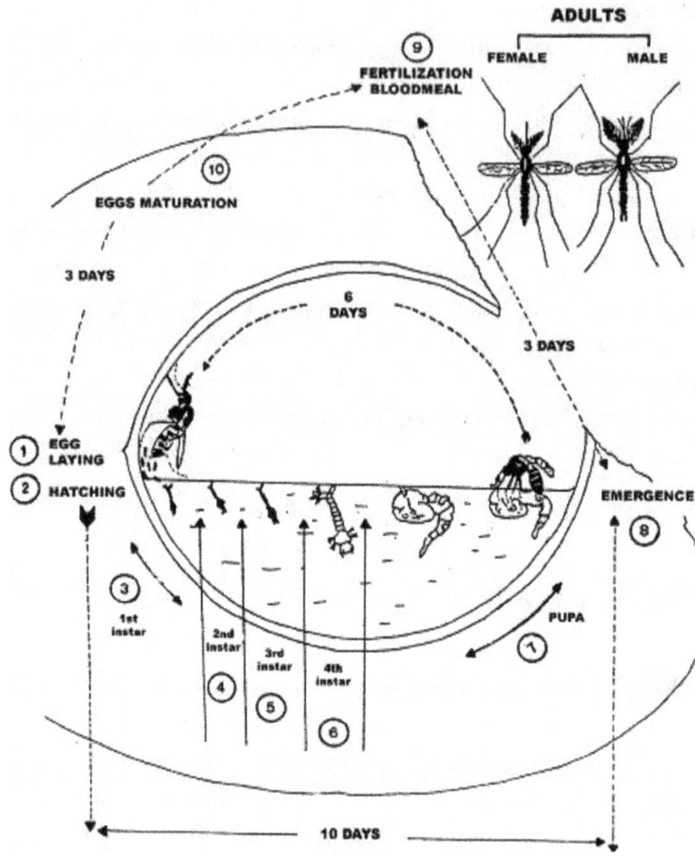

Figure 4. Lifecycle of *Aedes aegypti* (http:/www.ipnc.nc/FCKeditorFiles/Image/entomo_20.jpg).

causative agent of broadly analogous disease spectrum in humans [29–31]. It consists of ten proteins, out of which three proteins, capsid (C), membrane (M), and envelope (E), play structural role and seven (NS1, NS2A, NS2B, NS3, NS4A, NS4B and NS5) are identified as non-structural that direct DENV replication. Approximately 17% of these virions are lipid by weight which forms a lipid bilayer between E/M outer shell and the nucleocapsid core [32, 33].

Binding of dengue virus like most of the other viruses to its receptor is regulated by envelop protein (E). In mammalian cells, all the serotypes binds with nLc4Cer, DC-SIGN/L-SIGN, Heparan sulfate as well as Mannose receptors. Additionally DENV-2 serotype also show binding trend with HSP70/HSP90, CD14-associated protein, GRP78 and two other unknown protein receptors. On the other hand DENV 1–3 serotypes can also attach with Laminin receptor while DENV 2–4 serotypes are also found to bind with protein receptor which is unknown [34]. After binding with particular receptors through receptor-mediated endocytosis, virion fuses with acidic lysosomes. Then, the viral particle releases its RNA in the cytoplasm of host cell for the synthesis of viral proteins. After the synthesis of all the required proteins, viral RNA starts generating a minus strand, and then transcription of new plus stranded molecule occurs. Hundreds of copies of viral particles are generated from a single virus particle leading towards cellular damage and even death. RNA-dependent RNA polymerases (RdRps) encoded by the virus itself and other cellular factors catalyze the infection cycle of this virus

[35]. However the exact mechanism of vascular permeability and hemorrhagic fever is not clear. Studies are being oriented to understand these mechanisms specially focusing on the role played by T-cell immune response. High levels of interferon alpha were reported during secondary infection after 1–2 days of fever onset [36] while high concentration of soluble interleukin 2 receptor, interferon γ, soluble CD8 and soluble CD4 interleukin 2 were also described by researchers during the outset of vascular permeability [36, 37].

6. Clinical aspects

The most commonly occurring DENV infection transits through an asymptomatic or mildly symptomatic course [38]. Symptomatic dengue fever is usually accompanied by headache, malaise, retroorbital pain, arthralgia, and myalgia with a severity that honors "break-bone" fever alternative name of this disease. It lasts from three to 7 days. A small fraction of these patients evolve to the life-threatening clinical form of severe dengue, usually preceded by the appearance of warning signs (see below). All the four viral serotypes cause resembling disease symptoms.

In comparison to the previous 1997 version, the WHO revised classification of 2009. This makes more precision towards sensitivity and specificity of dengue cases. While being reported having changed dengue features with the passage of time during treatment; the dengue affected patients are categorized in Group A or Group B. More concern is recommended if symptoms becoming serious for next step of necessary hospitalization [39, 40]. As WHO 1997 version already includes plasma leakage and bleeding; but, however, the WHO 2009 classification entails target monitoring and organ impairment exhibiting the situation more clearly towards future dengue disease cure. Group C category of dengue patients has been explained in a better way in revised classification of WHO version 2009. This version, indeed is a practical guidance and very much helpful in dengue endemic areas especially where medical facilities are lacking. It is worth mentioning that WHO 2009 classification also highlights the other co-existing factors such as pregnancy, child and old age, diseases like diabetes and various social circumstances [41].

The WHO 2009 revised dengue classification stratifies disease into the following:

1. Without warning signs of dengue,
2. With warning signs of dengue (i.e., abdominal pain, vomiting, fluid accumulation, mucosal bleed, lethargic condition, liver enlargement >2 cm, and rapid decrease in platelet count), and
3. Severe symptoms of dengue.

Furthermore, three categories have been described in 2 WHO scheme of dengue-affected patients:

i. Group A includes patients without warnings signs,

ii. Group B includes patients with more than one warning sign, and annotated with certain coexisting conditions such as pregnancy, infancy, old age, obesity, diabetes, renal failure, and chronic hemolytic diseases), and with certain social circumstances,

iii. Group C includes patients with severe plasma leakage, severe bleeding leading towards extreme condition of organ impairment [41].

The classification is meant to make it realized that the group is clearly identified so that patients are going to be treated keeping in view the relevant category.

7. Diagnosis of dengue fever

Dengue infection symptoms are the major tool for its diagnosis. However, this is not a reliable method for the confirmation of dengue infection but laboratory studies are needed [42, 43]. Dengue virus in the initial stages may cause fever to dengue fever or later on more it can result in severe dengue. Common tools for the detection of dengue infection in laboratory tests include; an identification of the particular viral serotype, genomic sequences, viral antigen, genomic sequence, and/or antibodies. Major advances in the diagnosis of this infection include IgM captured ELISA, dengue specific monoclonal antibodies, viral RNA detection by nucleic acid amplification tests (NAAT), and viral isolation from mosquito cell lines and also live mosquitoes, all these are reported to have major advances in dengue diagnosis. Diagnosis involves two levels of detection. At level one, the patient is in acute febrile phase, where NS1 antigens and viral RNA can be detected, and at level two is the stage in which IgG and IgM antibodies are abundant in blood with the post febrile period [44]. Acute stages of dengue may be represented by flu like fever in which diagnosis is made possible by identifying viral RNA/proteins in the patient's blood. Dengue viral RNA can also be identified in early stage of infection using RT-PCR. This technique is quite reliable but unaffordable for the poor people [45, 46]. ELISA test is also being utilized to identify primary as well as secondary infection by utilizing dengue-specific monoclonal NS1 antibody to identify NS1 in victim's blood [47–49]. MACELISA assays in combination with NS1 Ag can be utilized for the detection of dengue viruses in earlier stages of infection [50]. Commonly used laboratory methods include immune-fluorescence tests, capture ELISAs, and hemagglutination assays [51]. Nonetheless, it is important to consider that serological tests can be misleading due to cross-reactivity while there is more that flavivirus circulating in the region.

8. Control of dengue fever

Vaccines against dengue are difficult to develop. Nonetheless, as for December of 2015, CYD-TDV vaccine was approved for human use, and to date it remains as the sole vaccine with this status. As for specific treatments none is available, however various anti-viral natural entities are being evaluated for the elimination of dengue virus [32, 47, 48, 52–54].

There are several methods used to control dengue infection. The first and most important preventive measure is the prevention of contact with infected mosquitoes. *Aedes* mosquitoes usually have biting preferences during daytime and its contact can be minimized in various ways, for example, proper management of stored water and wastes, use of insecticides to eradicate the mosquitoes, use of mosquito nets and coils as well as repellents, use of wearing which minimize the exposed body surface. Insecticide treated nets (ITNs) are also available in the market for the protection of people including young children, pregnant women, old people [55].

9. Control of vector *Aedes*

The best way to control dengue is to improve capabilities of mosquito abatement especially in the most populated areas where vector densities are high due to availability of hosts [18].

10. Public awareness

Public awareness counts in integrated pest management at a significant level, various examples can be sited from the literature when community efforts played a role for the eradication of disease agents. As *Aedes aegypti* was eliminated from countries various regions of the USA during the 1960s when relatively well funded eradication campaign supported by a high degree of political and community were involved. The effective collaboration of a well-educated society with the assistance of mosquito control well-trained staff will be the most compelling and economically reliable method for the removal of *Aedes albopictus* populations in rural and suburban regions [18].

11. Chemical control

The vector borne diseases are controlled worldwide, simply via controlling the vector. This thumb rule equally implies on dengue vector *Aedes* mosquitoes as well. Integrated Vector Management (IVM) mostly focuses on chemical control using insecticides; most frequently used are reported organophosphates and pyrethroids by WHO against dengue, malaria as well as yellow fever. These insecticides are affective against larvae, pupae and adults as well [25, 56, 57]. No new public health insecticides have been developed for mainstream vector control in disease-endemic countries (DECs) for the last three decades. Narrow range of public health insecticides necessitates new, safe, less expensive, environment friendly insecticides to replace those already being commercially used and mostly have been reported to develop resistance. Pyrethroid insecticides such as Permethrin, Deltamethrin, Cypermethrin, Cyhalothrin, etc. and DDVP organophosphate insecticides have been frequently used against mosquitoes and flies at household level. However, pyrethroid insecticides are reported to develop resistance. Hence, synergistic use of organophosphae and pyrethroid insecticides is being used now-a-days in order to combat this resistance menace [58]. New insecticides which are safe for health and environment as well demand investment. It is estimated that about US$70 million amount is required to develop a new insecticide. Public health insecticide market encompasses about US$151.2 million worldwide, hereby, shows the overall small size market. It is a dire need of time to engage commercial partners in the development of new insecticides. It has been suggested that both commercial and academic partners must collaborate and work together. In addition, community level health workers must be stimulated to locate and target the investment so that safe, cost-effective, user-friendly vector control insecticides can be developed.

12. Biological control

Although, chemical use in the form of synthetic insecticides remains promising factor for the control of insect vectors; however, indiscriminate and overuse pose insecticide resistance issues [58]. Moreover, various health and environmental concerns make the use of insecticide questionable. Thus, it is imagined that in future only those techniques will be accepted which may overcome the problems related to chemical insecticides. Recently, non-chemical methods have been summed-up into "biopesticides"; meaning thereby simply to kill the pest using material originated from living things [59]. Hence, it necessitates to explore biological control agents like various predators and parasites, that is, viruses, fungi, bacteria, etc. to look for a potent agent for the development of safe control program. Various pathogens and predators have been reported to use against mosquitoes as biological control agents. Recently, in Vietnam, copepods were used to control larvae of *A. aegypti.* At local level, the control program was launched very successfully and showed good results [61, 62]. In addition, a bacterium *Wolbachia pipientis* which is an obligate intracellular bacterium and vertically transmitted from mother to their offsprings and causes cytoplasmic incompatibility. It has been reported to present in 60% populations of insects in field conditions. Wolbachia infects the gonads and ensures transmission to the next host generation and orchestrates various reproductive manipulations in host. The symbiont can also cause feminization of genetic males, parthenogenesis and male killing, depending on the host species [63]. Thus, via females the Wolbachia spreads in the host populations and ultimately hinders its increase in number in future. It is reported that Wolbachia infections spread upto 100 km per annum. The Wolbachia strains were manifested and manipulated successfully in 1967 in Burma against filariasis vectors, where Wolbachia infected male *Culex quinquefasciatus* were released in wild populations. In principle, Wolbachia infection affects the sperm and prevents the further reproduction as a measure of local mosquito population control [65].

The sterile insect technique (SIT) is widely tested strategy in insects; wherein, males are treated with either sterilizing chemicals or exposed to γ-irradiation producing random dominant lethal mutations; means only one locus containing the DNA damage can cause dominant effect in the form of lethality. The SIT males when mate with normal females results non-viable offsprings leading to elimination of the populations in successive generations [65]. Another approach is RIDL (release of insects carrying a dominant lethal mutation) which is an improved version of SIT using transgenic technique and specifically focuses on female-killing. For instance, gene specifically expressing in the flight muscles were made transgenically expressed low and the resulting females in the offsprings would not be able to fly properly which causes its non-feeding on human blood meal which ultimately leads towards low fecundity [67]. Specific transgenic approaches have been proved successful also in pupae and adults [68, 69]. This RIDL techniques is being exploited and deployed by Oxitec® in Brazil and Malaysia and reproduced appreciable results [70]. Subsequently, *Bacillus thuringiensis israelensis* (*Bti*), methoprene and the insect growth hormone are also proven to be quite effective against *Aedes albopictus* in the laboratory as well as in the field [57, 71–75].

13. Botanical control

Plants as a whole and/or their certain parts plus various products originated from different plants have been incorporated in the control programs from long time ago. However, plant oils have been annotated with potentially good insecticidal properties [76, 77]. Plant extracts are reported as fumigant and caused ovicidal, larvicidal, and overall insecticidal activity against various insects. The plants derived insecticides; mostly mentioned as biopesticides are non-hazardous to the environment, cheap, and are considered safe to human as well as other animals. Black pepper extracts have been shown with significant potential as adulticide against *Aedes aegypti* and *Anopheles stephensi* [78].

It is thus, suggested that plant extracts have promising capability to control the mosquitoes. Being safe to human health and to the environment; these can be successfully incorporated in mosquito control programs [79]. In addition, a few plants extracts have been successfully tested against some viral diseases. Aforementioned wherein the life cycle of dengue virus; DENV makes an attachment with host via host receptors and envelope proteins; suggesting thereby that DENV infection can be controlled via inhibition of host-viral interactions using plants extracts. Moreover, NS2-NS3 protease and NS5 have also been reported as significant antiviral drug targets due to their impact on viral replication and other cellular processes as well [80, 81]. Several medicinal plants such as *Momordica charantia* and *Andrographis paniculata* have been reported in inhibiting the replication cycle of DENV. Few of the weed plants have been shown to cause insecticidal and enzyme inhibitory activities in insects [83, 84]. Further investigations are needed to develop potential dengue treatment [85].

14. Conclusion and future perspectives

Dengue viral disease is an emerging health concern in many regions of the world and has become a serious threat in many areas of the world including Southeast Asia and Pakistan. The control of the dengue is difficult as there is no vaccine available so far. Vaccine preparation against dengue requires a tetravalent vaccine but no such licensed compound has been prepared so far. However dengue viral envelope proteins can be targeted to make an effective drug against dengue as these proteins are involved in the entry of the virus into the host cell. Several medicinal plants have been identified so far which show significant inhibitory results against dengue but still there is a need of proper medicine which can show promising results. In future, exploration of interaction of *Aedes albopictus* and other mosquito species is required. *Toxorhynchites* mosquitoes should be searched out for their predatory role against *Aedes albopictus* and *Aedes aegypti*. Vectoral role of *Aedes albopictus* and *Aedes aegypti* must be regulated in and between countries. In addition, the predominant serotype in dengue outbreaks can be managed through respective vaccine especially against the documented serotype.

Author details

Muhammad Kashif Zahoor[1]*, Azhar Rasul[1], Muhammad Asif Zahoor[2], Iqra Sarfraz[1], Muhammad Zulhussnain[1], Rizwan Rasool[1], Humara Naz Majeed[3], Farhat Jabeen[1] and Kanwal Ranian[1]

*Address all correspondence to: kashif.zahoor@gcuf.edu.pk

1 Department of Zoology, Government College University Faisalabad, Pakistan

2 Department of Microbiology, Government College University Faisalabad, Pakistan

3 Department of Biochemistry, Government College Women University, Faisalabad, Pakistan

References

[1] Annonymous. Etymologia dengue. Emerging Infectious Diseases. 2006;**12**:893

[2] Mairuhu ATA, Wagenaar J, Brandjes DPM, van Gorp ECM. Dengue: An arthropod-borne disease of global importance. European Journal of Clinical Microbiology & Infectious Diseases. 2004;**23**:425-433

[3] Hotta S. Experimental studies on dengue. I. Isolation, identification and modification of the virus. The Journal of Infectious Diseases. 1952;**90**:1-9

[4] Gubler DJ. Dengue and dengue hemorrhagic fever: Its history and resurgence as a global public health problem. In: Gubler DJ, Kuno G, editors. Dengue and Dengue Hemorrhagic Fever. Wallingford, UK: CAB International; 1997. pp. 1-22

[5] Rush B. An account of the bilious remitting fever: As it appeared in Philadelphia in the summer and autumn of the year 1780. The American Journal of Medicine. 1951;**11**(5):546-550

[6] Siler JF, Hall MW, Hitchens AP. Dengue: Its history, epidemiology, mechanisms of transmission, etiology, clinical manifestations, immunity and prevention. Philippine Journal of Science. 1926;**29**:1-304

[7] Bancroft TL. On the etiology of dengue fever. Australasian Medical Gazette. 1906;**25**:17-18

[8] Kimura R, Hotta S. On the inoculation of dengue virus into mice. Nippon Igaku. 1944;**3379**:629-633

[9] World Health Organization. Weekly Epidimological Monitor. 2013;**6**:37

[10] World Health Organization. World Malaria Report. Geneva: World Health Organization. 2009a

[11] World Health Organization. Dengue and dengue haemorrhagic fever. In: Fact Sheet No117. Geneva: World Health Organization; 2009b

[12] Idrees S, Ashfaq UA. A brief review on dengue molecular virology, diagnosis, treatment and prevalence in Pakistan. Idrees and Ashfaq Genetic Vaccines and Therapy. 2012;**10**:6

[13] Hanna JN, Ritchie SA, Phillips DA, Serafin IL, Hills SL, van den Hurk AF. An epidemic of dengue 3 in far North Queensland, 1997-1999. The Medical Journal of Australia. 2001;**174**: 178-182

[14] Cobelens FG, Groen J, Osterhaus AD, Leentvaar-Kuipers A, Wertheim-van Dillen PM, Kager PA. Incidence and risk factors of probable dengue virus infection among Dutch travellers to Asia. Tropical Medicine & International Health. 2002;**7**:331-338

[15] Messer WB, Gubler DJ, Harris E, Sivananthan K, de Silva AM. Emergence and global spread of a dengue serotype 3, subtype III virus. Emerging Infectious Diseases. 2003;**9**: 800-809

[16] Hastead SB. Dengue fever and dengue Hemorrhagic fever. In: Kliegman RM, Behrman RE, Jenson HB, Stanton BF, editors. Nelson Textbook of Pediatrics. 18th ed. Philadelphia, USA: WB Saunders; 2007. pp. 1412-1414

[17] Halstead SB. Etiologies of the experimental dengue of Siler and Simmons. The American Journal of Tropical Medicine and Hygiene. 1974;**23**:974-982

[18] Gratz NG. Critical review of the vector status of *Aedes albopictus*. Medical and Veterinary Entomology. 2004;**18**:215-227

[19] Fontenille D, Toto JC. *Aedes* (Stegomyia) *albopictus* (Skuse), a potential new dengue vector in southern Cameroon. Emerging Infectious Diseases. 2001;**7**:1066-1067

[20] World Health Organization, Special Programme for Research, Training in Tropical Diseases, World Health Organization. Department of Control of Neglected Tropical Diseases, World Health Organization. Epidemic, & Pandemic Alert. Dengue: guidelines for diagnosis, treatment, prevention and control. World Health Organization. 2009. http://apps.who.int/iris/bitstream/handle/10665/44188/9789241547871?sequence=1

[21] Jacobs MG, Robinson PJ, Bletchly C, Mackenzie JM, Young PR. Dengue virus nonstructural protein 1 is expressed in a glycosyl-phosphatidylinositol-linked form that is capable of signal transduction. The FASEB Journal. 2000;**14**:1603-1610

[22] Gibbons RV, Vaughn DW. Dengue: An escalating problem. BMJ. 2002;**324**:1563-1566

[23] Kow CY, Koon LL, Yin PF. Detection of dengue viruses in field caught male *Aedes aegypti* and *Aedes albopictus* (Diptera: Culicidae) in Singapore by type-specific PCR. Journal of Medical Entomology. 2001;**38**(4):475-479

[24] Rey JR, O'Meara GF, O'Connell SM, Cutwa-Francis MM. Factors affecting mosquito production from storm water drains and catch basins in two Florida cities. Journal of Vector Ecology. 2006;**31**(2):334-343

[25] Curtis CF, Jana-Kara B, Maxwell CA. Insecticide treated nets: Impact on vector populations and relevance of initial intensity of transmission and pyrethroid resistance. Journal of Vector Borne Diseases. 2003;**40**:1-9

[26] Tripathi P, Kumar R, Tripathi S, Tambe JJ, Venkatesh V. Descriptive epidemiology of dengue transmission in Uttar Pradesh. Indian Pediatrics. 2008;**45**:315-318

[27] Raheel U, Faheem M, Riaz MN, Kanwal N, Javed F, Sahar N, et al. Dengue fever in the Indian subcontinent: An overview. Journal of Infection in Developing Countries. 2011;**5**(4):239-247

[28] Guzman MG, Kouri G. Dengue and dengue hemorrhagic fever in the Americas: Lessons and challenges. Journal of Clinical Virology. 2003;**27**:1-13

[29] Wang WK, Sung TL, Lee CN, Lin TY, King CC. Sequence diversity of the capsid gene and the nonstructural gene NS2B of dengue-3 virus in vivo. Virology. 2002;**303**:181-191

[30] Ross TM. Dengue virus. Clinics in Laboratory Medicine. 2010;**30**:149-160

[31] Wang E, Ni H, Xu R, Barrett AD, Watowich SJ, Gubler DJ, et al. Evolutionary relationships of endemic/epidemic and sylvatic dengue viruses. Journal of Virology. **74**:3227-3234

[32] Kuhn RJ, Zhang W, Rossmann MG, Pletnev SV, Corver J, Lenches E, et al. Structure of dengue virus: Implications for flavivirus organization, maturation, and fusion. Cell. 2001;**108**:717-725

[33] Hanley KA, Lee JJ, Blaney JE Jr, Murphy BR, Whitehead SS. Paired charge-to-alanine mutagenesis of dengue virus type 4 NS5 generates mutants with temperature-sensitive, host range, and mouse attenuation phenotypes. Journal of Virology. 2002;**76**:525-531

[34] Hidari KI, Suzuki T. Dengue virus receptor. Tropical Medicine and Health. 2011;**39**:37-43

[35] Filomatori CV, Lodeiro MF, Alvarez DE, Samsa MM, Pietrasanta L, Gamarnik AV. A 5' RNA element promotes dengue virus RNA synthesis on a circular genome. Genes & Development. 2006;**20**:2238-2249

[36] Kurane I, Innis BL, Nimmannitya S, Nisalak A, Meager A, Janus J, et al. Activation of T lymphocytes in dengue virus infections. High levels of soluble interleukin 2 receptor, soluble CD4, soluble CD8, interleukin 2, and interferon-gamma in sera of children with dengue. The Journal of Clinical Investigation. 1991;**88**:1473-1480

[37] Kurane I, Innis BL, Nimmannitya S, Nisalak A, Meager A, Ennis FA. High levels of interferon alpha in the sera of children with dengue virus infection. The American Journal of Tropical Medicine and Hygiene. 1993;**48**:222-229

[38] George R, Lum LC. Clinical spectrum of dengue infection. In: Dengue and Dengue Haemorrhagic Fever. New York: CAB International. 1997. pp. 89-113

[39] Narvaez F, Gutierrez G, Pérez MA, Elizondo D, Nuñez A, Balmaseda A, et al. Evaluation of the traditional and revised WHO classifications of dengue disease severity. PLoS Neglected Tropical Diseases. 2011;**5**:e1397

[40] Lee IK, Liu JW, Yang KD. Fatal dengue hemorrhagic fever in adults: Emphasizing the evolutionary pre-fatal clinical and laboratory manifestations. PLoS Neglected Tropical Diseases. 2012;**6**:e1532

[41] World Health Organization. Dengue: Guidelines for Diagnosis, Treatment, Prevention and Control. Geneva: World Health Organization. 2009

[42] Burke DS, Nisalak A, Johnson DE, Scott RM. A prospective study of dengue infections in Bangkok. The American Journal of Tropical Medicine and Hygiene. 1988;**38**:172-180

[43] Endy TP, Chunsuttiwat S, Nisalak A, Libraty DH, Green S, Rothman AL, et al. Epidemiology of inapparent and symptomatic acute dengue virus infection: A prospective study of primary school children in Kamphaeng Phet, Thailand. American Journal of Epidemiology. 2002;**156**:40-51

[44] Libraty DH, Young PR, Pickering D, Endy TP, Kalayanarooj S, Green S, et al. High circulating levels of the dengue virus nonstructural protein NS1 early in dengue illness correlate with the development of dengue hemorrhagic fever. The Journal of Infectious Diseases. 2002;**186**:1165-1168

[45] Kuno G, Cropp CB, Wong-Lee J, Gubler DJ. Evaluation of an IgM immunoblot kit for dengue diagnosis. American Journal of Tropical Medicine and Hygiene. 1998;**59**:757-762

[46] Laue T, Emmerich P, Schmitz H. Detection of dengue virus RNA in patients after primary or secondary dengue infection by using the TaqMan automated amplification system. Journal of Clinical Microbiology. 1999;**37**:2543-2547

[47] Shu PY, Chen LK, Chang SF, Yueh YY, Chow L, Chien LJ, et al. Comparison of capture immunoglobulin M (IgM) and IgG enzyme-linked immunosorbent assay (ELISA) and nonstructural protein NS1 serotype-specific IgG ELISA for differentiation of primary and secondary dengue virus infections. Clinical and Diagnostic Laboratory Immunology. 2003;**10**:622-630

[48] Dussart P, Labeau B, Lagathu G, Louis P, Nunes MR, Rodrigues SG, et al. Evaluation of an enzyme immunoassay for detection of dengue virus NS1 antigen in human serum. Clinical and Vaccine Immunology. 2006;**13**:1185-1189

[49] Khan AH, Hayat AS, Masood N, NM S, Shaikh TZ. Frequency and clinical presentation of dengue fever at Tertiary Care Hospital of Hyderabad/Jamshoro. JLUMHS. 2010;**09**(2): 88-93

[50] Datta S, Wattal C. Dengue NS1 antigen detection: A useful tool in early diagnosis of dengue virus infection. Indian Journal of Medical Microbiology. 2010;**28**:107-110

[51] Butt N, Abbassi A, Munir SM, Ahmad SM, Sheikh QH. Haematological and biochemical indicators for the early diagnosis of dengue viral infection. Journal of the College of Physicians and Surgeons–Pakistan. 2008;**282-285**(80):18

[52] Chadwick D, Arch B, Wilder-Smith A, Paton N. Distinguishing dengue fever from other infections on the basis of simple clinical and laboratory features: Application of logistic regression analysis. Journal of Clinical Virology. 2006;**35**(2):147-153

[53] Singh K, Lale A, Eong OE, Chiu L, Chow V, Tambyah P, et al. A prospective clinical study on the use of reverse transcription-polymerase chain reaction for the early diagnosis of dengue fever. The Journal of Molecular Diagnostics. 2006;**8**:613-616

[54] http://www.denguevirusnet.com/treatment.html

[55] Jahan F. Dengue fever (DF) in Pakistan. Asia Pacific Family Medicine. 2011;**10**:1. https://doi.org/10.1186/1447-056X-10-1

[56] Zaim M, Jambulingam P. Global Insecticide Use for Vector Borne Disease Control. World Health Organization Communicable Disease Control, Prevention and Eradication, WHO Pesticide Evaluation Scheme (WHOPES). 2004. Geneva (No. WHO/CDS/WHOPES/GCDPP/2007.2)

[57] Ali A, Nayar JK, Xue R-D. Comparative toxicity of selected larvicides and insect growth regulators to a Florida laboratory population of *Aedes albopictus*. Journal of the American Mosquito Control Association. 1995;**11**:72-76

[58] Zaim M, Guillet P. Alternative insecticides: An urgent need. Trends in Parasitology. 2002;**18**(4):161-163

[59] Broadhurst M. The influence of the molecular basis of resistance on insecticide discovery. Philosophical Transactions of the Royal Society of London B: Biological Sciences. 1998;**353**(1376):1723-1728

[60] Amer A, Mehlhorn H. Repellency effect of forty-one essential oils against *Aedes, Anopheles*, and *Culex* mosquitoes. Parasitology Research. 2006;**99**:478-490

[61] Nam VS, Yen NT, Duc HM, Tu TC, Thang VT, Le NH, et al. Community-based control of Aedes aegypti by using Mesocyclops in southern Vietnam. The American Journal of Tropical Medicine and Hygiene. 2012;**86**(5):850-859

[62] Kay B, Nam VS. New strategy against *Aedes aegypti* in Vietnam. The Lancet. 2005;**365**(9459):613-617

[63] O'Neill SL, Hoffmann AA, Werren JH, editors. Influential Passengers: Inherited Microorganisms and Arthropod Reproduction. USA, Oxford University Press; 1998. ISBN: 9780198501732

[64] Charlat S, Hurst GD, Merçot H. Evolutionary consequences of Wolbachia infections. Trends in Genetics. 2003;**19**(4):217-223

[65] Turelli M, Hoffmann AA. Cytoplasmic incompatibility in *Drosophila simulans*: Dynamics and parameter estimates from natural populations. Genetics. 1995;**140**(4):1319-1338

[66] Alphey L, Benedict M, Bellini R, Clark GG, Dame DA, Service MW, et al. Sterile-insect methods for control of mosquito-borne diseases: An analysis. Vector-Borne and Zoonotic Diseases. 2010;**10**(3):295-311

[67] Fu G, Lees RS, Nimmo D, Aw D, Jin L, Gray P, et al. Female-specific flightless phenotype for mosquito control. Proceedings of the National Academy of Sciences. 2010;**107**(10):4550-4554

[68] Phuc HK, Andreasen MH, Burton RS, Vass C, Epton MJ, Pape G, et al. Late-acting dominant lethal genetic systems and mosquito control. BMC Biology. 2007;**5**(1):11

[69] Bargielowski I, Nimmo D, Alphey L, Koella JC. Comparison of life history characteristics of the genetically modified OX513A line and a wild type strain of *Aedes aegypti*. PLoS One. 2011;**6**(6):e20699

[70] Lacroix R, McKemey AR, Raduan N, Wee LK, Ming WH, Ney TG, et al. Open field release of genetically engineered sterile male *Aedes aegypti* in Malaysia. PLoS One. 2012;**7**(8):e42771

[71] Farghal AI, Roe RM, Apperson CS. Evaluation of two insect growth regulators alone and in combination with *Bacillus thuringiensis* var. *israelensis* against *Culex quinquefaciatus* and *Aedes albopictus* larvae in the laboratory Assiut. Journal of Agricultural Science. 1988;**19**:284-303

[72] Toma T, Kamiyama S, Fujihara S, Miyagi I. Effects of methoprene, a juvenile hormone analogue, on mosquito larvae from the Ryukyu Archipelago, Japan. Japanese Journal of Sanitary Zoology. 1990;**41**:99-103

[73] Basci RS, Wright GB, Willis FS. Control of *Aedes albopictus* larvae using time release larvicide formulations in Lousiana. Journal of the American Mosquito Control Association. 1994;**10**:1-6

[74] Sulaiman S, Jeffery J, Sohadi AR. Residual efficacy of triflumuron and methoprene against the dengue vector, *Aedes albopictus* (Skuse). Bulletin of the Society for Vector Ecology. 1994;**19**:111-114

[75] Becnel JJ, Garcia J, Johnson M. Effects of three larvicides on the production of *Aedes albopictus* based on the removal of pupal exuvi Aedes. Journal of the American Mosquito Control Association. 1996;**12**:499-502

[76] Adebayo TA, Gbolade AA, Olaifa JI. Comparative study of toxicity of essential oils to larvae of three mosquito species. Nigerian Journal of Natural Products and Medicine. 1999;**3**:74-76

[77] Gbolade AA, Oyedele AO, Sosan MB, Adewoyin FB, Soyelu O. Mosquito repellent activities of essential oils from two Nigerian Ocimum species. Journal of Tropical Medicinal Plants. 2000;**1**:146-148

[78] Trongtokit Y, Burivong P, Moore S, Hill N, Curtis CF. Plant Extracts in Prevention of Mosquito Attacks. Botanical Medicine in Clinical Practice. 2008. pp. 807-813

[79] Nawaz R, Rathor RH, Bilal H, Hassan SA, Khan IA. Adulticidal activity of *Olea vera, Linum usitatissimum* and *Piper nigera* against *Anopheles stephensi* and *Aedes aegypti* under laboratory conditions. Journal of Arthropod-Borne Diseases. 2011;**5**(2):2-9

[80] Chow VT, Yong RY, Ngoh BL, Chan YC. Automated type specific ELISA probe detection of amplified NS3 gene products of dengue viruses. Journal of Clinical Pathology. 1997;**50**:346-349

[81] Falgout B, Miller RH, Lai CJ. Deletion analysis of dengue virus type 4 nonstructural protein NS2B: Identification of a domain required for NS2B-NS3 protease activity. Journal of Virology. 1993;**67**:2034-2042

[82] Tang LI, Ling AP, Koh RY, Chye SM, Voon KG. Screening of anti-dengue activity in methanolic extracts of medicinal plants. BMC Complementary and Alternative Medicine. 2012;**12**:3

[83] Sultana K, Zahoor MK, Sagheer M, Nasir S, Zahoor MA, Jabeen F, Riaz B. Insecticidal activity of weed plants, *Euphorbia prostrata* and *Chenopodiastrum murale* against stored

grain insect pest *Trogoderma granarium* Everts, 1898 (Coleoptera: Dermestidae). Turkish Journal of Entomology. 2016;**40**(3):291-301

[84] Riaz B, Zahoor MK, Zahoor MA, Majeed HN, Javed I, Ahmed A, Jabeen F, Zulhussnain M, Sultana K. Toxicity, phytochemical composition and enzyme inhibitory activities of some indigenous weed plant extracts in fruit fly, *Drosophila melanogaster*. Evidence-Based Complementary and Alternative Medicine. 2018;**2018**. Article ID: 2325659. DOI: 10.1155/2018/2325659

[85] Talarico LB, Damonte EB. Interference in dengue virus adsorption and uncoating by carrageenans. Virology. 2007;**363**:473-485

6

New Tools for Dengue Diagnostics

Om Parkash, Punam Kumari, Vasu Deva, Sham Lal,
Javed Ahmed Ujjan, Syed Mehmood Qadir,
Fateh Muhammad Soomro, Rani Faryal and
Nisar Ahmed Kanhar

Abstract

Dengue caused by four antigenically distinct serotype remains a serious health concern around the world, particularly in the tropical areas. Clinical signs and symptoms of this disease are indistinguishable from other infectious disease; therefore, laboratory diagnosis is very crucial for confirming the disease that will be useful for the patient's management. In laboratory, dengue can be confirmed using cell culture, RNA detection, and serological detection based on ELISA and immunochromatographic test. However, each of these methods has certain practical limitations. Therefore, researchers from all over the world have been working to address these limitations. In this chapter, we will highlight the current research toward the development of novel point-of-care test for the diagnosis of dengue in acute and convalescent phase.

Keywords: dengue, diagnosis, microfluidic, RT-LAMP, biosensor

1. Introduction

Despite the significant advancement in medical sciences, dengue remains a serious public health concern in more than 100 countries, precisely in tropical and subtropical parts of the world. Dengue has alarming situation in Southeast Asia, South America, and Africa. Approximately, half of the world's population living in dengue endemic area is at the risk of getting dengue infection. Evidence shows that every year about 390 million dengue infection appears worldwide, of which 100 million cases are found to be symptomatic and require medical attention [1–3].

Clinical symptoms typically appear 4–7 days following the mosquito bite and may persist for 3–10 days. Clinical manifestation of dengue varies from asymptomatic to acute febrile illness with headache, vomiting, severe myalgia, rash, retro-orbital pain, and arthralgia [4–6]. Classically, dengue was categorized as dengue fever, dengue hemorrhagic fever, and dengue shock syndrome. Nevertheless, classification was revised by the WHO in 2009 and classified it as dengue with or without warning signs. This version of classification divides dengue into three clinical phases: febrile, critical, and recovery phases [7, 8]. In the febrile phase, patient develops high fever due to acute viremia, and this phase lasts for 2–7 days. Critical phase usually lasts for 2 days and is indicated by plasma leakage, hemorrhage, and low platelet number. If patients survive in critical phase, then they will recover from the disease at the third phase known as recovery/convalescent phase [9, 10].

The spherical and enveloped dengue virus (DENV) which belongs to the family *Flaviviridae* is the causative agent of dengue. This virus is 50 nm in diameter and contains about 11 kb positive-sense single-stranded RNA genome that codes for three structural proteins (capsid, membrane, and envelope) and seven nonstructural proteins [11, 12]. The DENV is transmitted to human by the bite of *Aedes aegypti* and *Aedes albopictus* mosquito which usually breed in the clean water in urban areas [13, 14]. Each serotype of DENV can cause dengue and trigger inimitable immune response in host which provides long-term immunity to that particular serotype but limited and partial immunity against three other serotypes [15, 16]. Although, the four DENV serotypes are antigenically different but genetically are identical as they share about 65% of their RNA sequences [17, 18].

2. Diagnosis of dengue

At this time, a tetravalent dengue vaccine has been developed but due to its lack of protection on non-exposed individuals, it is not an effective option. On the other hand, antiviral drugs for curing the dengue are not available; thus, accurate and timely diagnosis is of utmost importance for appropriate management of a patient suffering from severe dengue [19]. However, diagnosis of dengue based on clinical manifestation is quite complicated as the signs of dengue are very common in other febrile illness; therefore, diagnosis is very challenging using this approach [10, 20]. Thus, laboratory confirmation is needed for definite diagnosis. Laboratory confirmation of dengue can be obtained using several techniques such as virus isolation, polymerase chain reaction (PCR)-based detection of viral genome, nonstructural protein 1 (NS1) antigen detection, and serological detection of dengue-specific antibodies such as IgM and IgG [21]. Nevertheless, effective application of each diagnostic technique depends on the disease stages.

2.1. Recent advancement in the diagnosis of dengue

The WHO set "affordable, sensitive, specific, user-friendly, rapid, easy to handle and deliver to those who need them (ASSURED)" as the characteristics of an ideal point-of-care test for resource-limited countries [22, 23]. With the advancement of science and technology, several novel diagnostic platforms emerged for the diagnostic of infectious disease such as biosensor, microfluidic, loop-mediated isothermal amplification (LAMP), and so on. These diagnostic platforms were also explored by the researchers for developing a point-of-care test for the diagnosis of dengue. The below section will briefly give an insight into some of these platforms investigated for the diagnosis of dengue.

2.1.1. *Biosensor platform*

The criteria of point-of-care test resulted attractive for industry and researchers in order to develop and satisfy the qualification of ideal diagnostic test. Therefore, numerous researchers around the world have been working on biosensors in a search of potential point-of-care test as they offer several advantages such as high sensitivity and specificity, simple instrumentation, rapid assay outcome, portability and disposability of developed tools. Several researchers have reported biosensor for the diagnosis of dengue. In this section, we take a glance over current biosensor methods aimed to improve the diagnostic of dengue using different biomarkers.

2.1.1.1. *NS1 antigen detection*

Omar et al. reported an electrochemical immunosensor based on screen-printed carbon electrodes (SPCE) for the detection of dengue NS1 antigen. Anti-NS1-capturing antibodies were immobilized on BSA-modified working electrode of SPCE. The detection was based on the measurement of electron transfer resistance before and after the NS1 binding. The study demonstrated that the immunosensor successfully detected NS1 antigen with a limit of detection (LOD) of 0.3 ng/mL and the linear range was 1–200 ng/mL [24]. Pirich et al. worked on piezoelectric immunosensor to detect dengue NS1 antigen. For the enhanced binding of anti-NS1 antibodies, sensor surface was coated with a thin film of bacterial cellulose nanocrystals. The formation of antigen antibody complex was then analyzed using quartz crystal microbalance. The study showed that immunochip was able to detect dengue NS1 antigen from serum with a LOD of 0.32 μg/mL [25]. In another study, NS1 was detected using Langmuir–Blodgett and gold nanoparticles (AuNP) composite as a biosensing surface. The anti-NS1 antibodies were immobilized on the biosensing surface and then the sample containing NS1 antigen was pipetted on it. Subsequently, the biorecognition event between anti-NS1 antibody and NS1 antigen was detected through electrochemical impedance spectroscopy. The study showed that developed electrochemical immunosensor was capable to detect dengue with a LOD of 1.19 ng/mL in spiked serum sample [26].

2.1.1.2. *Detection of dengue IgM antibodies*

Jahanshahi et al. targeted the dengue IgM antibody as an analyte in an optical biosensor. In the assay, four serotypes of DENV were used as ligands for capturing IgM antibodies. The assay time of optical biosensor was just 10 minutes and required a minimum volume of 1 μl of sample to perform it. The sensitivity of developed sensor was ranging from 83 to 93% and specificity was 100% [27]. Ortega et al. reported a novel "Magnetic Paper-Based ELISA" for isotype IgM-dengue antibodies detection. In the assay, magnetite nanoparticles were deposited on cellulose paper sheet. The antihuman IgM-capturing antibodies were immobilized on nanoparticle using a cross-linker, namely polydopamine. The concentration of IgM antibodies captured by antihuman IgM antibodies was determined using Bradford assay and SDS gel electrophoresis. The study claimed to have 700 times lower LOD than conventional ELISA [28]. Ortega et al. reported an electrochemical immunoassay using lead sulfide quantum dots as detection label for enhancing the sensitivity of assay by conjugating with anti-IgM detection antibodies. The immunoassay was performed on ELISA microplate, and electrochemical response generated by acid dissolution of detection label was measured on SPCE. The differential pulse anodic stripping voltammetry was used to measure the electrochemical response. Using this technique, immunosensor successfully detected dengue IgM antibodies with a LOD of 130 ng [29]. Wong developed an immunosensor using long-range surface plasmon-polariton waveguides for the detection of dengue IgM antibodies. The developed immunosensor detected IgM antibodies from a serum sample with a LOD of ~22 pg/mm^2 [30]. Liu et al. fabricated a label-free immunosensor based on optical fiber long-period grating (LPG) for detecting dengue IgM antibodies. For the detection of IgM antibodies, the LPG was modified with a film of three layers containing poly(allylamine hydrochloride) and silica nanoparticles. Later, anti-IgM antibodies were immobilized via covalent binding on modified surface. Subsequently, when the sample containing analyte IgM antibodies was added, it caused an increase in refractive index of film coated on the surface of LPG leading to a wavelength shift. This wavelength shift suggested was due to the binding of IgM antibodies with anti-IgM antibodies. The optical biosensor developed in this study detected IgM antibodies with a detection limit of 15 pg/mm^2 [31].

2.1.1.3. Detection of dengue genome

On the other hand, some researchers focused on viral genome as a target analyte in the hunt of a point-of-care test. Chan et al. developed a genosensor using a silver nanocluster (Ag NC) as hybridization indicator of target DNA with probe DNA. In the assay, the target DNA was synthesized from dengue RNA extracted from a mosquito. Afterward, the target DNA was hybridized with dengue probe DNA and amplified using isothermal amplification. Following the amplification, the product was mixed with $AgNO_3$. Subsequently, the reduction agent $NABH_4$ was added to mixture to produce Ag NC which was observed using a UV light. This study showed that the developed genosensor could detect DENV genome with a LOD of 100 nM [32]. Jin et al. developed an electrochemical genosensor by modifying graphene oxide surface with SiO_2 particles for enhancing the electrochemical properties of the surface. The negatively charged oligonucleotide primer specific for dengue complementary DNA was immobilized on the graphene-oxide-modified surface. Afterward, the sample containing target complementary DNA was pipetted. It was found that the oligonucleotide primer hybridized with complimentary DNA indicating the presence of dengue DNA in the sample. EIS was carried out on three electrode cell using PBS solution, and impedance spectra were measured. The study claimed to detect dengue DNA with a LOD of 1 femto-molar concentration of viral genome [33].

Another genosensor was developed using silicon nanowire to carry out electrochemical-based assay. First of all, silicon nanowire surface was pretreated for immobilizing the probe DNA. Later, the target DNA was added on the surface. The hybridization between probe and target DNA was detected through variation in current, conductance, and resistance on genosensor because of negative charges which increased with the binding of probe and target DNA. The genosensor developed in this study successfully detected DNA with a LOD of 2.0 fM [34]. Ariffin et al. employed nickel(II) salphen complex as DNA hybridization indicator for developing optical genosensor to detect DENV DNA. The indicator was known as a DNA intercalating agent. Porous silica nanospheres (PSiNs) were fixed on round plastic supporting case as carrier matrix. PSiNs were pretreated with glutaric acid followed by immobilization of DNA probe. Subsequently, complementary DNA analyte intercalated with nickel (II) salphen complex was pipetted on PSiNs' surface. The fiber optic reflectance spectrophotometer was used to measure the reflectance intensity of hybridization of target DNA with probe DNA. The study demonstrated that genosensor was capable to detect dengue DNA with a LOD of 0.2 aM [35].

Multicolor triangular silver nanoparticles (TAgs) were used by Vinayagam et al. as detection labels for the detection of DENV RNA. TAgs were conjugated with capture probe and reporter probe which will hybridize with different regions of target RNA. Later, these capture and reporter probes were pooled with analyte RNA, and hybridization was promoted using NaCl. The reaction was left for 10 minutes at 37°C. In comparison to non-hybridization, the hybridization of probes with target RNA was more stable in the presence of NaCl and, thus, develops colors and determines the presence of dengue RNA [36]. Tripathy et al. reported a genosensor was based on Manganese (III) Oxide (Mn_2O_3) nanofibers modified glassy carbon electrode (GCE). The COOH group was introduced on the surface and activated via EDC/NHS cross-linker. The capture probe was then immobilized via NH2 group with COOH group on GCE. Subsequently, the sample containing target DNA was added, and electrochemical responses were measured against a standard calomel reference electrode. The study revealed that nanoscale genosensor successfully detected dengue DNA and LOD of the sensor was found to be 120 zeptomoles [37]. Rashid et al. worked on electrochemical genosensor that is developed on screen-printed gold electrode modified with silicon nanowires (SiNWs). SiNWs were deposited on SPGE using various chemical pretreatment. Following the deposition of SiNWs, the thiolate DNA probe were immobilized on sensing surface. Subsequently, the sample containing target DNA was pipetted to hybridize with probe DNA. The electrochemical response was measured in the presence of redox indicator using CV and DPV. It was found that the developed biosensor was able to detect dengue DNA with a LOD of 1.63×10^{-12} M [38].

2.1.2. RT-LAMP platform

Loop-mediated amplification (LAMP) is a modified version of PCR in which a uniform temperature ranging from 60 to 65°C is applied using a water bath for nucleic acid amplification and, thus, obviates the requirement of a thermocycler [39, 40]. This approach to nucleic acid amplification relies on strand displacement reaction that produces a self-complementary single-stranded loop structure for binding the primers and amplifies target with high specificity and rapidity [41, 42]. The resulting DNA product can be observed by measuring the turbidity produced from the precipitation of by-product magnesium pyrophosphate [43, 44]. In addition, the amplification product can be visualized using UV in the presence of fluorescent dyes which intercalate in double-strand DNA. The target DNA can be visualized either by the naked eyes or quantified by turbidimeter. In comparison to conventional PCR, LAMP is highly specific as it employs 4/6 primers that specifically recognize 6/8 distinct sequence of target DNA [45, 46]. Sahni et al. developed and evaluated RT-LAMP assay for the detection of dengue. In this study, 279 samples including 100 dengue positive, 100 dengue negative, and 79 samples from healthy person for negative control were evaluated for testing the sensitivity and specificity of the developed RT-LAMP assay and compared with conventional RT-PCR. The study showed that RT-PCR detected dengue in 77 samples while RT-LAMP showed good sensitivity and detected dengue in 83 samples. The diagnostic specificity analysis revealed the developed assay did not show any cross-reactivity [47]. In another study, a different approach was used to design dengue-specific primers for developing RT-LAMP assay. This study exploited a highly conserved dengue NS1 gene which study claimed to have >90% sequence similarity among different genotypes within each serotype. The assay was single step and carried out in four tubes, each one was specific for distinct dengue serotype. For the visualization of RT-LAMP product, Genie® II fluorometer was employed for real-time fluorescence detection. The sensitivity of RT-LAMP PCR was compared with CDC 1-4 real-time PCR. The study showed that the developed RT-LAMP was equally effective in discriminating dengue in the acute phase. The limit of detection of this nucleic acid amplifier was found to be 100 copies of viral RNA extracted from each serotype. The specificity of RT-LAMP evaluated using the RNA of four closely related *Flavivirus* is found to be very selective [48]. Dauner et al. developed pan-serotype dengue RT-LAMP and investigated the sensitivity of RT-LAMP using a panel of clinical samples confirmed by qRT-PCR. The study showed that pan-serotype RT-LAMP could discriminate dengue with a sensitivity of 86%. This study also visualized the amplification of target gene on lateral flow assay [49]. In one study Lau et al. employed hydroxynaphthol blue (HNB) dye for the colorimetric visualization of RT-LAMP-amplified product through the naked eye, thus, making the assay simpler as it does not require specific tool to interpret the LAMP product. The assay was developed in a single tube as multiplex RT-LAMP to detect any of the dengue serotype present in the sample. Serotype-specific primers were developed using 3′ noncoding region gene sequences for DENV 1–4. The study revealed that RT-LAMP was able to discriminate all four dengue serotypes with high sensitivity and short assay time of 45 minutes [50]. Hu et al. reported a RT-LAMP technique which employed primers designed from 3′UTR, a highly conserved gene in dengue. The 3′UTR sequence of dengue genome was obtained from GenBank, and its multiple sequence alignment was achieved using Clustal X. 2.0. In this study, RT-LAMP evaluated using mixture of clinical and reference samples containing all four serotypes of dengue. It was demonstrated that multiplexed RT-LAMP detected all the four serotypes and showed high sensitivity as this method was able to detect as low as 10 copies of viral RNA. In addition, virus found to be selective as it did not amplify the RNA of any closely related *Flavivirus* when tested with developed multiplexed RT-LAMP [51]. Lopez et al. developed RT-LAMP using a novel approach for designing LAMP primers that aimed to match the sequence of all circulating dengue virus throughout the world. This study used fast-growing sequence databases having 932 entries of complete dengue genome sequence, and, thus, covered a huge diversity reported at that time. A mixture of four final reaction primers was achieved using a blend principal component analysis of the full dengue virus genome, and LAMP primers were designed through LAVA software. The developed RT-LAMP is found to be selective and did not cross-react with other types of *Flavivirus*. The assay for DENV1 and DENV2 were validated using blood and serum samples obtained from different regions [40].

2.1.3. Microfluidic platform

Lab-on-chip (LoC) technology allows the real-time detection of target analyte by integrating multiple laboratory process (such as biological sample preparation, processing, and analyzing) on a microprocessor chip into a completely automated and controlled analytical device [52–54]. Usually, LoC exploit the microfluidic platform owing to its ability to handle very small volume of bodily fluid, less than pico-liters, in micrometer scale channels with dimensions of tens to hundreds of micrometers [55, 56]. In addition, LoC based on microfluidics offers several other advantages such as miniaturization, short assay time, portability, user-friendly, and amenable for multiple detections of target analytes [57, 58]. Since 2000, this technology has been widely used in the field of diagnosis for developing a point-of-care test [59]. Weng et al. incorporated microfluidic platform with ELISA assay for reducing the detection time of the assay and lowering the sample volume and developed suction type microfluidic immunosensing chip for the identification of DENV. Microfluidic chip designed in this study contained a multifunctional micro-transport unit for the transportation and mixing of reagents. To reduce nonspecific protein binding polydimethylsiloxane, the material used for the fabrication of microfluidic surface was modified. The study demonstrated that microfluidic-based immunochip was able to detect dengue using a small volume of 12 μL of dengue sample. The developed assay demonstrated high sensitivity with a LOD of 10^3 PFU/mL and short assay time of half an hour and makes more rapid test than ELISA which usually takes 3–4 hours for detection [60]. Hosseini et al. develop a hybrid platform by combining microsphere and microfluidic disk for the detection of dengue virus. Microspheres were selected as they offer large specific surface area, and microspheres designed with functional group were integrated into microfluidic disk to promote biorecognition event. For the maximum utilization of microspheres' specific surface area for bimolecular interaction, micromixing system was fitted in microfluidic disk. The detection principle of this assay was based on sandwich ELISA technique. Utilization of this hybrid platform reduced the long incubation period from several hours to 5 minutes and demonstrated high sensitivity by detecting as low as few units of dengue virus [61]. Aeinehvand et al. employed centrifugal microfluidic platforms for the detection of DENV. Microballoon mixer was introduced that works by its expansion and contraction and yields steady periodical reciprocating flow. Implementation of micromixer reduced the mixing time of liquids from about 3 hours to 23 s. This study revealed that centrifugal microfluidic platforms developed in this study successfully detected dengue virus and shows better sensitivity than traditional ELISA [62]. Thiha et al. miniaturized sandwich ELISA method on lab-on-compact disk (LOCD) for the detection of dengue IgG antibody. LOCD was established by integrating microfluidic platform on a compact disk-like structure for performing the entire lab-based procedures, while the centrifugal force of spinning disk was employed for transporting the fluid from one chamber to another. The main reason behind choosing this LOCD platform was the low cost, rapid detection, fully automation, and multiplex detection of target analytes. In addition, this platform provides high surface area to volume ratio and micromixing facility which enhance the biosensing of the assay in terms of sensitivity and specificity. After the successful development of the assay, it was evaluated by detecting dengue IgG antibody from the several hospitalized patients. The study claimed that LOCD successfully detected dengue IgG antibodies with 95% sensitivity and 100% specificity [63]. Using the microfluidic dielectrophoresis platform, Iswardy et al. developed a bead-based immunofluorescence assay for the detection of dengue virus. During the assay development, mouse anti-*Flavivirus*-capture antibodies were modified with beads, and DENV was modified with fluorescence label. The principle of this assay was based on employing the DEP to capture modified beads in the microfluidic chip which will later interact with modified DENV to form immune complex on these beads. Fluorescence microscopy was used to detect fluorescent signals, and later these signals were quantified by Image J freeware. It was found that incorporation of microfluidic platform speeds up the immuno-reactions and target analyte was detected in a short period of 5 minutes. Interestingly, this assay used ~15 μL of dengue sample to test the dengue virus presence. The study showed that the developed assay was able to detect DENV with a LOD of 10^4 PFU/mL [64].

2.1.4. Novel paper-based diagnostic devices

Paper offers several unique advantages than conventional device materials such as power-free liquid transport through capillary force and evaporation, high surface area to volume ratio, and storing reagent in active form within the fiber network [65, 66]. Lo et al. combined RT-LAMP with paper-based diagnostic devices for the detection of dengue virus. First, cDNA was amplified using RT-LAMP at 63°C. Later, the amplified products were mixed with detection probes and then moved in paper-based test zone constructed on paper-based diagnostic device. Afterwards, the fluorescent signals were examined and analyzed by image recoding system and Image J. The developed assay demonstrated high sensitivity in paper-based diagnostic device with a LOD of 31.75 μg/mL of amplified products [67]. Zhang et al. worked on to improve the flow of salivary fluid in paper-based immunoassay. This study believes that paper-based immunoassay is more often compromised due to the formation of aggregates between conjugates and specimen and, thus, inhibits the labeled target molecule to reach at test line. To resolve this issue, this study developed a stacking flow immunoassay to detect dengue-specific IgG antibody in salivary fluid. The stacking flow architecture was aimed to bypass the sample pretreatment step which is often required for testing the salivary fluid. To achieve this goal, two different paths were designed for guiding the sample and reagents separately in the test strip. According to study, application of this tactic prevented the interference of salivary substances with particle-based sensing system, and these substances were omitted before making any contact with the detection reagents, therefore, resulting in low background. Moreover, study showed equipping the strip with flow regulator enables the uniform flow in the strip which produces even test line. It was found the developed immunoassay successfully detected the dengue IgG antibodies which are important biomarker for the secondary dengue infection [68]. As we know that low sensitivity is a great disadvantage of lateral flow assay. In one study, Kumar et al. worked on to improve the sensitivity of a paper-based assay for the detection of NS1 antigen. They exploited tapered nitrocellulose membrane and gold decorated graphene oxide sheets as the detection labels for enhancing the sensitivity of the assay. The study showed that lateral flow could detect dengue NS1 antigen with a LOD of 4.9 ng/mL using this novel format [69]. Theillet et al. developed laser-cut paper-based diagnostic device for detecting the dengue NS1 antigens and IgM antibodies. Laser cutting is a substitute pattern for producing paper analytical devices (PAD). The important aspect about this method is that any layer material could be patterned, irrespective of the fragility or thickness size of the layer. Moreover, the reproducibility pattern using laser cutting is outstanding. Laser cutting also provides the facility of modulating fluidics inside the paper channel. The purpose of using porous and hydrophilic glass-fiber paper was the motion of fluid specimen via passive capillarity. During the assay development, PADs were modified with anti-NS1-capture antibodies and EDIII antigen to capture the NS1 antigen and dengue-specific IgM antibodies, respectively. Later the plasma samples obtained from patients having acute dengue were tested on PAD as well as on LFA, for comparing the sensitivity. Detection with this type of paper-based device is found to be successful for both NS1 antigen and IgM antibody. LOD for the NS1 antigen was 25 ng/mL and it was comparable with commercial LFA [70].

3. Conclusion

In this chapter, we discussed the advanced diagnostic methods for the diagnosis of dengue. In terms of analytical sensitivity and rapidity, these novel methods showed remarkable achievements. However, most of these studies ignored the specificity criteria of diagnostic test. Specificity is a very important aspect of diagnostic test which discriminates true negative from false positive and true-positive from false-negative detection of an infectious disease. So, this aspect should be also investigated along with the sensitivity of the diagnostic test. In addition, diagnostic sensitivity and specificity should be also investigated using well-referenced samples. Moreover, all the four serotypes should be tested to see whether this method is equally effective for all serotypes. Testing of these parameters of diagnostic test will give much broad picture to analyze its potential for evolving as a point-of-care test.

Acknowledgements

Om Parkash is extremely grateful to his father Rano Mal and mother Devi for motivating and supporting to write this chapter.

Conflict of interest

The authors declare no conflict of interest.

Author details

Om Parkash[1*], Punam Kumari[2], Vasu Deva[2], Sham Lal[1], Javed Ahmed Ujjan[1], Syed Mehmood Qadir[3], Fateh Muhammad Soomro[1], Rani Faryal[3] and Nisar Ahmed Kanhar[1]

*Address all correspondence to: om.aprembhagat@gmail.com

1 Institute of Microbiology, Shah Abdul Latif University, Khairpur, Pakistan

2 Liaqat Medical University of Health Sciences, Jamshoro, Pakistan

3 Quaid-i-Azam University, Islamabad, Pakistan

References

[1] Rowe SL et al. The rise of imported dengue infections in Victoria, Australia, 2010-2016. Tropical Medicine and Infectious Disease. 2018;**3**(1):9

[2] Leta S et al. Global risk mapping for major diseases transmitted by *Aedes aegypti* and *Aedes albopictus*. International Journal of Infectious Diseases. 2018;**67**:25

[3] Stanaway JD et al. The global burden of dengue: An analysis from the global burden of disease study 2013. The Lancet Infectious Diseases. 2016;**16**(6):712-723

[4] Waggoner JJ et al. Characterization of dengue virus infections among febrile children clinically diagnosed with a non-dengue illness, Managua, Nicaragua. The Journal of Infectious Diseases. 2017;**215**(12):1816-1823

[5] Adam A et al. Clinical profile and warning sign finding in children with severe dengue and non-severe dengue. In: IOP Conference Series: Earth and Environmental Science. IOP Publishing; 2018

[6] de Souza Pereira BB et al. Prolonged viremia in dengue virus infection in hematopoietic stem cell transplant recipients and patients with hematological malignancies. Transplant Infectious Disease. 2017;**19**(4):e12721

[7] Kuo H-J, Lee I-K, Liu J-W. Analyses of clinical and laboratory characteristics of dengue adults at their hospital presentations based on the World Health Organization clinical-phase framework: Emphasizing risk of severe dengue in the elderly. Journal of Microbiology, Immunology, and Infection. 2017. DOI: 10.1016/j.jmii.2016.08.024

[8] Morra ME et al. Definitions for warning signs and signs of severe dengue according to the WHO 2009 classification: Systematic review of literature. Reviews in Medical Virology. 2018;**28**:e1979

[9] Cheng N-M et al. Isolation of dengue virus from the upper respiratory tract of four patients with dengue fever. PLoS Neglected Tropical Diseases. 2017;**11**(4):e0005520

[10] Tai A et al. Dengue fever in travellers: Are we missing warning signs of severe dengue in a non-endemic setting? The Medical Journal of Australia. 2016;**204**(7):267

[11] Meng F et al. Unstructural biology of the dengue virus proteins. The FEBS Journal. 2015;**282**(17):3368-3394

[12] Carocci M, Kuhn JH, Yang PL. Flaviviruses: Introduction to dengue viruses. In: Global Virology I-Identifying and Investigating Viral Diseases. New York City, United States: Springer; 2015. pp. 403-424

[13] Medeiros AS et al. Dengue virus in *Aedes aegypti* and *Aedes albopictus* in urban areas in the state of Rio Grande do Norte, Brazil: Importance of virological and entomological surveillance. PLoS One. 2018;**13**(3):e0194108

[14] Whitehorn J et al. Comparative susceptibility of *Aedes albopictus* and *Aedes aegypti* to dengue virus infection after feeding on blood of viremic humans: Implications for public health. The Journal of Infectious Diseases. 2015;**212**(8):1182-1190

[15] Whitehead SS, Subbarao K. Which dengue vaccine approach is the most promising, and should we be concerned about enhanced disease after vaccination? The risks of incomplete immunity to dengue virus revealed by vaccination. Cold Spring Harbor Perspectives in Biology. 2018;**10**(6):a028811

[16] Beatty PR et al., editors. Dengue virus NS1 triggers endothelial permeability and vascular leak that is prevented by NS1 vaccination. Science Translational Medicine. 2015;**7**(304):304ra141

[17] Yung C-F et al. Dengue serotype-specific differences in clinical manifestation, laboratory parameters and risk of severe disease in adults, Singapore. The American Journal of Tropical Medicine and Hygiene. 2015;**92**(5):999-1005

[18] Metz SW et al. Dengue virus-like particles mimic the antigenic properties of the infectious dengue virus envelope. Virology Journal. 2018;**15**(1):60

[19] Low JG et al. Dengue antiviral development: A continuing journey. In: Hilgenfeld R, Vasudevan SG, editors. Dengue and Zika: Control and Antiviral Treatment Strategies. Singapore: Springer Singapore; 2018. pp. 319-332

[20] García-Ruíz D et al. Detection of dengue, West Nile virus, rickettsiosis and leptospirosis by a new real-time PCR strategy. Springerplus. 2016;**5**(1):671

[21] Centre for Disease Control and Prevention. Laboratory guidance and diagnostic testing. 2017, August 3 [cited 2018 4 July]. Available from: https://www.cdc.gov/dengue/clinical-lab/laboratory.html

[22] Sanjay ST et al. A paper/polymer hybrid microfluidic microplate for rapid quantitative detection of multiple disease biomarkers. Scientific Reports. 2016;**6**:30474

[23] Liang T, Fu E. High-performance paper microfluidic malaria test for low-resource settings. In: Frugal Innovation in Bioengineering for the Detection of Infectious Diseases. Cham, Switzerland: Springer; 2018. pp. 39-55

[24] Omar NAS et al. Development of an optical sensor based on surface plasmon resonance phenomenon for diagnosis of dengue virus E-protein. Sensing and Bio-Sensing Research. 2018;**20**:16-21

[25] Pirich CL et al. Piezoelectric immunochip coated with thin films of bacterial cellulose nanocrystals for dengue detection. Biosensors and Bioelectronics. 2017;**92**:47-53

[26] Solanki S et al. Langmuir–Blodgett Nanoassemblies of the MoS_2–Au composite at the air–water interface for dengue detection. ACS Applied Materials & Interfaces. 2018;**10**(3): 3020-3028

[27] Jahanshahi P et al. Rapid immunoglobulin M-based dengue diagnostic test using surface Plasmon resonance biosensor. Scientific Reports. 2014;**4**:3851

[28] Ortega G, Pérez-Rodríguez S, Reguera E. Magnetic paper–based ELISA for IgM-dengue detection. RSC Advances. 2017;**7**(9):4921-4932

[29] Ortega GA, Zuaznabar-Gardona JC, Reguera E. Electrochemical immunoassay for the detection of IgM antibodies using polydopamine particles loaded with PbS quantum dots as labels. Biosensors and Bioelectronics. 2018;**116**:30-36

[30] Wong WR. Long Range Surface Plasmon Based Biosensor for Dengue Virus Detection. University of Malaya; 2015

[31] Liu L et al. Highly sensitive label-free antibody detection using a long period fibre grating sensor. Sensors and Actuators B: Chemical. 2018;**271**:24-32

[32] Chan SK et al. Dengue serotyping with a label-free DNA sensor. Analytical Methods. 2018;**10**(2):214-222

[33] Jin S-A et al. Impedimetric dengue biosensor based on functionalized graphene oxide wrapped silica particles. Electrochimica Acta. 2016;**194**:422-430

[34] Nuzaihan MNM et al. Electrical detection of dengue virus (DENV) DNA oligomer using silicon nanowire biosensor with novel molecular gate control. Biosensors and Bioelectronics. 2016;**83**:106-114

[35] Ariffin E et al. Optical DNA biosensor based on square-planar ethyl Piperidine substituted nickel(II) Salphen complex for dengue virus detection. Sensors. 2018;**18**(4):1173

[36] Vinayagam S et al. DNA-triangular silver nanoparticles nanoprobe for the detection of dengue virus distinguishing serotype. Spectrochimica Acta Part A: Molecular and Biomolecular Spectroscopy. 2018;**202**:346-351

[37] Tripathy S et al. Electrospun manganese (III) oxide nanofiber based electrochemical DNA-nanobiosensor for zeptomolar detection of dengue consensus primer. Biosensors and Bioelectronics. 2017;**90**:378-387

[38] Rashid JIA et al. A novel disposable biosensor based on SiNWs/AuNPs modified-screen printed electrode for dengue virus DNA oligomer detection. IEEE Sensors Journal. 2015;**15**(8):4420-4427

[39] Fernández-Soto P et al. A loop-mediated isothermal amplification (LAMP) assay for early detection of *Schistosoma mansoni* in stool samples: A diagnostic approach in a murine model. PLoS Neglected Tropical Diseases. 2014;**8**(9):e3126

[40] Lopez-Jimena B et al. Development and validation of four one-step real-time RT-LAMP assays for specific detection of each dengue virus serotype. PLoS Neglected Tropical Diseases. 2018;**12**(5):e0006381

[41] Sahoo PR et al. Loop mediated isothermal amplification: An innovative gene amplification technique for animal diseases. Veterinary World. 2016;**9**(5):465-469

[42] Phillips EA et al. Strand displacement probes combined with isothermal nucleic acid amplification for instrument-free detection from complex samples. Analytical Chemistry. 2018;**90**(11):6580-6586

[43] Sengar GS et al. RT-LAMP assay: An alternative approach for profiling of bovine heat shock protein 70 gene in PBMC cultured model. Molecular Biology Reports. 2017;**44**(3): 281-287

[44] Faggioli F, Luigi M, Boubourakas IN. Viroid amplification methods: RT-PCR, real-time RT-PCR, and RT-LAMP. In: Viroids and Satellites. London, UK: Elsevier; 2017. pp. 381-391

[45] Liu W et al. Establishment of an accurate and fast detection method using molecular beacons in loop-mediated isothermal amplification assay. Scientific Reports. 2017;**7**:40125

[46] Gadkar VJ et al. Real-time detection and monitoring of loop mediated amplification (LAMP) reaction using self-quenching and De-quenching Fluorogenic probes. Scientific Reports. 2018;**8**(1):5548

[47] Sahni AK et al. Reverse transcription loop-mediated isothermal amplification (RT-LAMP) for diagnosis of dengue. Medical Journal Armed Forces India. 2013;**69**(3):246-253

[48] Neeraja M et al. Rapid detection and differentiation of dengue virus serotypes by NS1 specific reverse transcription loop-mediated isothermal amplification (RT-LAMP) assay in patients presenting to a tertiary care hospital in Hyderabad, India. Journal of Virological Methods. 2015;**211**:22-31

[49] Dauner AL et al. Development of a pan-serotype reverse transcription loop-mediated isothermal amplification assay for the detection of dengue virus. Diagnostic Microbiology and Infectious Disease. 2015;**83**(1):30-36

[50] Lau Y-L et al. Colorimetric detection of dengue by single tube reverse-transcription-loop-mediated isothermal amplification. PLoS One. 2015;**10**(9):e0138694

[51] Hu S-f et al. Development of reverse-transcription loop-mediated isothermal amplification assay for rapid detection and differentiation of dengue virus serotypes 1-4. BMC Microbiology. 2015;**15**(1):265

[52] Pires NMM et al. Recent developments in optical detection technologies in lab-on-a-chip devices for biosensing applications. Sensors. 2014;**14**(8):15458-15479

[53] Jung W et al. Point-of-care testing (POCT) diagnostic systems using microfluidic lab-on-a-chip technologies. Microelectronic Engineering. 2015;**132**:46-57

[54] Su W et al. Microfluidic platform towards point-of-care diagnostics in infectious diseases. Journal of Chromatography A. 2015;**1377**:13-26

[55] Jayamohan H, Sant HJ, Gale BK. Applications of microfluidics for molecular diagnostics. In: Microfluidic Diagnostics. New York City, United States: Springer; 2013. pp. 305-334

[56] Wu J et al. Lab-on-chip technology for chronic disease diagnosis. npj Digital Medicine. 2018;**1**(1):7

[57] Foudeh AM et al. Microfluidic designs and techniques using lab-on-a-chip devices for pathogen detection for point-of-care diagnostics. Lab on a Chip. 2012;**12**(18):3249-3266

[58] Weigl B, Domingo G, Steele M. Microfluidic diagnostic technologies for global public health. Clinical Chemistry and Laboratory Medicine. 2007;**45**:S72

[59] Sharma S et al. Point-of-care diagnostics in low resource settings: Present status and future role of microfluidics. Biosensors. 2015;**5**(3):577

[60] Weng C-H et al. A suction-type microfluidic immunosensing chip for rapid detection of the dengue virus. Biomedical Microdevices. 2011;**13**(3):585-595

[61] Hosseini S et al. Microsphere integrated microfluidic disk: Synergy of two techniques for rapid and ultrasensitive dengue detection. Scientific Reports. 2015;**5**:16485

[62] Aeinehvand MM et al. Biosensing enhancement of dengue virus using microballoon mixers on centrifugal microfluidic platforms. Biosensors and Bioelectronics. 2015;**67**:424-430

[63] Thiha A, Ibrahim F. A colorimetric enzyme-linked immunosorbent assay (ELISA) detection platform for a point-of-care dengue detection system on a lab-on-compact-disc. Sensors. 2015;**15**(5):11431

[64] Iswardy E et al. A bead-based immunofluorescence-assay on a microfluidic dielectrophoresis platform for rapid dengue virus detection. Biosensors and Bioelectronics. 2017;**95**:174-180

[65] Hu J et al. Advances in paper-based point-of-care diagnostics. Biosensors and Bioelectronics. 2014;**54**:585-597

[66] Cate DM et al. Recent developments in paper-based microfluidic devices. Analytical Chemistry. 2014;**87**(1):19-41

[67] Lo S-J et al. Molecular-level dengue fever diagnostic devices made out of paper. Lab on a Chip. 2013;**13**(14):2686-2692

[68] Zhang Y, Bai J, Ying JY. A stacking flow immunoassay for the detection of dengue-specific immunoglobulins in salivary fluid. Lab on a Chip. 2015;**15**(6):1465-1471

[69] Kumar S et al. Tapered lateral flow immunoassay based point-of-care diagnostic device for ultrasensitive colorimetric detection of dengue NS1. Biomicrofluidics. 2018;**12**(3):034104

[70] Theillet G et al. Laser-cut paper-based device for the detection of dengue non-structural NS1 protein and specific IgM in human samples. Archives of Virology. 2018;**163**:1757-1767

7

Cell Biology of Virus Infection: The Role of Cytoskeletal Dynamics Integrity in the Effectiveness of Dengue Virus Infection

Elizabeth Orozco-García, Andrea Trujillo-Correa and Juan Carlos Gallego-Gómez

Abstract

The cell biology of viral infections is the focus of this research, in which the role of the cytoskeleton in dengue virus (DENV) replication in cell cultures was evaluated by means of Nocodazole and Cytochalasin D treatments before and after of DENV infection. The potential contribution of cytoskeleton elements with/without the treatment of depolymerizing agents was evidenced and quantified by the subcellular distribution of viral proteins, virions produced, and viral protein quantification. The cytoskeleton is involved in DENV replication because treatments with actin microfi-laments and microtubule depolymerizing agents in non-cytotoxic concentrations, affected DENV2 replication in Vero cells and decreased both the viral protein expression and infectious virion production, when compared with non-treated cells. The actin and microtubules are partly involved in DENV2 replication, since the treatment does not completely blocked viral replication, suggesting that these components are necessary but not sufficient alone for DENV2 replication in Vero cells. The structural and functional role of actin and the microtubules in replication are postulated here, opening new perspectives for understanding the architecture of the replicative complex and viral morphogenesis processes, due to the role of the cytoskeleton in the organization, recruitment, and function of the cellular elements necessary for the assembly of viral factories.

Keywords: Cell biology, infection, dengue virus, cytoskeleton, viral replication

1. Introduction

The cell biology of viral infection, as a new scientific approach, considers the cell as the structural and functional unit of viral infection. Within this new research program there are four topics:

1. Virus and the cytoskeleton.
2. Virus and endomembrane systems.
3. Virus and signal cascades.
4. Virus and the nucleus–nuclear envelope [1].

There are a lot of publications already covering these four points of the cell biology of virus infection; however, here we will focus only on the role of the cytoskeleton on DENV infection. Although many years ago these studies could be classified as "virus–host cell interactions" as it was usually considered in many virology journals, since the onset of the new millennium and the advent of converged methodologies/fields of research it is possible to take another view of viral infections. Recent developments in confocal microscopy hardware, image capture and collection with augmented resolution using charge-coupled device (CCD) cameras, digital image processing, improvements in the genetic engineering of green fluorescent protein (GFP) and the chemistry of fluorophores, together with the increased capacity of computational tools for taking thousands of images, have created innovative conditions permitting the understanding of viral infections as a whole [2, 3]. Several researchers consider viruses as tools, or molecular scalpels, which are very useful for dissecting complex molecular and cellular mechanisms [4]. This chapter will consider the cycle of Virus Dengue Serotype 2 (DENV2) as a series of steps in which the virus takes control of the cytoskeleton from host cells [5].

The possibility of real-time visualization of viral infections was reached by means of genetic manipulation of the cells and viruses – cells with fluorescent subcellular compartments and viruses with fluorescent tags [6, 7]; this will be not considered here since the main goal of our approach is to study complete virions within host cells. In this context, molecular studies of isolated viral proteins in a cellular environment are not considered under the cell biology of viral infections discipline, however, those approaches are important if they are following previous research in cell biology of viral infections, because these reductionist studies can offer details regarding the identification of molecular actors in the complex cellular environment of viral infection.

On the other hand, the study of intracellular invaders [5], considering not only viruses but also bacteria, fungi, and protozoan parasites, which aims to find a cellular platform for microbiology research with the eukaryotic host cell as the main actor, is defined as cellular microbiology [8]. Since viruses are obligated parasites, they entirely depend on the cellular machinery to carry out its replication cycle; in this sense for enveloped viruses the intracellular–vesicle trafficking and the cytoskeleton play a decisive role, mainly because both of them offer structural and functional platforms where many RNA viruses are assembled and whose morphogenesis occurs in the cytoplasm of known viral factories [9, 10]. From this viewpoint, DENV will be considered as one experimental system for studying the cell biology of viral infections – its complex interactions could throw light on the search for disease therapies.

Dengue is emerging globally as the most important arboviral disease threatening human populations. It is caused by the *Flavivirus* DENV [11, 12], which is a small and enveloped virus with a single-stranded, positive-sense RNA, which can be translated into a single polyprotein by a host cell and viral proteins [1, 13], and is transmitted to humans by *Aedes* genus mosquitoes [14-17]. There are nearly 2.5 billion people at risk of infection with DENV in tropical and subtropical countries. It is endemic in more than 100 countries and about 100 million cases of dengue fever are estimated annually, with over 500,000 cases being the potentially fatal dengue hemorrhagic fever [12]. Dengue virus is therefore associated with high socio-economic impacts [18, 19].

The availability of vaccines and drugs for RNA viruses has become a much greater challenge than expected, because RNA viruses evolution/mutation rates continue to elude both, vaccine design and drug effectiveness, generating extensive drug-resistant mutants, and therefore over time creating far more virulent strains [20-23]. Therefore, searching for answers inside the cell may offer an alternative method to combat the virus. Recently Villar and collaborators [24], in a big clinical trial implicating several Latin American countries, have shown important protection percentages (greater than 60%), representing an important advance in the fight against the first viral infection in Colombia. In spite of these encouraging clinical responses in patients given the tetravalent vaccine for dengue, it is necessary to wait for several years in order to evaluate the impact of this vaccine has in changing the epidemiological data of the disease. Since such vaccines take time to develop or be assessed, hope could come in the form of the development of antiviral drugs directed to cellular/molecular targets in host cells.

In this way, the cell biology of viral infections [1] has matured considerably in recent years, with cytoskeleton–virus interactions being of particular interest, because it plays both a structural and functional roles in several steps of the viral replication cycle [25, 26], connecting the cell with its environment and participating decisively in the spreading of the virus to neighboring uninfected cells [27]. The virus cannot be transported into the cell by diffusion like small molecules can, therefore, the cytoskeleton and other intracellular structures become a barrier to these [28]. This is why many viruses have shown that viral infection can cause extensive and sophisticated cytoskeletal rearrangements [10, 29-31] and alterations in the endomembrane system, something required for the replication and assembly of new virions [10, 32]. All of this leads to a cytopathic effect, which is widely known and distinctive for viral infection in cellular cultures [32]. This structural and functional intimate interaction between intracellular pathogens and the cell, involves the three elements of the cytoskeleton (actin, microtubules, and intermediate filaments) [30, 33, 34].The involvement of the cytoskeleton in viral infection has been studied for over 30 years [35], and has been found to be involved throughout the life cycle of different viruses. There are many descriptions of its involvement for adenovirus [36], human and equine herpes virus [37], HIV [38], HTLV-1 [27], Rous Sarcoma Virus [39], poliovirus [40], Epstein–Barr Virus [41], human respiratory syncytial virus [42], SV40 [43], Vaccinia virus [44, 45], poliedrosis [46], papiloma [47], and pseudorabies [48]. The replication cycle of DENV has been extensively studied with particular regard to early events such as binding, fusion, uncoating, and intracellular transport of viral proteins [28, 49, 50]. On the other hand, the relationships between the replication of DENV and the cytoskeleton host cell are not fully characterized, although data in some literature, concerning influenza and other viruses, support their existence [13, 51-56].

A structural and functional integration of vesicle trafficking and cytoskeletal/endomembrane systems in viral replication and morphogenesis represents the viral factories redefinition [10, 57, 58]. It has been postulated that trafficking occurs in microtubule motor proteins (entry via dynein and exit through kinesin [59]), something which explains the translocation of proteins between the two routes in the microtubule organizing center (MTOC) [59]. Specifically, with respect to DENV, cytoskeleton and endo/exocytosis have not been studied comprehensively [60], especially where there is dependence between vimentin intermediate filaments and the DENV infection, in which microtubules now were apparently necessary. Intercalating fluorophores were used to label the envelopes of virions associated with cholesterol isolated DENV [50, 61]; tracking was achieved in the early events of cell entry, but this did not shed new light on the endomembrane system and cytoskeleton. It has also been reported that DENV entry by endocytosis, which is pH dependent and mediated by clathrin [62], and the involvement of actin microfilaments and microtubules in mosquito cells DENV had infected was important because the inhibition of these cytoskeleton components decreased infection by 80%. The small Rho GTPases are a protein family which among other cellular functions, govern cytoskeleton reorganization [63]. When isoprenylation of Rho GTPases was blocked, using statins, the incidence of HIV[64] and DENV [65, 66] infection was reduced via alteration of the virus assembly pathway in the rough endoplasmic reticulum.

The interactions between specific viral components and different molecular complexes of the host cell are fundamental in determining the infection rate. By such reasoning, cell biological characterization of the host–pathogen interactions, and knowledge of the possible role of the basic components of the cytoskeleton, microtubules, and actin microfilaments, allow the elucidation of some mechanisms involved in the pathogenesis of DENV. This allows the identification of new potential host targets that could be used to design efficient and rational antiviral therapies.

The applied focus of the cell biology of viral infections is to searching for antiviral therapies based in cellular targets, which have special importance, because the mutation rates of cellular genes are several thousands of times smaller than the antivirals directed to the specific viral proteins. To illustrate this there are several reports of antiviral candidates blocking cellular targets in the host (Src kinase), like the works of Yang and collaborators [67, 68], and some reports from our working group where the HMG-CoA was blocked by lovastatin on assays *in vitro* and *in vivo* [65, 69]. Additionally, we have found out that ubiquitin–proteasome and cytoskeletal elements seem altered after dengue infected cells were treated with curcumin [70]. However, the most relevant finding in this approach is that one protein (IFITM, interferon-induced transmembrane protein) could be altered for blocking different viruses belonging to several families [71].

In order to determine the contribution of the two cytoskeleton elements (actin and microtubules) in DENV replication, a series of experimental assays was completed using Cytochalasin

D and Nocodazole concomitantly using a high preservation/fixation method on the cytoskeleton in order to analyze cellular images taken using fluorescent microscopy in combination with viral titration and quantification of viral proteins. This gave a better understanding of the participation of the cytoskeleton on the functional and structural issues of DENV replication. The data shown here are in agreement with previous reports from several authors confirming distinct roles in the viral infections of DENV [72-76]. The high quality of the subcellular resolution of cytoskeleton elements in this research actually reinforces their role in these structures in DENV replication.

2. Results and discussion

2.1. Preservation/ fixation of the cytoskeleton in infected cells

To understand the cytoskeletons involvement in the DENV replication cycle and virus–host cell interaction, it is necessary to make appropriate preservations with minimal levels of perturbations to the cell morphology. To test which components of the cytoskeleton (microtubules and actin microfilaments) play a role in DENV infection, a method for preserving and fixing the cytoskeleton should be implemented [39, 40], because the conventional preparations for fluorescence microscopy with methanol/acetone, have a very dramatic effect on the cell by flushing (emptying) most of its cellular contents; thus, the information obtained from ultrastructural studies depends on the type of fixation, among other things, and therefore the level of structure conservation [77-79]. In several cell lines it was demonstrated (Fig. 1) that methanol/acetone treatment preserves microtubules but depolymerizes microfilaments and disrupts both mitochondrial and nuclear morphology. PFA-PBS preserves the general cytoarchitecture, but compromises the quality of microstructural detail. PFA-CBS was found to be the best method to fix and preserve cellular microarchitecture (actin, tubulin), without inducing any cellular change.

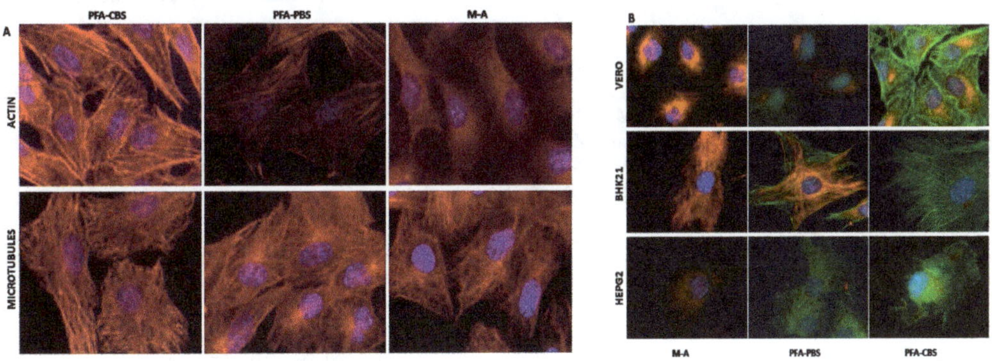

Figure 1. Fluorescence microscopy optimization for visualizing cellular elements. The methanol-acetone (MA) standard protocol does not preserve actin filaments. A comparison between PFA-PBS and PFA-CBS did not demonstrate wide differences in the most notable structures, however, only PFA-CBS method revealed some cellular components which were stabilized satisfactorily. It was found that the optimal concentration for cytoskeletal element visualization was with 3.8% PFA-CBS to fix the cells and antibodies or fluorophores dilutions in CBS of +5% FBS.

2.2. Non-cytotoxic concentrations of cytoskeleton depolymerizing agents

The integrity and functionality of cytoskeleton elements are necessary for their hypothesized role in DENV infections, for which there functionality was evaluated by means of depolymerizing agents. These agents are not entirely harmless to the cells, something which was determined by means dosage ranges having low cytotoxicity (10–20% cytotoxicity) Fig. 2 (a, b). In Fig. 2 (c), the pattern and distribution of cytoskeleton and nucleus components are normal, with no condensation or fragmentation observed. Cellular alterations due to a toxic injury were not evident in these concentrations.

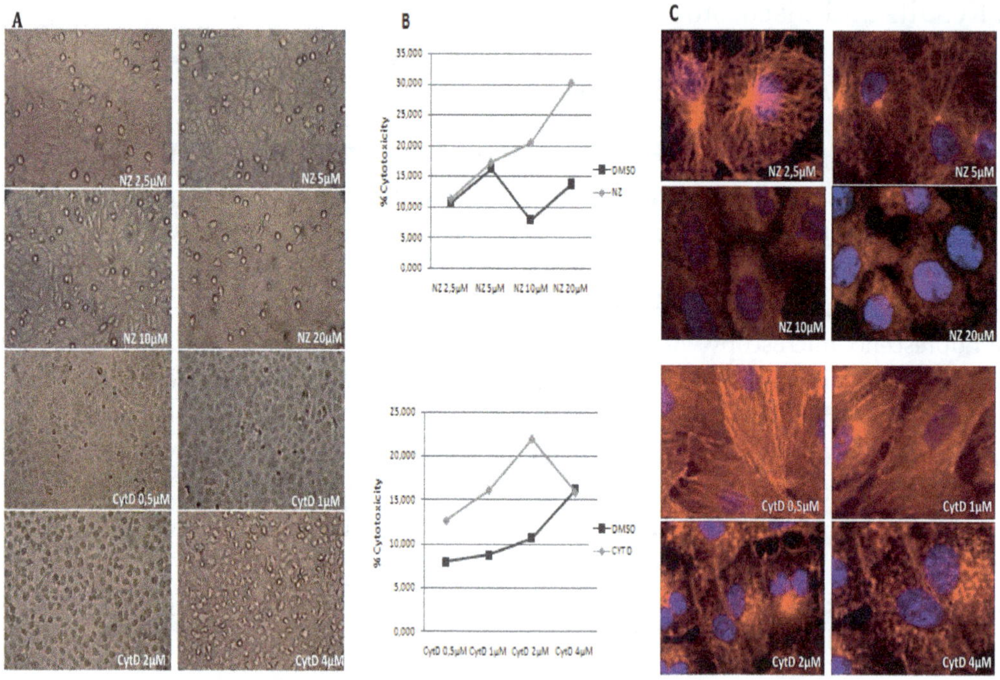

Figure 2. Cytotoxicity assays for cytoskeleton depolymerizing agents. Cytotoxicity assays were performed by cell viability measuring by the method of MTT [3-[4,5 dimetiltiazole-2yl)-2,5 diphenyl tetrazolium bromide), to determine NZ and CytD concentrations that were below the toxic level to cells. We were able to observe the NZ (a, c, e) and CytD (b, d, f) effect in Vero cells. It was found that NZ 10 µM and 4 µM CytD had a cytotoxicity of about 20% and 15%, respectively.

2.3. Relationship between DENV2 and the cytoskeleton

In order to determine some relationship between viral particles and cytoskeletal elements in several steps of the replicative cycle of DENV, Vero cells were infected with DENV2, and processed 18 hours post infection (hpi) by fluorescence microscopy. The fluorescence signal coincident between actin, Fig. 3 (a, b), or the microtubules (c–f), and the viral protein, matching the envelope protein with stress fibers (b) for actin, and microtubules (d), suggests some potential structural relationship, which has an involvement of these cytoskeleton elements within some steps of the DENV infectious cycle.

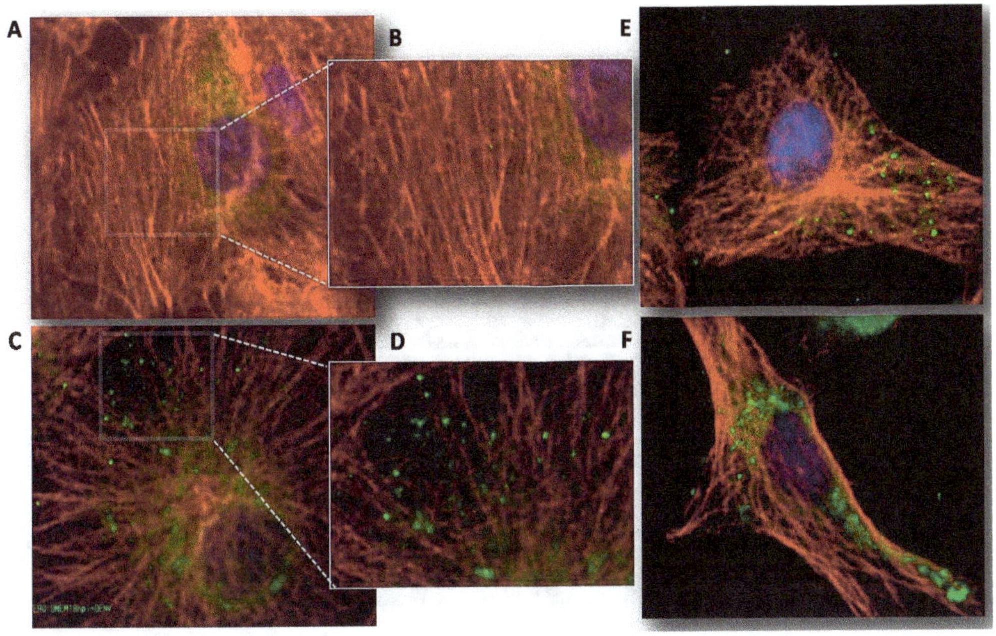

Figure 3. DENV2–cytoskeleton interaction. Vero cell DENV2 infected, viral particles interact with actin (a–b); viral particles interact with microtubules (c–f), were used Phalloidin-Alexa 594 for detect actin or Mab antiβ III Tubulin-Cy3 for microtubules, polyclonal antibody anti-Envelope + antiR IgG Alexa Fluor® 488 for viral envelope protein and Hoechst 33258 for nuclei.

2.4. Subcellular distribution pattern of viral protein altered by depolymerization of microtubules (treatment with nocodazole, NZ)

To investigate the effect of the interrupted cytoskeleton on the viruses replication cycle, Vero cells were treated with NZ before, or after, DENV2 infections. As shown in Fig. 4 (a) and Fig. 5 (a), mock-infected cells without treatment using microtubule depolymerizing agent, NZ, had structures and patterns of observed microtubules traditionally described, i.e., long filaments which are flexible and winding that occupy almost the entire space of the cytosol which emerge from the perinuclear region and are consistent with the MTOC. In contrast, cells that were treated with NZ, Fig. 4 (a), had microtubules which were completely depolymerized, as evidenced by a very fine spotted pattern when observed – something which was not observed the perinuclear region of the MTOC.

Infected cells without treatment with NZ showed a subcellular pattern distribution of diffuse staining of the viral envelope protein, with some small dotted clumps. In order to understand whether microtubules are required for viral entry, treatment was performed 6 hours before infection with NZ (5μM and 10μM), and then with DENV2 at a multiplicity of infection (MOI) of 5 for 1 hour. The inoculum was retired, washings were performed with PBS, and cells were fixed at 24 hpi. The results obtained by fluorescence microscopy indicated that there was a great decrease in the number of infected cells, Fig. 4 (a). In contrast to this, when the cells were infected and post-treated with NZ, significant alterations were produced in this distribution pattern, showed the envelope protein in vesicles as being distributed throughout the cyto-

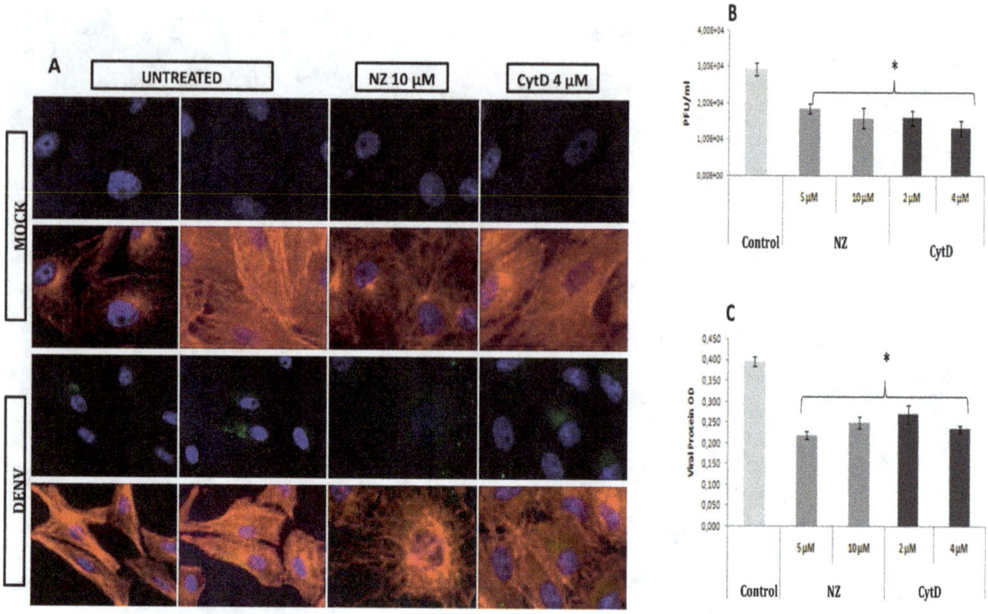

Figure 4. Effects of treatment with NZ and CytD prior to DENV2 infection Vero cells were treated with NZ 5 at 10 μM and CytD 2 at 4 mM, 6 hours before infection to determine if these elements were necessary for virus entry. In both treatments a decrease in infected cells was observed using fluorescence microscopy (a). For NZ and CytD there was an inhibition of about 50% in PFU compared to the control (b), and also a significant decrease of viral protein (c). Were used monoclonal anti-β III Tubulin-Cy3 to detect microtubules, Phalloidin-Alexa 594 for detect actin, polyclonal anti-Envelope + antiR IgG Alexa 488 for viral envelope protein and Hoechst 33258 for nuclei.

plasm, with an apparent subcellular distribution compatible with a Golgi complex Fig. 5 (a). This is because microtubule depolymerization–induced NZ treatment leads to Golgi apparatus disintegration, since the DENV maturation processes used the secretory route in this organelle. In all treatments with NZ, the nucleus was observed with a normal structure.

2.5. Subcellular distribution patterns of viral protein altered by actin depolymerization (treatment with CytD)

To investigate the effect of the interrupted cytoskeleton on the virus replication cycle, Vero cells were treated with cytochalasin D (CytD) before or after infection with DENV2. The mock-infected cells without the depolymerizing agent, CytD, showed a normal pattern with long and parallel fibrils distributed throughout the cytosol, mainly stress fibers, Fig. 4(a) and Fig. 5 (a). This is dramatically reduced after treatment with CytD, resulting in actin depolymerization, and leaving it in a spotted pattern of coarse grains, producing some larger groupings. In the case of actin microfilaments, in DENV2 infected cells, somewhat different findings arose compared with those observed with microtubules. In cells without CytD treatment, remodeling of actin microfilaments was clear, where cells were characterized by *filopodia* formation and many cells were observed with actin tails. These two actin conformations may be related to actin remodeling by Rho GTPases signaling pathway effectors. The envelope viral protein showed two subcellular distribution patterns, one being a diffuse pattern which was very fine

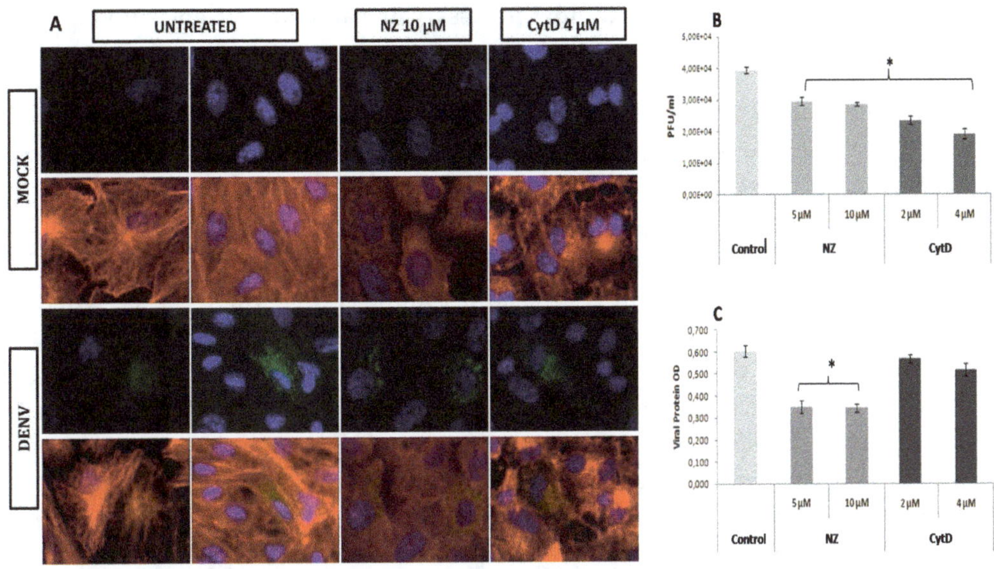

Figure 5. Effects of treatment with NZ and CytD after DENV infection. Vero cells were infected with DENV for 1 hour, the inoculum was removed and washed with PBS, after this the cells were treated with NZ 5–10 μM and CytD 2–4 mM, for 24 hours, in order to determine if these elements were necessary during the replicative cycle of DENV. In both treatments there was a decrease in infected cells when viewed using fluorescence microscopy (a), which was confirmed by the reduction of PFU in the supernatant of the treated cells (b) and viral protein concentration (c). Were used monoclonal anti-β III Tubulin-Cy3 to detect microtubules, phalloidin 594 for actin, polyclonal anti-Envelope + antiR IgG Alexa 488 for viral envelope protein and Hoechst for nuclei

and distributed in the perinuclear region throughout the cytosol, while the other pattern showed a few small clumps of viral protein. According to previous findings in vaccinia virus [45] and DENV [45, 65] the first patters is called "non-assembled viral protein" and the second "assembled viral protein."

In order to understand actin's role in whether microtubules are required for viral entry, the treatment was performed 6 hours before infection with CytD (2μM and 4μM) then with DENV-2 at a MOI of 5 for 1 hour. The inoculum was retired, washings were performed with PBS, and cells were fixed at 24 hpi. To depolymerize actin filaments with CytD in DENV2 infected cells, the subcellular distribution pattern of these cells was altered similarly to uninfected cells. The results obtained by fluorescence microscopy indicated that there was a decrease in the number of infected cells, Fig. 4 (a), with observations using fluorescence microscopy showing a clear accumulation in the perinuclear region that matched the viral factory. In contrast, when cells were infected and post-treated with CytD, significant alterations in this distribution pattern were produced, although the two patterns of distribution of "assembled" viral protein and "non-assembled" changed very little, since they remained in both cells infected with DENV2 and treated with CytD, and in those infected without CytD, Fig. 5 (a). Nevertheless, it is notable that the amount of viral protein "assembled" was markedly reduced in CytD treated cells, suggesting the great role of actin integrity in viral assembly. In all treatments with CytD, the nucleus was observed with a normal structure, Fig. 5 (a).

2.6. The dynamic integrity of microtubules necessary to maintain efficiency of viral replication

To assess if microtubule dynamic integrity has any functional impact on the viral replication process, DENV2-infected cells were pre- or post-treated with 5μM and cell ELISA, after which supernatants were collected in order to quantify viral infectious particle production and intracellular viral protein. NZ pre-treatment, in addition to causing a decrease in the number of infected cells, also produced a decrease in the number of plaque forming units (PFU) quantified in the supernatant with respect to a control group, where the percentage of inhibition od PFUs was 37% for NZ 5 μM and 46% for 10 μM, Fig. 4 (b), and the amount of viral protein in infected cells was reduced to 43% and 37%, respectively, Fig. 4 (c). NZ post-treatment produced a decrease in the number of infectious particles with respect to the control group (infected cells, DMSO), measured by plaque assay (PFU), between 25% and 28% for 5μM and 10uM of this depolymerizing agent, Fig. 5 (b), consistent with a decreased viral protein of 42% approximately for both NZ concentrations, Fig. 5 (c). Together, these results suggest a role is played by microtubules in the assembly, and export, of infectious viral particles. It is probable that, if cellular structures are not properly preserved, not possible observe changes associated with the infection. In this work, we note that altering microtubule dynamics has a direct effect on infection with DENV2, contrary to what was reported by [60].

2.7. Integrity of actin filaments has a greater role in viral protein production than microtubule integrity

To assess if actin dynamic integrity has any functional impact on the viral replication process, DENV2-infected cells were pre- or post-treated with 2μM and 4mM of CytD, after which supernatants were collected for quantifying the viral infectious particle production, and cell ELISA measured intracellular viral protein expressed. In CytD 2–4 μM pre-treated cells, a clear diminution of viral infectious particles was observed, 35–43%, Fig. 4 (b), and viral protein 47–56%, Fig. 4 (c). Interestingly, CytD post-treatment produced a significant decrease in the number of infectious particles production with respect to a control group (infected cells, DMSO), which were measured by plaque assay (PFU), detecting a reduction in viral titer of approximately 37% for CytD 2 μM and 50% for 4 μM, Fig. 5 (b). Actin filament depolymerization produced an insignificant decrease in the amount of viral protein, with non-statistical differences with respect to the control cells, Fig. 5 (c). This suggests that actin may be involved not only in virus entry, but also in any step of virus maturation and, since depolymerized can alter the assembly of viral infectious particles and/or delay the output of these, reflected in a decrease of PFUs and in an intracellular accumulation of viral protein. Thus, although the depolymerization of microtubules and actin filaments reduces the production of infectious viral particles, actin filaments appear to have the most relevant role in this process.

Most recently authors found out that the cytoskeleton is not really necessary for diverse virus replication, specifically for these viruses: Sindbis virus (SINV; family Togaviridae), vesicular stomatitis virus (VSV; family Rhabdoviridae), and Herpes simplex virus (family Herpesviridae) [80]. Although these interesting data suggest a non-conventional role of the cytoskeleton, it must be taken into account that the images are only partially showing the phenomena, because the fine elements of the cytoskeleton (i.e., actin and microtubules), apparently demonstrated some artificial effects due to their preservation/fixation conditions.

There is an important role played by cytoskeleton elements in the assembly and morphogenesis of several viruses, reported in classical works [81] and more recent papers [30, 82, 83], which partially explains the data shown here. The replication complex and the viral factories are cellular structures from viral origins, but these complex structures need macromolecular and cellular constituents. In viral factories membranes and cytoskeleton elements are recruited as part of their constituents, because it is necessary to limit viral activities in this limited space [32]. In this sense, it is logical to attribute the important role of actin and microtubules in the viral assembly process, which in the case of some kind of blocking might produce a reduction in viral particle production.

Although there are some works about the role of the cytoskeleton on DENV infection, in which the participation of filopodia in DENV entry, as well as the function of Rho GTPases in regulation, is confirmed – a process by means of a cross-talk between Rac1 and Cdc42 [74, 76] – the preservation/fixation techniques in those specimens were not the best. Therefore, there are some doubts about the real participation of these elements in the dengue viral infections, because once the cells are significantly damaged the possibility for making the ulterior steps of the infectious cycle are difficult. However, the early stages of viral infections, like those shown by means of filopodia, are undoubtedly because the fine elements are well preserved.

In this vein, there is a collection of data, via images, proteins, and production of virions, demonstrating that the cytoskeleton plays an essential function in the viral replication processes. The viruses can be considered as probes for dissecting cellular signaling, cytoskeleton reorganization, and endocytosis [83, in this sense the research with dengue viruses could be considered similarly – with the actin microfilaments used for the viral assembly process since the disruption of these elements causes envelope viral protein aggregation. Images of "non-assembled" viral proteins have not been shown in others works. This pattern described here is compatible with other viruses [45, 84]. One such piece of work shows that altering actin remodeling by inhibition of a HMG-CoA reductase produces a scattered punctuated fluorescence pattern in viral protein after the treatment of lovastatin, which is compatible with an impaired assembly process. In agreement with these findings, we have shown the DENV2 infected cells treated with lovastatin, produce a clustering of envelope viral protein which also is attributed to some difficulties in the viral assembling process [65].

Consistent with this interpretation, the amounts of viral protein which had accumulated after the inhibition of actin filaments with cytochalasin D treatment was higher in comparison with the microtubules inhibited in the same conditions. If the "non-assembled" protein is reflecting some difficulty in this case [45, 65, 84], the potential role of actin microfilaments is implied in the viral assembly and/or maturation process of DENV. The indirect connection of actin microfilaments, Rho GTPases, with DENV assembly [65] had been used for clinical trials [85], based on the pleiotropic effects of inhibition of HMG-CoA by means of lovastatin [66]. The findings shown here offer new perspectives in the viral replication and morphogenesis of DENV, since at present there is lack of knowledge about the role played by actin in the viral factories and/or in the replication complex. On the other hand, the advantages of the technical approach shown here have been evidenced with other work, in which curcumin is able to alter the DENV2 replication process by blocking several cellular processes such as ubiquitin-proteasome and those of the cytoskeleton [72].

In spite of the diverse roles microtubules and actin microfilaments have in the different viral steps of replication for diverse viruses, more recently it was found that the replicative complex has intermediate filaments of vimentin which have a close, and structural, relationship with the non-structural protein 4A of DENV, forming part of their replication complex [86].

3. Conclusions

There has been an increased interest in recent years in understanding the cellular mechanisms that viruses exploit in the host cell, "Cell Biology of Viral Infection" is a new discipline that seeks to understand these intricate mechanisms [1]. Hence, in order to describe the participation of the cellular elements in DENV2 infection it is necessary to preserve the fine structure of cell morphology as closely as possible by avoiding any generation of artifacts.

In this work we have demonstrated the involvement of the cytoskeleton during DENV replication. It was determined that depolymerized microtubules and actin microfilaments generate disturbances in the DENV2 lifecycle, which causes a reduction in the production of infectious viral particles and in the intracellular expression of the viral envelope protein, as well as an altered subcellular distribution pattern of the viral protein envelope. This effect was more significant in the depolymerization of microtubules that in actin microfilaments. It has been reported that viral infections alter the global host proteomic in response to these, including cytoskeletal proteins [87-89]. However, although a role for the involvement of these proteins in viral infection is hypothesized, a route through which this occurs has yet to be identified.

4. Methods

4.1. Cell lines and virus

Aedes albopictus mosquito C6/36HT cells and epithelial Vero cell line (American Type Culture Collection CCL-81™) were grown in Dulbecco's Eagle's minimum essential medium (DMEM, GIBCO) supplemented with 2% or 10% fetal bovine serum (FBS, GIBCO), with 100 U/ml penicillin/100 µg/ml streptomycin and 0.25 µg/mL Amphotericin B. The cells were grown at 34°C with 5% CO_2 (C6/36HT) and 37°C with 5% CO_2 (Vero). DENV2 (New Guinea strain) was generously donated by María Elena Peñaranda and Eva Harris from the Sustainable Sciences Institute (SSI), San Francisco, California. The viruses were propagated in C6/36HT cells at low multiplicity of infection (MOI: 0,01 PFU/cell) and stored at -80ºC until used. Viral titers were detected by plaque assay, using a Vero cell monolayer culture under 1% methylcellulose overlay medium.

4.2. Antibodies and chemicals

The serum from rabbits against the envelope protein of DENV (polyclonal anti-DENV) was donated by Dr. Eva Harris and Robert Beatty (University of California, Berkeley, CA, USA). The secondary antibody coupled to peroxidase and anti-β-tubulin monoclonal coupled to Cy3 were purchased from Sigma-Aldrich Chemical Co. (St. Louis, MO, USA). Mycotoxin phalloidin conjugated with Alexa Fluor-488 or Alexa Fluor 594 and acetylated tubulin were purchased from Molecular Probes Invitrogen Life Technologies (Carlsbad, CA, USA). CytD, NZ, and 3-(4,5-dimethyl thiazol-2yl)-2,55-diphenyltetrazolium bromide (MTT) were purchased from the Sigma-Aldrich Chemical Co. (St. Louis, MO, USA). FluorSave was purchased from Calbiochem.

4.3. MTT assay

Cell viability was measured by MTT assay [90] to determined NZ and CytD concentrations that were below cytotoxic levels. Cells were seeded, 25,000 cells/well, in 96-well plates and allowed to adhere for 24 hours at 37ºC in 5% CO_2; cells were exposed to MTT (0.5mg/ml) for 4 hours, acid isopropanol (100μl) was then added to solubilize the formazan crystals produced. The culture dishes were incubated for 30 minutes and the absorbance was measured at 570nm in a Benchmark reader (Bio-Rad Laboratories, Hercules, CA). Vero cells were treated with 6 concentrations of these cytoskeleton-depolymerizing agents (NZ: 1.25, 2.5, 5, 10, 20 and 40μM) and (CytD: 0.25, 0.5, 1, 2, 4 and 8μM) for several periods (3, 6, 12, and 24 hours). The NZ and CytD were chosen at two concentrations (5μM and 10μM) and (2μM and 4mM) with a lower cytotoxicity (10% and 15%), but a preserved ability to depolymerize microtubules and inhibit actin polymerization, respectively. These agents were added to cultures 1 hour post-infection (hpi) with DENV.

4.4. Viral infection and treatments

In order to determine the cytoskeletal depolymerizing agent's effects on DENV2 replication, experiments were undertaken as follows. Confluent Vero cell monolayers were grown on 24 (1×10^5) and 96 (2.5×10^4) multi-wells, in DMEM with 2% FBS, at 37°C and 5% CO_2. Cells were infected in the absence of FBS at an MOI of 5 PFU/cell, after a 1-hour adsorption period at 4ºC, the viral inoculum was replaced with maintenance DMEM and incubated at 37ºC. Infected cells were incubated in the presence of NZ, CytD, or DMSO for the indicated times. These cells were maintained for 24 hours after infection and treatment. As a cytoskeleton infection control, we performed the same procedure without DENV under the same conditions. Coverslips for immunofluorescence (IF) were placed in 24 multi-wells. The cell monolayers were fixed and processed to visualize the viruses and cytoskeleton components by confocal fluorescence microscopy. Monolayers and culture supernatants were collected to determine the effect of CytD and NZ in viral protein production by cell ELISA. Additionally, the supernatants also were used to quantify the cytoskeleton blockage effect in infectious viral particle production by means of titration by plaque assay.

4.5. Titration by plaque assays

For quantification of infectious viral particles, the virus was titrated by plaque assays using supernatants of Vero cells infected with DENV2 and treated under different conditions, as described in [91, 92]. Briefly, cells were plated, $5x10^4$ cells/well, on 24-well plates, in DMEM 2% FBS at 37°C in 5% CO_2, and inoculated with serial dilutions of viral collected supernatants from 10^{-1} to 10^{-5} in DMEM without FBS. At 1 hpi the inoculum was removed, washed, had DMEM 2% FBS and finally 1.5% of carboximetilcelulose (SIGMA) added to it. After 8 days post-infection (dpi), the cells were fixed with paraformaldehyde (PFA) at 4% in PBS and revealed with crystal violet. The plaque number was recorded in order to calculate the PFU/ml. Two independent experiments were performed, each in duplicate.

4.6. Cell ELISA

Viral protein was quantified by a spectrophotometric cell ELISA, which is a modification of fluorometric ELISA previously described by [65]. To this immunodetection of viral protein in infected cells, Vero cells ($2.5x10^4$ cells) were submitted to different experimental strategies and were fixed for 30 minutes with 4% paraformaldehyde (PFA), washed three times with PBS, and permeabilized for 30 minutes with 0.1% Triton X-100. Endogenous peroxidase was quenched with 0.3% H_2O_2 in 10% methanol and, non-specific sites were saturated with a blocking buffer (10% FBS in PBS). Then the anti-DENV2 diluted (1:500) blocking buffer was incubated for 1 hour at 37°C. After washing with PBS, this was incubated for 30 minutes with a secondary antibody, anti-mouse IgG conjugated with HRPO. Finally after washing with PBS, chromogenic substrate SIGMA ® FAST OPD (St. Louis, MO, USA) was added to reveal the reaction and its absorbance was read at 405nm in the Benchmark reader (Bio-Rad Laboratories, Hercules, CA, USA). To normalize the data, the total protein concentration in each well was determined by Bradford assay, interpolating absorbance data in a calibration curve with known concentrations of bovine serum albumin. Two independent experiments were performed with 3 replicates for each assay.

4.7. Fluorescence microscopy

In order to use the best preservation and fixation protocol for assays linked to the research, three fixations were assessed: paraformaldehyde 3.7% in phosphate buffered saline (PFA-PBS), paraformaldehyde 3.7% in cytoskeletal buffered sucrose (PFA-CBS), and Methanol-Acetone 1-1 (M-A). Vero cells were cultured in 24 multi-well plates with glass cover slips, at a density of $4.5x10^4$ cells/well in DMEM 2% FBS. After 24 hours monolayers were fixed with different treatments. For the PFA-CBS treatment the medium was discarded, washed with CBS at 37°C, and fixed with PFA-CBS over 30 minutes at 37°C in 5% CO_2. For the PFA-PBS treatment the medium was discarded, washed with PBS, and fixed with PFA-PBS over a period of 30 minutes. For the M-A treatment the medium was discarded, washed with PBS, and fixed with methanol-acetone over a period of 30 minutes at 4°C.

To evaluate the cytoskeleton blocking effects of CytD and NZ in DENV-2 infection, 24 hours after treatment Vero cell monolayers were rinsed once at 37ºC with CBS [10 mM PIPES (pH

6.9) (1,4-piperazinebis-ethane sulfonic acid), 100 mM NaCl, 1.5 mM MgCl2, and 300 mM sucrose. The cells were then permeabilized and simultaneously fixed with PFA-CBS for 30 minutes at 37ºC. To avoid auto-fluorescence the cells were placed in 50mM NH^4Cl for 10 minutes, then were permeabilized with 0.3% Triton X-100 and had their non-specific sites blocked with 5% FBS in CBS. For detection of viral protein and cytoskeleton, cells were incubated with primary monoclonal anti-DENV antibody (1:500) and Alexa 488 conjugated secondary antibody. After that, cells were incubated with anti-phalloidin 594 or anti-β tubulin Cy3 and Hoechst 33258. Following washing with CBS, slides were mounted with mounting medium and examined under a confocal fluorescent microscope (Olympus IX-81 DSU). The micrographs were recorded using an Olympus CCD camera and processed with Image Pro Plus software (from Media Cybernetics).

4.8. Statistical analysis

Data are presented as means ± SD. In all cases, they represent at least three independent determinations. The significance of the results was calculated by Student's t test. In this case, p values < 0.05 were considered significant with respect to controls.

Acknowledgements

This research was supported by COLCIENCIAS grant 111554531592 from the Colombian government. JCGG was the recipient of a Full-Time Professor Program (Exclusive Dedication) for the Medicine Faculty at University of Antioquia for 2014–2015.

Author details

Elizabeth Orozco-García[1], Andrea Trujillo-Correa[2] and Juan Carlos Gallego-Gómez[1*]

*Address all correspondence to: juanc.gallegomez@gmail.com

1 Translational and Molecular Medicine Group, Medellín Medical Research Institute, Faculty of Medicine, Universidad de Antioquia, Medellín, Colombia

2 Institute of Biology, Faculty of Exact and Natural Sciences, Universidad de Antioquia, Medellín, Colombia

The authors declare that they have no competing interests.
AITC contributed to the experimental design, carried out the experiments. EOG worked on analysis interpretation of data, and drafted the manuscript. JCGG conceived the study, participated in its design, and coordinated and finalized the manuscript. All the authors read and approved the final version of the manuscript.

References

[1] Sodeik B, Hannover Medical School DoV, CarlâNeubergstrasse 1, Hannover 30625, Germany, Schramm B, EMBL CBaBP, Meyerhofstrasse 1, Heidelberg 69117, Germany, Suomalainen M, University of Helsinki HI, Department of Virology, PO Box 21, Helsinki FINâ00014, Finland, et al. Meeting Report: EMBO Workshop â˜Cell Biology of Virus Infectionâ™, September 25â"29, 2004, EMBL, Heidelberg, Germany. Traffic. 6(4):351-6.

[2] Radtke K, Dohner K, Sodeik B. Viral interactions with the cytoskeleton: a hitchhiker's guide to the cell. Cell Microbiol. 2006;8(3):387-400.

[3] Stephens DJ, Allan VJ. Light microscopy techniques for live cell imaging. Science. 2003;300(5616):82-6.

[4] Sanderson CM, Smith GL. Cell motility and cell morphology: how some viruses take control. Expert Rev Mol Med. 1999;1999:1-16.

[5] Cellular Microbiology. 2nd ed: ASM Press; 2004. 593 p.

[6] Schudt G, Kolesnikova L, Dolnik O, Sodeik B, Becker S. Live-cell imaging of Marburg virus-infected cells uncovers actin-dependent transport of nucleocapsids over long distances. Proc Natl Acad Sci U S A. 2013;110(35):14402-7.

[7] Lippincott-Schwartz J, Patterson GH. Development and use of fluorescent protein markers in living cells. Science. 2003;300(5616):87-91.

[8] Stephens RS, Sansonetti P, Sibley D. Cellular microbiology - a research agenda and an emerging discipline. Cell Microbiol. 1999;1(1):1-2.

[9] Risco C, Castro IFd, Sanz-Sánchez L, Narayan K, Grandinetti G, Subramaniam S. Three-Dimensional Imaging of Viral Infections. Annual Review of Virology. 2014;1:453-73.

[10] Novoa RR, Calderita G, Arranz R, Fontana J, Granzow H, Risco C. Virus factories: associations of cell organelles for viral replication and morphogenesis. Biol Cell. 2005;97(2):147-72.

[11] Farrar J, Focks D, Gubler D, Barrera R, Guzman MG, Simmons C, et al. Towards a global dengue research agenda. Trop Med Int Health. 12. England2007. p. 695-9.

[12] Guzman MG, Halstead SB, Artsob H, Buchy P, Farrar J, Gubler DJ, et al. Dengue: a continuing global threat. Nature Reviews Microbiology. 2010;8.

[13] Mukhopadhyay S, Kuhn RJ, Rossmann MG. A structural perspective of the flavivirus life cycle. Nat Rev Microbiol. 2005;3(1):13-22.

[14] Gubler DJ, Clark GG. Dengue/dengue hemorrhagic fever: the emergence of a global health problem. Emerg Infect Dis. 1995;1(2):55-7.

[15] Gubler DJ. Dengue and dengue hemorrhagic fever. Clin Microbiol Rev. 1998;11(3): 480-96.

[16] Guzman MG, Kouri G. Dengue diagnosis, advances and challenges. Int J Infect Dis. 2004;8(2):69-80.

[17] Guzman M, Kouri G, Diaz M, Llop A, Vazquez S, Gonzalez D, et al. Dengue, one of the great emerging health challenges of the 21st century. Expert Rev Vaccines. 2004;3(5):511-20.

[18] Halstead SB, Suaya JA, Shepard DS. The burden of dengue infection. Lancet. 2007;369(9571):1410-1.

[19] Shepard DS, Coudeville L, Halasa YA, Zambrano B, Dayan GH. Economic Impact of Dengue Illness in the Americas. Am J Trop Med Hyg. 2011;84(2):200-7.

[20] Mendez JA, Usme-Ciro JA, Domingo C, Rey GJ, Sanchez JA, Tenorio A, et al. Phylogenetic history demonstrates two different lineages of dengue type 1 virus in Colombia. Virol J. 2010;7:226.

[21] Usme-Ciro JA, Mendez JA, Tenorio A, Rey GJ, Domingo C, Gallego-Gomez JC. Simultaneous circulation of genotypes I and III of dengue virus 3 in Colombia. Virol J. 2008;5:101.

[22] Isaguliants MG, Belikov SV, Starodubova ES, Gizatullin RZ, Rollman E, Zuber B, et al. Mutations conferring drug resistance affect eukaryotic expression of HIV type 1 reverse transcriptase. AIDS Res Hum Retroviruses. 2004;20(2):191-201.

[23] Mendez JA, Usme-Ciro JA, Domingo C, Rey GJ, Sanchez JA, Tenorio A, et al. Phylogenetic reconstruction of dengue virus type 2 in Colombia. Virol J. 2012;9:64.

[24] Villar L, Dayan GH, Arredondo-Garcia JL, Rivera DM, Cunha R, Deseda C, et al. Efficacy of a tetravalent dengue vaccine in children in Latin America. N Engl J Med. 2015;372(2):113-23.

[25] Smith GA, Enquist LW. Break ins and break outs: viral interactions with the cytoskeleton of Mammalian cells. Annu Rev Cell Dev Biol. 2002;18:135-61.

[26] Miller S, Krijnse-Locker J. Modification of intracellular membrane structures for virus replication. Nat Rev Microbiol. 2008;6(5):363-74.

[27] Igakura T, Stinchcombe JC, Goon PK, Taylor GP, Weber JN, Griffiths GM, et al. Spread of HTLV-I between lymphocytes by virus-induced polarization of the cytoskeleton. Science. 2003;299(5613):1713-6.

[28] Luby-Phelps K. Cytoarchitecture and physical properties of cytoplasm: volume, viscosity, diffusion, intracellular surface area. Int Rev Cytol. 2000;192:189-221.

[29] Wileman T. Aggresomes and pericentriolar sites of virus assembly: cellular defense or viral design? Annu Rev Microbiol. 2007;61:149-67.

[30] Taylor MP, Koyuncu OO, Enquist LW. Subversion of the actin cytoskeleton during viral infection. Nat Rev Microbiol. 2011;9(6):427-39.

[31] Risco C, Rodriguez JR, Lopez-Iglesias C, Carrascosa JL, Esteban M, Rodriguez D. Endoplasmic reticulum-Golgi intermediate compartment membranes and vimentin filaments participate in vaccinia virus assembly. J Virol. 2002;76(4):1839-55.

[32] Netherton C, Moffat K, Brooks E, Wileman T. A guide to viral inclusions, membrane rearrangements, factories, and viroplasm produced during virus replication. Adv Virus Res. 2007;70:101-82.

[33] Mercer J, Schelhaas M, Helenius A. Virus entry by endocytosis. Annu Rev Biochem. 2010;79:803-33.

[34] Heath CM, Windsor M, Wileman T. Aggresomes Resemble Sites Specialized for Virus Assembly. J Cell Biol. 2001;153(3):449-56.

[35] Bonneau AM, Darveau A, Sonenberg N. Effect of viral infection on host protein synthesis and mRNA association with the cytoplasmic cytoskeletal structure. J Cell Biol. 1985;100(4):1209-18.

[36] Belin MT, Boulanger P. Processing of vimentin occurs during the early stages of adenovirus infection. J Virol. 1987;61(8):2559-66.

[37] Norregard Nielsen L, Forchhammer J, Dabelsteen E, Jepsen A, Stubbe Teglbjaerg C, Norrild B. Herpes simplex virus-induced changes of the keratin type intermediate filament in rat epithelial cells. J Gen Virol. 1987;68 (Pt 3):737-48.

[38] Liu B, Dai R, Tian CJ, Dawson L, Gorelick R, Yu XF. Interaction of the human immunodeficiency virus type 1 nucleocapsid with actin. J Virol. 1999;73(4):2901-8.

[39] Notter MF, Balduzzi PC. Cytoskeletal changes induced by two avian sarcoma viruses: UR2 and Rous sarcoma virus. Virology. 1984;136(1):56-68.

[40] Elliott J, Jones MD, Griffin BE, Krauzewicz N. Regulation of cytoskeletal association by a basic amino acid motif in polyoma virus middle T antigen. Oncogene. 1998;17(14):1797-806.

[41] Friedrich RE, Bartel-Friedrich S, Lobeck H, Niedobitek G, Arps H. Epstein-Barr virus DNA, intermediate filaments and epithelial membrane antigen in nasopharyngeal carcinoma. Anticancer Res. 2000;20(6d):4909-16.

[42] Horvath AR, Kellie S. Regulation of integrin mobility and cytoskeletal association in normal and RSV-transformed chick embryo fibroblasts. J Cell Sci. 1990;97 (Pt 2): 307-15.

[43] Nunbhakdi-Craig V, Craig L, Machleidt T, Sontag E. Simian virus 40 small tumor antigen induces deregulation of the actin cytoskeleton and tight junctions in kidney epithelial cells. J Virol. 2003;77(5):2807-18.

[44] Mallardo M, Schleich S, Krijnse Locker J. Microtubule-dependent Organization of Vaccinia Virus Core-derivd Early mRNAs into Distinct Cytoplasmic Structures. Mol Biol Cell. 2001;12(12):3875-91.

[45] Gallego-Gomez JC, Risco C, Rodriguez D, Cabezas P, Guerra S, Carrascosa JL, et al. Differences in virus-induced cell morphology and in virus maturation between MVA and other strains (WR, Ankara, and NYCBH) of vaccinia virus in infected human cells. J Virol. 2003;77(19):10606-22.

[46] Roncarati R, Knebel-Morsdorf D. Identification of the early actin-rearrangement-inducing factor gene, arif-1, from Autographa californica multicapsid nuclear polyhedrosis virus. J Virol. 1997;71(10):7933-41.

[47] Selinka HC, Giroglou T, Sapp M. Analysis of the infectious entry pathway of human papillomavirus type 33 pseudovirions. Virology. 2002;299(2):279-87.

[48] Van de Walle GR, Favoreel HW, Nauwynck HJ, Van Oostveldt P, Pensaert MB. Antibody-induced internalization of viral glycoproteins in pseudorabies virus-infected monocytes and role of the cytoskeleton: a confocal study. Vet Microbiol. 2002;86(1-2): 51-7.

[49] Mackenzie JM, Jones MK, Westaway EG. Markers for trans-Golgi Membranes and the Intermediate Compartment Localize to Induced Membranes with Distinct Replication Functions in Flavivirus-Infected Cells†. J Virol. 1999;73(11):9555-67.

[50] van der Schaar HM, Rust MJ, Waarts BL, van der Ende-Metselaar H, Kuhn RJ, Wilschut J, et al. Characterization of the early events in dengue virus cell entry by biochemical assays and single-virus tracking. J Virol. 2007;81(21):12019-28.

[51] Berghall H, Wallen C, Hyypia T, Vainionpaa R. Role of cytoskeleton components in measles virus replication. Arch Virol. 2004;149(5):891-901.

[52] Douglas MW, Diefenbach RJ, Homa FL, Miranda-Saksena M, Rixon FJ, Vittone V, et al. Herpes simplex virus type 1 capsid protein VP26 interacts with dynein light chains RP3 and Tctex1 and plays a role in retrograde cellular transport. J Biol Chem. 2004;279(27):28522-30.

[53] Lakadamyali M, Rust MJ, Babcock HP, Zhuang X. Visualizing infection of individual influenza viruses. Proc Natl Acad Sci U S A. 2003;100(16):9280-5.

[54] Leopold PL, Kreitzer G, Miyazawa N, Rempel S, Pfister KK, Rodriguez-Boulan E, et al. Dynein- and microtubule-mediated translocation of adenovirus serotype 5 occurs after endosomal lysis. Hum Gene Ther. 2000;11(1):151-65.

[55] Martinez-Moreno M, Navarro-Lerida I, Roncal F, Albar JP, Alonso C, Gavilanes F, et al. Recognition of novel viral sequences that associate with the dynein light chain LC8 identified through a pepscan technique. FEBS Lett. 2003;544(1-3):262-7.

[56] Ng ML, Hong SS. Flavivirus infection: essential ultrastructural changes and association of Kunjin virus NS3 protein with microtubules. Arch Virol. 1989;106(1-2):103-20.

[57] Ward BM. The Taking of the Cytoskeleton One Two Three: How Viruses Utilize the Cytoskeleton During Egress. Virology. 2011;411(2):244-50.

[58] Netherton CL, Wileman T. Virus factories, double membrane vesicles and viroplasm generated in animal cells. Current Opinion in Virology. 2011;1(5):381-7.

[59] Pierini R, Cottam E, Roberts R, Wileman T. Modulation of membrane traffic between endoplasmic reticulum, ERGIC and Golgi to generate compartments for the replication of bacteria and viruses. Semin Cell Dev Biol. 2009;20(7):828-33.

[60] Chen W, Gao N, Wang JL, Tian YP, Chen ZT, An J. Vimentin is required for dengue virus serotype 2 infection but microtubules are not necessary for this process. Arch Virol. 2008;153(9):1777-81.

[61] van der Schaar HM, Rust MJ, Chen C, van der Ende-Metselaar H, Wilschut J, Zhuang X, et al. Dissecting the cell entry pathway of dengue virus by single-particle tracking in living cells. PLoS Pathog. 2008;4(12):e1000244.

[62] Mosso C, Galvan-Mendoza IJ, Ludert JE, del Angel RM. Endocytic pathway followed by dengue virus to infect the mosquito cell line C6/36 HT. Virology. 2008;378(1): 193-9.

[63] Heasman SJ, Ridley AJ. Mammalian Rho GTPases: new insights into their functions from in vivo studies. Nat Rev Mol Cell Biol. 2008;9(9):690-701.

[64] del Real G, Jimenez-Baranda S, Mira E, Lacalle RA, Lucas P, Gomez-Mouton C, et al. Statins Inhibit HIV-1 Infection by Down-regulating Rho Activity. J Exp Med. 2004;200(4):541-7.

[65] Martinez-Gutierrez M, Castellanos JE, Gallego-Gomez JC. Statins reduce dengue virus production via decreased virion assembly. Intervirology. 2011;54(4):202-16.

[66] Rothwell C, Lebreton A, Young Ng C, Lim JY, Liu W, Vasudevan S, et al. Cholesterol biosynthesis modulation regulates dengue viral replication. Virology. 2009;389(1-2): 8-19.

[67] Yang CC, Tsai MH, Hu HS, Pu SY, Wu RH, Wu SH, et al. Characterization of an efficient dengue virus replicon for development of assays of discovery of small molecules against dengue virus. Antiviral Res. 2013;98(2):228-41.

[68] Chu JJH, Yang PL. c-Src protein kinase inhibitors block assembly and maturation of dengue virus. Proc Natl Acad Sci U S A. 2007;104(9):3520-5.

[69] Martinez-Gutierrez M, Correa-Londono LA, Castellanos JE, Gallego-Gomez JC, Osorio JE. Lovastatin delays infection and increases survival rates in AG129 mice infected with dengue virus serotype 2. PLoS One. 2014;9(2):e87412.

[70] Padilla SL, Rodriguez A, Gonzales MM, Gallego GJC, Castano OJC. Inhibitory effects of curcumin on dengue virus type 2-infected cells in vitro. Arch Virol. 2014;159(3): 573-9.

[71] Brass AL, Huang IC, Benita Y, John SP, Krishnan MN, Feeley EM, et al. The IFITM proteins mediate cellular resistance to influenza A H1N1 virus, West Nile virus, and dengue virus. Cell. 2009;139(7):1243-54.

[72] Padilla-S L, Rodríguez A, Gonzales MM, Gallego-G JC, Castaño-O JC. Inhibitory effects of curcumin on dengue virus type 2-infected cells in vitro. Arch Virol. 2013.

[73] Yang J, Zou L, Hu Z, Chen W, Zhang J, Zhu J, et al. Identification and characterization of a 43 kDa actin protein involved in the DENV-2 binding and infection of ECV304 cells. Microbes Infect. 2013;15(4):310-8.

[74] Zamudio-Meza H, Castillo-Alvarez A, Gonzalez-Bonilla C, Meza I. Cross-talk between Rac1 and Cdc42 GTPases regulates formation of filopodia required for dengue virus type-2 entry into HMEC-1 cells. J Gen Virol. 2009;90(Pt 12):2902-11.

[75] Shrivastava N, National Institute of Virology P, India, Sripada S, National Institute of Virology P, India, Kaur J, National Institute of Virology P, India, et al. Insights into the Internalization and Retrograde Trafficking of Dengue 2 Virus in BHK-21 Cells. PLOS ONE. 2011;6(10).

[76] Wang JL, Zhang JL, Chen W, Xu XF, Gao N, Fan DY, et al. Roles of Small GTPase Rac1 in the Regulation of Actin Cytoskeleton during Dengue Virus Infection. PLoS Negl Trop Dis. 2010;4(8).

[77] Cande WZ, Lazarides E, McIntosh JR. A comparison of the distribution of actin and tubulin in the mammalian mitotic spindle as seen by indirect immunofluorescence. J Cell Biol. 1977;72(3):552-67.

[78] Connolly JA, Kalnins VI, Cleveland DW, Kirschner MW. Immunoflourescent staining of cytoplasmic and spindle microtubules in mouse fibroblasts with antibody to tau protein. Proc Natl Acad Sci U S A. 1977;74(6):2437-40.

[79] Szechyńska-Hebda M, University W, Sciences IoPPPAo, Wędzony M, Sciences IoPPPAo, Dubas E, et al. Visualisation of microtubules and actin filaments in fixed BY-2 suspension cells using an optimised whole mount immunolabelling protocol. Plant Cell Reports. 2006;25(8):758-66.

[80] Matthews JD, Morgan R, Sleigher C, Frey TK. Do viruses require the cytoskeleton? Virol J. 2013;10:121.

[81] Genty N, Bussereau F. Is cytoskeleton involved in vesicular stomatitis virus reproduction? J Virol. 1980;34(3):777-81.

[82] Hyde JL, Gillespie LK, Mackenzie JM. Mouse norovirus 1 utilizes the cytoskeleton network to establish localization of the replication complex proximal to the microtubule organizing center. J Virol. 2012;86(8):4110-22.

[83] Jeffree CE, Brown G, Aitken J, Su-Yin DY, Tan BH, Sugrue RJ. Ultrastructural analysis of the interaction between F-actin and respiratory syncytial virus during virus assembly. Virology. 2007;369(2):309-23.

[84] Ravi LI, Liang L, Wong PS, Brown G, Tan BH, Sugrue RJ. Increased hydroxymethyl-glutaryl coenzyme A reductase activity during respiratory syncytial virus infection mediates actin dependent inter-cellular virus transmission. Antiviral Res. 2013;100(1):259-68.

[85] Whitehorn J, Van Vinh Chau N, Truong NT, Tai LT, Van Hao N, Hien TT, et al. Lovastatin for adult patients with dengue: protocol for a randomised controlled trial. Trials. 2012;13:203.

[86] Teo CS CJ. Cellular Vimentin Regulates Construction of Dengue V... [J Virol. 2014] - PubMed - NCBI J Virol.2014. Available from: http://www.ncbi.nlm.nih.gov/pubmed/.

[87] Frontiers: Global host proteomic responses to virus infection: Frontiers Media SA; 2014.

[88] Zhang M, Zheng X, Wu Y, Gan M, He A, Li Z, et al. Differential proteomics of Aedes albopictus salivary gland, midgut and C6/36 cell induced by dengue virus infection. Virology. 2013;444(1-2):109-18.

[89] Pando-Robles V, Oses-Prieto JA, Rodriguez-Gandarilla M, Meneses-Romero E, Burlingame AL, Batista CV. Quantitative proteomic analysis of Huh-7 cells infected with Dengue virus by label-free LC-MS. J Proteomics. 2014;111:16-29.

[90] Mosmann T. Rapid colorimetric assay for cellular growth and survival: application to proliferation and cytotoxicity assays. J Immunol Methods. 1983;65(1-2):55-63.

[91] Meiklejohn G, England B, Lennette. Propagation of dengue virus strains in unweaned mice. Am J Trop Med Hyg. 1952;1(1):51-8.

[92] Fujita N, Tamura M, Hotta S. Dengue virus plaque formation on microplate cultures and its application to virus neutralization (38564). Proc Soc Exp Biol Med. 1975;148(2):472-5.

8

The Burden of Dengue Illness and its Economics Costs in the Americas: A Review on the Most Affected Countries

Raúl Castro Rodríguez,
Jorge Armando Rueda-Gallardo and
Manuel Felipe Avella-Niño

Abstract

According to the Pan American Health Organization (PAHO) reports, the annual average number of dengue cases in the Americas has been 1,579,658 in the last 8 years (2010–2017), affecting the population's welfare. The high level in dengue cases does not only have an impact from an epidemiological perspective but also from an economical perspective as the treatment cost that must be borne. The aim of this chapter is to review the situation as reported in the American countries with the highest number of cases, focusing on the burden of the disease (measured in DALYs and number of cases) and its total treatment cost, which includes direct (medical and non-medical) costs and indirect costs. We calculate the total treatment cost per DALY for the epidemic year (2015). The results show that Mexico has the highest cost per DALY (US$ 17,703) followed by Brazil (US$ 11,218), Colombia (US$ 4,540), and the Dominican Republic (US$ 1,157). Additionally, after adjusting for total health expenditure, we found all the countries exhibit a similar share of total treatment cost over health expenditure (0.16% in average).

Keywords: dengue, disease outbreaks, epidemiologic measurements, disability adjusted life year, economics costs

1. Introduction

Dengue is a viral infection endemic to tropical regions, which is transmitted by *Aedes aegypti* and *Aedes albopictus* mosquitoes. It usually presents a cyclic behavior with peaks separated by

3–5 years [1–3]. Even though this illness has been present for many years in tropical countries, the main prevention strategy is controlling the vector that carries the infection. Nowadays, vector control and prevention programs are the only strategies in the hands of public officials to handle and reduce dengue incidence.

In the 1970s, because of the vector control campaign against yellow fever, dengue was close to be eliminated, but then it showed a reinvasion that has been present to this day [4]. The constant presence of the illness (and the mosquitoes) is related with the suboptimal conditions of trash collection, piped water supplies and uncontrolled urban development [5]. Another possible cause is climate change [6]. Warming temperatures have expanded the endemic territories of the *A. aegypti* and *A. albopictus* mosquitoes allowing them to be present in larger areas [7], which added to the low efficacy of vector control strategies and create the perfect scenario for the number of dengue cases to rise. Unfortunately, the programs aimed to control the mosquito population have low success rates which are reflected in the consistent high number of dengue cases in the last decade.

In recent years, there has been enough interest from the pharmaceutical industry to develop a dengue vaccine that could act as a preventive strategy against the infection [8–10]. Nevertheless, most dengue vaccine strategies are still in their final stages before implementation [11].

Figure 1 shows the evolution of the reported dengue cases in the Americas for the period 2010–2017, from which it can be observed a drastic decline in the year 2017 after 2 years of high levels of dengue cases. Particularly, 2015 corresponds to the year with the highest number of cases in the region, which suggest it was an epidemic year. Given the cyclic behavior of the disease, the year 2017 could be interpreted as an interepidemic year.

The World Health Organization (WHO) recommends conducting an economic analysis for infectious disease to estimate the cost borne by the society, especially in low- and middle-income countries. These studies provide information to the governments that help them design policies and allocate public resources that achieve a positive impact on public health. The most common and recommended type of analysis is the cost-effectiveness analysis (CEA), which

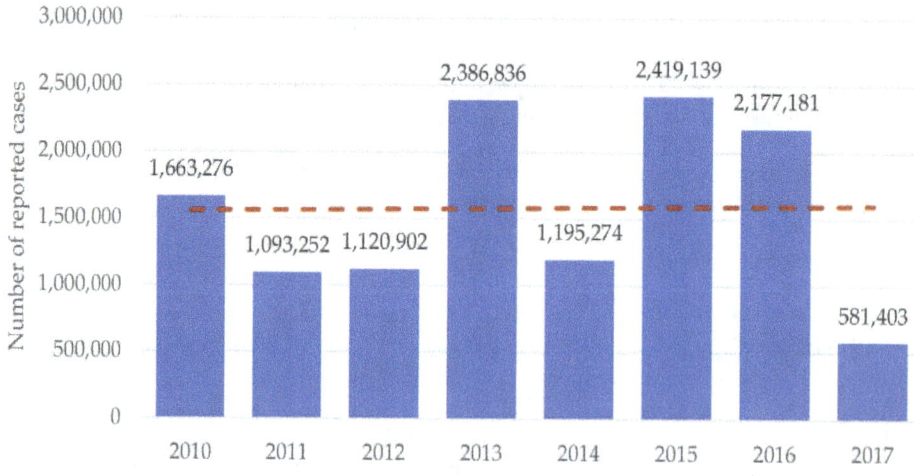

Figure 1. Evolution of reported dengue cases in the Americas (2010–2017). Source: PAHO.

compares different healthcare interventions estimating the economic costs and health gains (usually measured as Disability-Adjusted Life Years) of each intervention and hence identifies strategies with the potential of yielding the greatest health improvement for the least resources used [12]. The aforesaid type of analysis consists of two main elements, the burden estimation in the status quo scenario or current condition and the estimation in the intervention scenario. From this perspective, the analysis conducted in this chapter presents the burden estimation in the status quo scenario.

As well as Latin-American and Caribbean countries, Asian countries have also been affected by dengue. Epidemiological studies conducted for Myanmar show that DALYs per million of inhabitants lost ranged between 90 and 97 in the 1990s [13], while in Thailand, the burden was estimated at 427 DALYs per million in the early 2000s. The latter allow us to have a frame of reference about the burden of dengue. Due to the increasing number of cases in Americas and Asia [14–16] and the economic cost that society must borne to treat (medical and out-of-pocket costs) and control the disease (prevention and promotion, surveillance and control activities), dengue continues to be a public health priority, especially in the regions previously mentioned. This chapter aims to present a recent picture of the treatment costs, generated by the disease and borne by the healthcare system and households, and its burden on the public health in relevant countries for each one of the main territories of the Americas.

The following sections contain: the explanation of the criteria used to select the group of countries for which the total economic cost and burden of the disease were calculated (Countries selection); the methodology used for estimating the DALY and the total economic cost, as well as the necessary adjustment in the cost figures (Materials and methods); the main results for the year 2015 (Results) and finally a brief discussion on the current levels of incidence of dengue as a comparison between 2015 and 2017 in terms of total costs and burden. By estimating the burden for 2015, which corresponds to the year with the highest number of reported dengue cases, according to PAHO, we can estimate the impact that dengue has on public health and health expenditure in an epidemic year. In contrast, having the results for 2017 not only shows a more recent level of the burden but also serve as a comparison of the disease's impact between epidemic and inter-epidemic years. It is worth noting that even though the figures used in this chapter correspond to official figures collected by PAHO, underreport in the information health systems is an element that could hide the real burden[1].

2. Countries selection

To select the countries reviewed, we consider two main elements. The total number of dengue cases in each country according to Pan American Health Organization (PAHO) reports and the availability of information regarding total and average economic costs (per patient). Additionally,

[1] Although it is challenging to estimate a robust level for underreport, attempts have been made. In Brazil the underreport expansion factor for total dengue cases have been estimated in 1.6, while in Nicaragua this estimation goes as high as 28. Additionally, the estimation for the underreport factor specific for severe dengue cases ranges from 1.4 to 3 [20].

we aimed for having a relevant[2] country for each one of the main territories of the Americas as described by PAHO: Central America and Mexico, Andean, Southern Cone, and the Caribbean[3] (**Map 1**). Given that dengue cases recorded in North America usually correspond to non-endemic cases, we exclude from this chapter the information related to the USA and Canada.

To obtain robust figures for each country and avoid making a selection based on a particular year, we used the aggregated figures, by adding the total number of reported cases and death for the period 2014–2017. Based on the total number of reported dengue cases and deaths, we

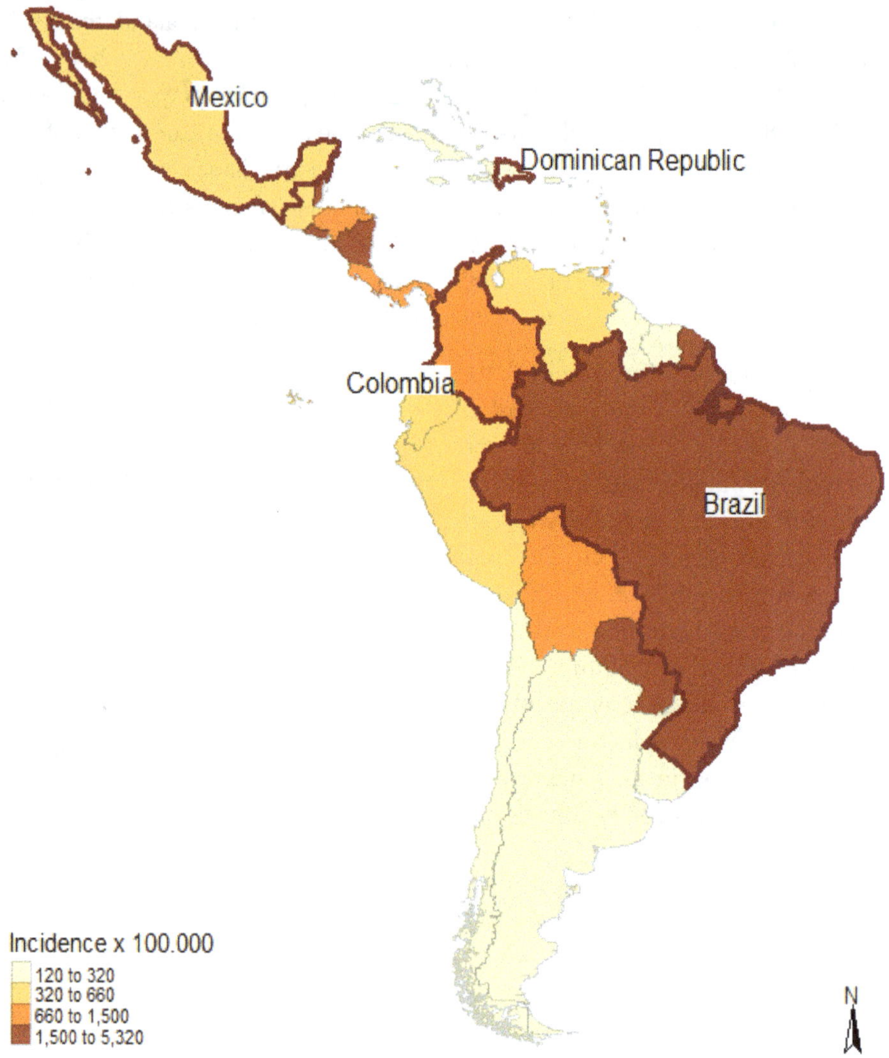

Map 1. Incidence per 100,000 inhabitants in Americas (2014–2017). Source: PAHO. 2017.

[2]We consider a country as relevant based on the burden of the disease in terms of reported dengue cases and dengue related deaths.

[3]As Caribbean territory we considered both Latin Caribbean and Non-Latin Caribbean.

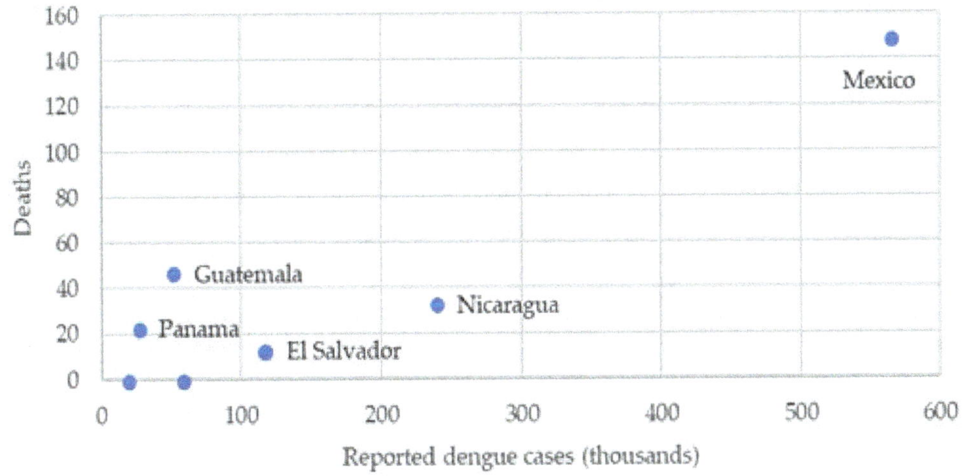

Figure 2. Dengue cases and mortality in Central America and Mexico territory (2014–2017). Source: PAHO. 2017.

selected Mexico as the representative country of the Central America and Mexico territory (**Figure 2**). Mexico has the highest number of dengue deaths (149) as well as the highest number of reported dengue cases (564,498). Another benefit of reviewing the Mexican case is the availability of information regarding total and per patient economic cost through a micro-costing approach [17]. Similarly, for the Andean territory, we observed that the country with the highest number of reported dengue cases (337,018) and deaths (318) is Colombia (**Figure 3**). For this country, the cost for patient was calculated using a micro-costing approach that employed the administrative records of the national healthcare system and a household survey conducted by the authors [18].

In the Southern Cone territory (**Figure 4**), we observe Brazil as the country with the highest number of dengue cases (3,992,664) and deaths (2,048). The latter is particularly expected since

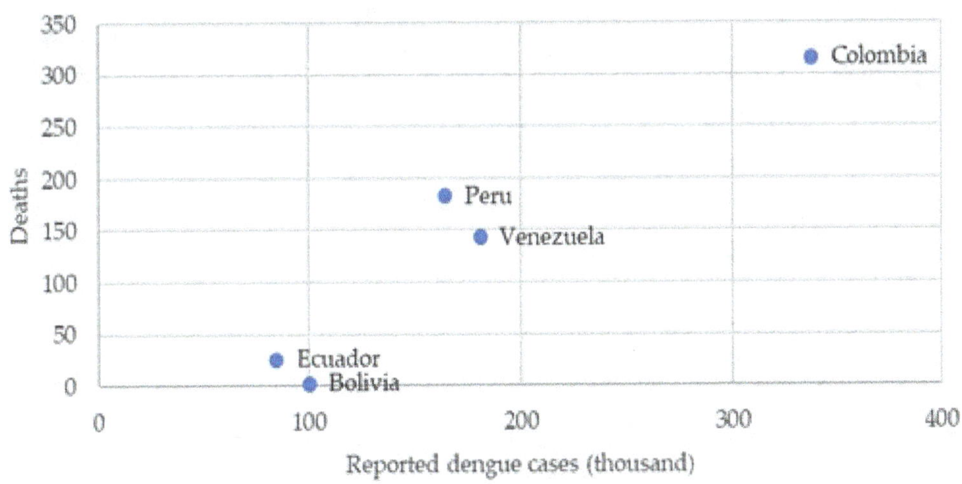

Figure 3. Dengue cases and mortality in Andean territory (2014–2017). Source: PAHO. 2017.

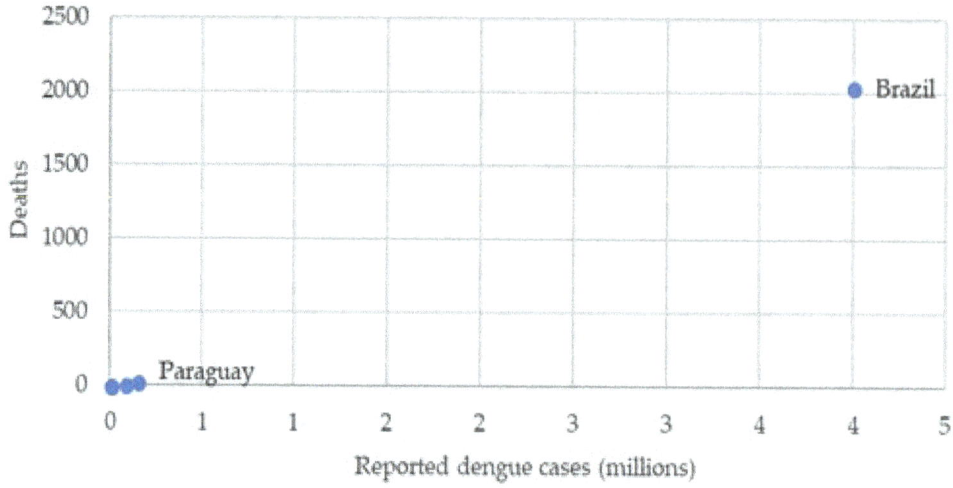

Figure 4. Dengue cases and mortality in Southern Cone territory (2014–2017). Source: PAHO. 2017.

not only Brazil has the largest population in the region (Southern Cone and Andean territory), but also the other countries in this territory are sub-tropical (Paraguay) and non-tropical (Chile, Argentina and Uruguay). The advantage of reviewing the Brazilian case is the large evidence of total and per patient economics costs which has been estimated using micro-costing, bottom-up approach from administrative records, household survey and interviews [19].

Finally, for the Caribbean territory, we found that, based on the information from PAHO, between 2014 and 2017, the country with the highest number of dengue cases (31,326) and deaths (209) is the Dominican Republic (**Figure 5**). In contrast to Brazil, Colombia and Mexico, no published study, which quantifies the cost of the disease per patient considering the same cost structure framework commonly found in the literature (direct and indirect costs), was

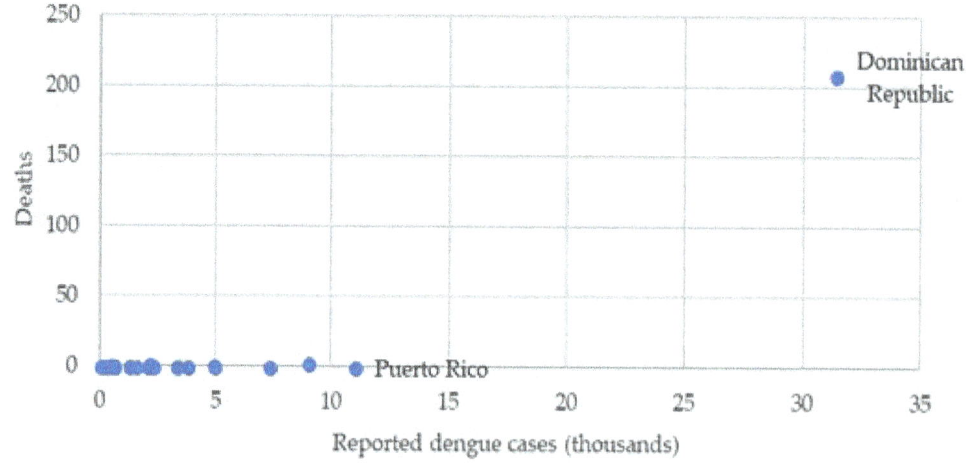

Figure 5. Dengue cases and mortality in the Caribbean territory (2014–2017). Source: PAHO. 2017.

found. Thus, we used the costs per patient estimated by Shepard [20] by extrapolating the results from other countries and considering the differences in purchasing power and income[4].

3. Materials and methods

To assess the economic cost of the disease, we used the results found for Brazil, Colombia, the Dominican Republic, and Mexico. To maintain cost structure homogeneity, we exploited the common methodological framework used in the literature, which is employed in the papers reviewed. There are three main cost categories used to quantify the economic burden of a disease: direct medical cost, direct non-medical cost, and indirect cost.

Direct medical cost comprises the cost borne by the healthcare unit (professional services, medical inputs, medical drugs, laboratory test). Additionally, direct non-medical cost corresponds to the value expended during a dengue episode and comprises food, lodging and travel expenses. Finally, indirect cost includes the productivity loss[5] (by patient and caregivers).

Even though the authors researched a common topic, there are some methodological differences that are worth noting to make a correct comparison between the results. In contrast to Mexico [17], Colombia [18] and Brazil [19] estimate the direct cost per patient grouping the medical and non-medical component in the same category, thus their figures could only be compared to the sum of medical and non-medical direct cost[6] from Mexico and Colombia.

Although the three studies present their results in dollars, nominal adjustment[7] was needed[8], for this we use the GDP deflator calculated by the World Bank for each country. Once the appropriate per patient is defined, the total number of reported dengue cases is required to estimate the total cost in each country; for this, we took the information reported by PAHO for

[4]More details about the methodology employed by the authors can be found in [20].

[5]Productivity loss corresponds to a monetary estimate of the days of work lost by the patient as well as caregivers.

[6]Direct non-medical costs include out-of-pocket expenses borne by the patient.

[7]Nominal adjustment accounts for price changes due to inflation between years. This adjustment allows for proper comparison between figures from different years.

[8]To nominally adjust the cost figures the GDP deflator was used for two different years (i, j).

$$GDP_{nominal,i} = \left(1 + \Delta\%_{real}^{i,j}\right) \times \left(1 + \Delta\%_{nominal}^{i,j}\right) \times GDP_{nominal,j}$$

$$GDP_{real,i} = \left(1 + \Delta\%_{real}^{i,j}\right) \times GDP_{real,j}$$

$$\Longrightarrow \frac{GDP_{nominal,i}}{GDP_{real,i}} = \left(1 + \Delta\%_{nominal}^{i,j}\right) \times \frac{GDP_{nominal,j}}{GDP_{real,j}}$$

$$\Longrightarrow \Delta\%_{nominal}^{i,j} = \frac{def_i}{def_j} - 1$$

$$def_i = \frac{GDP_{nominal,i}}{GDP_{real,i}}$$

the year 2015[9]. Considering potential lack of homogeneity among countries regarding laboratory confirmation practices and policies, we used total reported cases instead of laboratory confirmed cases for our analysis; we allow for this since reported dengue cases also received treatment and PAHO definition for reported cases only includes people "who has a fever or history of fever for 2-7 days duration, two or more symptoms of dengue and one serological test positive or epidemiological nexus with confirmed dengue case 14 days before onset of symptom." Even though using reported dengue cases, we are allowing for a potential overestimation of the economic burden, it is worth noting that by using DALY figures from WHO, we avoid this potential bias in the burden of the disease. It might also be noted that by using this approach, the results we found could be interpreted as an upper bound for the economic burden of the disease. To calculate the total treatment cost, we make the following assumption, and severe cases are considered to receive hospitalized treatment while nonsevere dengue cases[10] are considered to receive ambulatory treatment. From now on, we will refer only to ambulatory cases and hospitalized cases.

Total treatment cost was calculated for both ambulatory and hospitalized cases as presented in Eq. (1).

$$TC = AD \times PPC_{ambulatory} + HD \times PPC_{hospitalized} \tag{1}$$

where TC represents total cost, AD number of ambulatory dengue cases, HD number of hospitalized dengue cases, and PPC per patient cost.

$$PPC_i = DMC_i + DnMC_i + IC_i, \quad i \in \{ambulatory, hospitalized\} \tag{2}$$

where DMC represents direct medical cost, $DnMC$ direct non-medical cost and IMC indirect cost. In other words, the total cost of the disease is equal to the number of dengue cases times the cost per patient, for both ambulatory and hospitalized cases. The total treatment cost per patient corresponds to the sum of direct medical cost per patient, direct non-medical cost per patient and indirect cost per patient.

As estimates for the burden of the disease, measured as the number of Disability Adjusted Life Years (DALY)[11], we use the figures from the World Health Organization (WHO) for the year

[9] We considered the last published report that includes the information from the whole year. PAHO gathers epidemiological information from official reports made by the countries themselves. Thus, PAHO figures represent the official number of reported dengue cases, death and incidence. This mechanism has been working since 1980 and nowadays counts with systems of mandatory notification across the national territories.

[10] The number of ambulatory dengue cases is equal to the total number of reported cases minus the total number of hospitalized cases; both figures are used as reported by PAHO.

[11] According to WHO, one Disability Adjusted Life Years can be thought of as one lost year of "healthy" life. The sum of these DALYs across the population can be thought of as a measurement of the gap between current health status and an ideal health situation where the entire population lives to an advanced age, free of disease and disability and are calculated as the sum of the Years of Life Lost (YLL) due to premature mortality in the population and the Years Lost due to Disability (YLD) for people living with the health condition or its consequence.

2015; we preferred DALYs as measurement of the disease's burden because it allows to express numerically the burden of the disease as years based on a set of standard weights [21].

Additionally, to estimate the number of DALYs for 2017, which is presented in the discussion section, we used the following approach. Using the DALY estimates of WHO for 2015 and the number of cases of dengue reported by PAHO, we calculated the ratio of DALY per reported dengue case, which we then used to calculate the burden of the disease for 2017.

$$rDALY = \# \frac{DALY_{2015-WHO}}{\#Cases_{2015-PAHO}} \tag{3}$$

$$DALY_{2017} = rDALY \times \#Cases_{2017-PAHO} \tag{4}$$

This approach relies on one underlying assumptions, mortality rates do not change dramatically from 2015 to 2017[12]. It is noteworthy that following this approach, we benefit from the WHO information about DALY estimation parameters, reduce bias (noise) from lack of specific data needed to estimate the burden of the disease[13] and get highly comparable estimations from a homogeneous methodology.

4. Results

After nominally adjusting the figures, the cost per patient found by the authors for Brazil, Colombia, the Dominican Republic, and Mexico are shown in **Table 1**. Since the authors used the same cost structure in their estimation process, we can separate the total cost into their main categories (direct medical and non-medical cost and indirect cost). The figures are presented in 2017 prices, which allows for comparison. **Table 1** shows the total cost per patient disaggregated.

In the four countries reviewed, Mexico is the one with the most expensive treatment cost per patient in ambulatory care, even when their indirect cost is the lowest. For ambulatory cases, in contrast to Brazil, Colombia, and the Dominican Republic, the direct medical cost in Mexico is larger than the direct non-medical cost and the indirect cost (even when combined). For hospitalized cases, Mexico keeps having the most expensive treatment cost per patient, with direct costs that more than double the direct costs of the other countries.

The latter shows that Mexico has the most expensive dengue treatment per patient, regardless of the type of care (ambulatory US$ 501 or hospitalized US$ 1,475). On the other hand, the less expensive treatment for ambulatory (US$ 189) and hospitalized (US$ 488) cases would be in Brazil.

---

[12]We do not find this assumption to be particularly strong.

[13]Recalling the method used to estimate the total cost of the disease it is noteworthy that the latent risk of overestimation is not present in the estimation of the burden of the disease (DALY), as it is estimated by extrapolating the results of 2005 using the ratio of DALY per reported dengue case.

	Brazil	Colombia	The Dominican Republic	Mexico
Cost per ambulatory patient				
Direct medical	$70	$75	$75	$281
Direct non-medical		$33	$14	$102
Indirect	$119	$219	$136	$118
Total	$189	$327	$224	$501
Cost per hospitalized patient				
Direct medical	$258	$368	$366	$1,123
Direct non-medical		$59	$152	$193
Indirect	$230	$345	$366	$159
Total	$488	$771	$883	$1,475

Source: Martelli, et al. (2015) [19], Castro, et al. (2015) [18], Undurraga, et al. (2014) [17], Shepard, et al. (2011) [20]. Prices 2017.

Table 1. Treatment cost per patient by country (nominally adjusted 2017 dollars).

Since the number of cases presented in **Table 2** is not corrected by country-specific population, they cannot be directly compared between themselves; nevertheless, we can observe that more than half the total number of de dengue cases in the Americas in 2015 are located in Brazil (69.1%) and although the population of Brazil is less than twice the population of Mexico, its number of dengue cases exceeds twice the number dengue cases of the latter. This exhibits a concerning situation for the public health in Brazil. Once we controlled for the population of each country, we found that in 2015, the lowest incidence rate corresponds to the Dominican Republic and the highest to Brazil. Although the Dominican Republic has the lowest incidence rate, its mortality rate is much higher than that of the other countries.

Once we have defined the total number of dengue cases for each country and its corresponding treatment cost, it is possible to calculate the total cost following Eqs. (1) and (2). **Table 3** exhibits the total treatment cost for the year 2015 (in 2017 prices). In absolute terms, the highest economic cost corresponds to Brazil, which, as was shown before, has the less expensive treatment cost per patient, hence the extent of the total cost is mainly due to the high incidence

	Brazil	Colombia	The Dominican Republic	Mexico
Number of cases				
Ambulatory dengue	1,647,439	95,023	15,194	214,129
Hospitalized dengue	1,569	1,421	1,854	5,464
Deaths	863	155	107	42
Incidence per 10.000 inhabitants	80.6	20.0	17.1	18.1
Mortality rate (%)	0.05	0.16	0.63	0.02

Source: PAHO. 2015. Week 52. IMF.

Table 2. Number of cases, death and epidemiological by country (2015).

	Brazil	Colombia	The Dominican Republic	Mexico
Total ambulatory (US Dollars)	310,672,689	31,052,056	3,411,045	107,351,329
Total hospitalized (US Dollars)	766,211	1,096,202	1,637,140	8,060,036
Total cost (US Dollars)	**311,438,900**	**32,148,258**	**5,048,184**	**115,411,366**
Total DALY	**49,500**	**16,200**	**9,600**	**12,100**
Population	204,469,667	48,202,951	9,980,185	121,006,250
DALY per million inhabitants	**242**	**336**	**962**	**100**

Source: PAHO. 2015. Week 52. Martelli, et al. (2015) [19], Castro, et al. (2015) [18], Undurraga, et al. (2014) [17], Shepard, et al. (2011) [20]. Prices 2017.

Table 3. Total annual treatment cost and DALYs lost per million inhabitants by country (2015). 2017 dollars.

in the country. In terms of burden of the disease, measured as DALY, Brazil keep having the highest figures in absolute terms (49,500 DALYS), followed by Colombia (16,200 DALYS).

Having DALY in absolute terms does not allow for a proper comparison, therefore, we adjusted the results by dividing them by the country-specific population. Hence, we could express the burden of the disease as the number of DALY per million inhabitants, which is now perfectly comparable between countries. Now, Brazil is not the country with the highest burden relative to its population size, but the Dominican Republic (336 DALYS per million inhabitants), followed by Colombia, which remains in second place (962 DALYS per million inhabitants).

As well as adjusting the DALY by the population, it is also important to adjust the total treatment cost relative to some economic measure that allows to compare figures between countries in a proper manner. One alternative is to present the results as share of the total Gross Domestic Product (GDP) of each country, but this approach has two disadvantages. First, the resulting figures are too small, which by multiplying them by a factor makes the interpretation more difficult, and second, it does not consider GDP composition. Instead, we have used the total health expenditure estimated by the World Bank (WB) to adjust the total treatment cost. **Table 4** exhibits the total health expenditure by country in US billion dollars for 2015 (in 2017 prices).

Once adjusted, the total annual cost is very similar among countries. Notably, Colombia and Mexico spend nearly the same proportion (0.18%) of their health expenditure in dengue treatment, and Brazil has a lower share than the latter (0.16%). Given the country selection criteria used, one could assert that the average share of total cost caused by dengue treatment

	Brazil	Colombia	The Dominican Republic	Mexico
GDP (US Dollars billions)	2,142	297	67	1,093
Health expenditure (US Dollars billions)	191	18	4	64
Health expenditure (% of GDP)	8.9	6.2	6.2	5.9

Source: World Bank. IMF.

Table 4. Total health expenditure (2015). 2017 dollars.

in health expenditure in an epidemic year is 0.16% for the countries with the highest number of cases (**Table 5**). Although this result cannot be perfectly extrapolated to all the countries of the Americas, it could be interpreted as an upper bound for the size of the economic burden of dengue in the region.

Figure 6 shows the normalized treatment cost[14] and burden for each country. We can observe that while the Dominican Republic is the country with the highest number of DALY adjusted by population, it has the lowest cost per each DALY lost because of the disease. In contrast, Mexico has the highest cost per DALY lost, but the lowest number of DALY adjusted by population.

Finally, **Table 6** exhibits the 2015 total economic cost per DALY adjusted for purchasing power parity (PPP). There appears to be high variance in the total treatment cost, with its ranges from $1,157 in the case of the Dominican Republic to $17,703 for Mexico. It is noteworthy that Mexico, in relative terms, always presents the highest treatment cost. This result is consistent whether we analyze the total treatment cost per patient, the share of total annual cost over the total health expenditure or the total treatment per DALY adjusted for PPP.

	Brazil	Colombia	The Dominican Republic	Mexico
Total ambulatory (%)	0.16	0.17	0.08	0.17
Total hospitalized (%)	0.00	0.01	0.04	0.01
Total cost (%)	**0.16**	**0.18**	**0.12**	**0.18**

Source: PAHO. 2015. Week 52. Martelli, et al. (2015) [19], Castro, et al. (2015) [18], Undurraga, et al. (2014) [17], Shepard, et al. (2011) [20]. Prices 2017.

Table 5. Total annual treatment cost as share of the total health expenditure (2015).

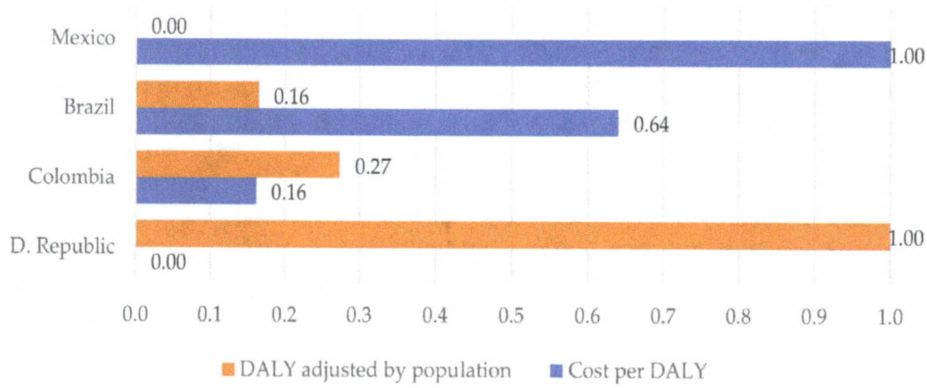

Figure 6. Normalized results. 2015. Source: PAHO. 2015. Week 52. Martelli, et al. (2015) [19], Castro, et al. (2015) [18], Undurraga, et al. (2014) [17], Shepard, et al. (2011) [20]. Prices 2017.

[14]Variable definition: level of current health expenditure expressed as a percentage of GDP. Estimates of current health expenditures include healthcare goods and services consumed during each year. This indicator does not include capital health expenditures such as buildings, machinery, innovation and technology and stocks of vaccines for emergency or outbreaks.

	Brazil	Colombia	The Dominican Republic	Mexico
Total ambulatory (PPP Dollars)	$11,190.5	$4,385.6	$782.0	$16,466.4
Total hospitalized (PPP Dollars)	$27.6	$154.8	$375.3	$1,236.3
Total cost (PPP Dollars)	**$11,218.1**	**$4,540.4**	**$1,157.3**	**$17,702.7**

Source: PAHO. 2015. Week 52. Martelli, et al. (2015) [19], Castro, et al. (2015) [18], Undurraga, et al. (2014) [17], Shepard, et al. (2011) [20]. Prices 2017.

Table 6. 2015 Total economic cost per DALY (2017 PPP dollars).

The variance in the results could be explained by the income gap between countries. If we consider the GDP per capital as proxy for the median income of each country, it makes sense that Mexico and Brazil have the highest cost per case and DALY since their GDP (US$ 9,033 and US$ 10,476 respectively) is close to 50% higher than the GDP per capita of Colombia and the Dominican Republic (US$ 6,161 and US$ 6,713 respectively).

5. Discussion

According to the review made by Shepard [22], who estimate the burden at a global scale for the year 2013, Latin-American and the Caribbean regions exhibit the highest treatment cost per case. From this perspective, our review presents the burden of the disease for the most affected countries, in terms of reported cases, of the region with the most expensive treatment cost. The latter is particularly relevant if we considered the estimates of the share of total treatment cost over the total health expenditure presented because our results could be interpreted as an upper bound for relative economic burden of dengue.

As mentioned before, in this section, we will discuss how the total treatment cost and the burden change in 2017, which we consider to be an inter-epidemic year given the low number of cases relative to previous years (2010–2017) (**Table 7**).

	Brazil	Colombia	The Dominican Republic	Mexico
Total ambulatory (US Dollars)	47,458,401	8,494,113	285,339	44,878,911
Total hospitalized (US Dollars)	184,593.94	220,629	77,707	553,169
Total treatment cost (US Dollars)	**47,642,995**	**8,714,742**	**363,046**	**45,432,079**
Total DALY	**7,599**	**2,481**	**259**	**7,554**
Population	207,680,999	49,293,878	10,172,243	123,517,856
DALY per 1 million inhabitants	**37**	**50**	**25**	**61**

Source: PAHO. 2017. Week 52. Martelli, et al. (2015) [19], Castro, et al. (2015) [18], Undurraga, et al. (2014) [17], Shepard, et al. (2011) [20]. Prices 2017.

Table 7. 2017 Economic and DALY lost per million inhabitants by country (2017 dollars).

To estimate the total number of DALY for the year 2017, we calculated the ratio between dengue cases and DALY for 2015 with the WHO and PAHO figures and extrapolate the results as discussed in section "Materials and methods." Population has been updated too, to correspond to the year 2017. DALY adjusted for population present a dramatic decline of 76.53% in average due to the decrease in total number of dengue cases. Additionally, the total treatment cost of the disease decreased 77.8% in average (from 2015 to 2017), being Dominica Republic the country with the highest reduction rate (92.8%). It is worth saying that the change in the figures is closely tied to the change in the number of dengue cases since the cost per patient remained the same (**Table 8**).[15]

As result of the decline in the number dengue cases in 2017, the share of the total costs decreased to almost a fifth of the share in 2015 (**Figure 7**).

	Brazil	Colombia	The Dominican Republic	Mexico
GDP (US Dollars billions)	2,081	307	75	1,142
Health expenditure (% of GDP)	8.9	6.2	6.2	5.9
Health expenditure (US Dollars billions)	185	19	5	67
Total ambulatory (%)	0.03%	0.04%	0.01%	0.07%
Total hospitalized (%)	0.00%	0.00%	0.00%	0.00%
Total cost (%)	**0.03%**	**0.05%**	**0.01%**	**0.07%**

Source: PAHO. 2017. Week 52. Martelli, et al. (2015) [19], Castro, et al. (2015) [18], Undurraga, et al. (2014) [17], Shepard, et al. (2011) [20]. Prices 2017.

Table 8. Total health expenditure and 2017 total economic cost as share of the total health expenditure (2017 dollars).

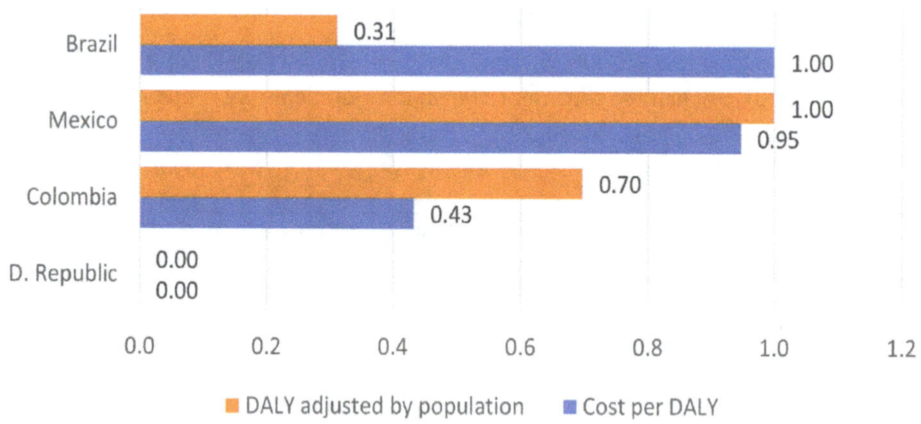

Figure 7. Normalized results. 2017. Source: PAHO. 2017. Week 52. Martelli, et al. (2015) [19], Castro, et al. (2015) [18], Undurraga, et al. (2014) [17], Shepard, et al. (2011) [20]. Prices 2017.

[15] Cost per patient do not vary since they are expressed in 2017 dollar are correspond to the figures obtained in the respective studies reviewed.

Normalized results for 2017 show that, in contrast to 2015, the Dominican Republic exhibits both the lowest total treatment cost per DALY and DALY per million of inhabitants, which suggest an improvement for the Caribbean country, especially considering the noneconomic burden. On the other hand, Mexico went from having the lowest number of DALY adjusted for population to having one of the highest.

One important limitation about this review and potentially other burden analyses is the accuracy of the epidemiological information. As the number of total dengue cases, severe and non-severe, corresponds to reported cases, one cannot assume that they correspond to the effective number of cases. Reported (or febrile) cases can overestimate the total actual burden of the disease. On the other hand, one should consider that by using laboratory confirmed cases, bias in the other direction is introduced, since not only that figure would be affected by laboratory confirmation policies and practices but also by underreport. After reviewing the latter, we decided to use reported cases and allow for potential overestimation in the economic burden. Thus, our results should be considered as upper bound estimates of the economic burden[16] and not completely accurate figures.

The results found have three interesting implications for further studies and reviews. Economic burden of dengue should follow a structured costing framing, which allows for proper comparison between results and better estimation of treatment cost per case. The data and sources used in this chapter could serve as inputs in future cost-effectiveness analysis (CEA); once economic cost per cases has been covered, the remaining element to conduct a CEA would be the approximate reduction in dengue cases due to the use of a prevention technology. Finally, the similar results in terms of relative economic burden suggest that 0.16%[17] could be interpreted as an upper bound of the total treatment cost of dengue as share of total health expenditure.

Author details

Raúl Castro Rodríguez*, Jorge Armando Rueda-Gallardo and Manuel Felipe Avella-Niño

*Address all correspondence to: rcastro@uniandes.edu.co

Department of Economics, Universidad de los Andes, Bogotá D.C., Colombia

References

[1] Martín J, Brathwaite O, Zambrano B, Solórzano J, Bouckenooghe A, Dayan G, Guzman M. The Epidemiology of Dengue in the Americas over the last Three Decades: a Worrisome Reality. The American Journal of Tropical Medicine and Hygiene. 2010;**82**(1):128-135

[16] Burden measured as DALY is not affected by overestimation since WHO figures are used.

[17] 0.16% is the mean share for the four countries reviewed during a period of high incidence in the region with the most expensive treatment cost per case.

[2] Suaya J, Shepard D, Siqueira J, Martelli C, Lum L, Huat Tan L, Kongsin S, Jiamton S, Garrido F, Montoya R, Armien B, Huy R, Castillo L, Caram M, Sah B, Sughayyar R. Cost of Dengue Cases in Eight Countries in the Americas and Asia: A Prospective Study. The American Jounal of Tropical Medicine and Hygiene. 2009;**80**(5):846-855

[3] World Health Organization. Dengue Guidelines for Diagnosis, Treatment, Prevention and Control. World Health Organization; 2009

[4] Gubler D. Epidemin dengue/dengue hemorrhagic fever as a public health, social and economic problem in the 21st century. TREND in Microbiology. 2002;**10**(2):100-103

[5] Fernández-Salas I, Danis-Lozano R, Casas-Martínez M, Ulloa A, Guillermo J, Teresa CF, Ordóñez E, Quiroga A, Torres-Monzón JA, González D, Esteban E. Historical inability to control Aedes aegypti as a main contributor of fast dispersal of chikungunya outbreaks in Latin America. Antiviral Research. 2015;**124**:30-42

[6] Naish S, Dale P, Mackensie J, McBride J, Mengersen K, Tong S. Climate change and dengue: a critical and systematic review of quantitative modelling approaches. BMC Infectious Diseases. 2014;**14**(167)

[7] Ebi KL, Nealon J. Dengue in a changing climate. Environmental Research. 2016

[8] Sabchareon A, Wallace D, Sirivichayakul C, Limkittikul K, Chanthavanich P, Jiwaiyavej V, Dulyachai W, Pngsaa K, Wartel A, Moueau A, Saville M, Bouckenooghe A, Viviani S. Protective Efficacy of the Recombinant, Live-Attenuated, CYD Tetravalent Dengue Vaccine in Thai schoolchildren: a Randomised, Controlled Phase 2b Trial. The Lancet. 2012; **380**(9853):1559-1567

[9] Villar L, Dayan G, Arredondo-García J, Rivera D, Cunha R, Deseda C, Reynales H, Costa M, Morales-Ramíez J, Carrasquilla G, Rey L, Dietze, Reynaldo. Efficacy of a Tetravalent Dengue Vaccine in Children in Latin America. The New England Journal of Medicine. 2015;**372**:113-123

[10] Carrasco L, Lee L, Lee V, Eong E, Shepard D, Thein T, Gan V, Cook A, Lye D, Ng LC, Leo YS. Economic Impact of Dengue Illness and the Cost-Effectiveness of Future Vaccination Programs in Singapore. PLOS Negleted Tropical Diseases. 2011;**5**(12)

[11] Halstead. Dengue vaccine development: a 75% solution? The Lancet. 2012;**380**(9853): 1535-1536

[12] WHO. Cost-effectiveness analysis for health interventions. World Health organization; 2018. [Online]. Available: http://www.who.int/heli/economics/costeffanalysis/en/. [Accessed June 15, 2018]

[13] Beatty M, Beutels P, Meltzer M, Shepard D, Hombach J, Hutubessy R, Dessis D, Coudeville L, Dervaux B, Wichmann O, Margolis H, Kuritsky J. Health Economics of Dengue: A Systematic Literatue Review and Expert Panel's Assessment. American Journal of Tropical Medicine and Hygiene. 2011;**84**(3):473-488

[14] Hotez P, Bottazzi M, Franco-Paredes C, Ault S, Peiago M. The Neglected Tropical Diseases of Latin America and the Caribbean: A Review of Disease Burden and Distribution and a Roadmap for Control and Elimination. PLOS Negleted Tropical Diseases. 2008;**2**(9):1-11

[15] Castro Rodríguez R, Carrasquilla G, Porras A, Galera-Gelvez K, Lopez J, Rueda-Gallardo JA. The Burden of Dengue and the Financial Cost to Colombia, 2010–2012. The American Journal of Tropical Medicine and Hygiene. 2016;**94**(5):1065-1072

[16] Tapia-Conyer R, Méndez-Galván J, Gallardo-Rincón, Héctor. The growing burden of dengue in Latin America. Journal of Clinical Virology. 2009;**46**

[17] Undurraga E, Betancourt-Cravioto M, Ramos-Castañeda J, Martínez-Vega R, Méndez-Galván J, Gubler D, Guzmán M, Halstead S, Harris E, Kuri-Morales P, Tapia-Conyer R. Economic and Disease Burden of Dengue in Mexico. PLoS Neglected Tropical Diseases. 2015;**9**(3):1-26

[18] Castro Rodríguez R, Galera-Gelvez K, López Yescas JG, Rueda-Gallardo J. Costs of Dengue to the Health System and Individuals in Colombia from 2010 to 2012. The American Journal of Tropical Medicine and Hygiene. 2015;**92**(4):709-714

[19] Turchi Martelli C, Junior J, Parente M, Amancio A, Oliveira C, Braga C, Pimenta F, Cortes F, Lopez J, Bahia L, Mendes M, Machado M, Filha N, Constenla D, Vierira W. Economic Impact of Dengue: Multicenter Study Across Four Brazilian regions. PLoS Neglected Tropical Diseases. 2015;**9**(9):1-19

[20] Shepard D, Coudeville L, Halasa Y, Zambrano B, Dayan G. Economic Impact of Dengue Illness in the Americas. The American Journal of Tropical Medicine and Hygiene. 2011; **84**(2):200-2007

[21] Sassi F. Calculating QALYs, comparing QALY and DALY calculations. Health Policy and Planning. 2006

[22] Shepard D, Undurraga E, Halasa Y, Stanaway J. The global economic burden of dengue: a systematic analysis. Lancet. 2016

9

Urban Ecology and the Effectiveness of *Aedes* Control

Wladimir J. Alonso and Benjamin J.J. McCormick

This study is dedicated to the memory of the researcher, colleague and friend Ellis Mackenzie.

Abstract

Past initiatives to control *Aedes* mosquitoes were successful, in part because they implemented draconian top-down control programs. To achieve similar results now, explicit recognition of the complexity in urban ecologies in terms of land ownership, law enforcement and accessibility for control interventions are required. By combining these attributes, four classes of spaces, along with corresponding control strategies, are suggested to better target *Aedes* species population control efforts. On one end of the spectrum there are accessible and accountable spaces (e.g. backyards and closely managed public facilities), where interventions can rely predominantly on bottom-up strategies with the local population playing the principle role in the implementation of actions, but with government coordination. On the other end of the spectrum are inaccessible and unaccountable spaces, which require top-down and extensive approaches. By identifying these and the intermediate classes of space, government and private resources can be allocated in a more efficient customized manner. Based on this new framework, a set of actions is proposed that might be implemented in dengue and other *Aedes*-borne crises. The framework considers existing limitations and opportunities associated with modern societies–which are fundamentally different from those associated with the successful control of *Aedes* species in the past.

Keywords: *Aedes*, mosquitoes control, prevention, dengue, community action, urban health, policy

1. Introduction

Urban pest species are highly effective and opportunistic in their use of the physical, legal and administrative interstices of the landscape we inhabit, and *Aedes* mosquitoes are a case in point. Any inaccessible nook or cranny, any vacant land or neglected facility permits adult mosquitoes to hide and, in as little water as might accumulate in the lid of a bottle, find ideal breeding places. *Aedes* mosquitoes take advantage of the heterogeneous urban ecologies through "skip oviposition," laying a few eggs, spread across the largest possible number of sites. It is an especially well suited strategy for urban environments with abundant, but sparse and even temporary breeding sites [1].

The control of *Aedes* mosquitoes is failing in most tropical regions [1–3], and human diseases transmitted by this vector, like dengue, chikungunya, yellow fever and Zika, are among the top public health priorities [4, 5]. The strategies for suppressing mosquito populations below a threshold at which they no longer support viral amplification [6–10] has focused on two strategies [7, 11, 12]: (a) negating larval development opportunities by eliminating breeding places and the sites of immature stages; and (b) killing adults by fumigation with insecticides. More recently biomolecular and biogenetic approaches have also been suggested, although their effectiveness under field conditions are uncertain [13, 14]. Therefore new approaches are urgently needed, especially in urban landscapes [15].

Here we propose that an important strategic aspect that is currently overlooked in *Aedes* control programs: recognition of the complexity of urban ecologies in terms of land ownership, enforcement and accessibility for control interventions. We suggest that a systematic strategy that accounts for this physical complexity is essential to best implement *Aedes* control.

2. Physical and legal accessibility for control purposes

In the current absence of safe and economically sustainable methods to sterilize or kill whole populations of adult mosquitoes, and especially ones that might be deployed on a scale and speed required to impact an epidemic, control over potential breeding and resting sites (PBRP) continues to play a pivotal role in the strategies against *Aedes*.

We suggest tackling this challenge by framing it based on these two variables that are especially relevant to the control of PBRPs: accessibility and accountability. The first relates to how easily breeding sites can be accessed for cleaning and intervention purposes. Although most PBRPs can be readily managed by private citizens (e.g., plant pots, fountains, household refuse and sidewalks), some are physically difficulty to locate or access for control purposes (e.g., roof gutters, cracks in houses or water-containing holes in trees). The second factor relates to how the stewardship of land is distributed between individuals, companies or the state. Even though all PBRPs are, in theory, under some legal responsibility (private residence, public buildings and tended public spaces), neglected public spaces (particularly in developing nations) and areas with uncertain ownership are under *de facto* diffuse or a non-accountable authority and frequently result in a state of abandonment (e.g. vacant lands, neglected public parks, open sewage).

The interaction between these physical and legal factors yields an actionable categorization of areas for vector control (**Figure 1**) that goes beyond the traditional system of "domestic, peridomestic and public spaces" [16], which is limited to types of habitat. The framework

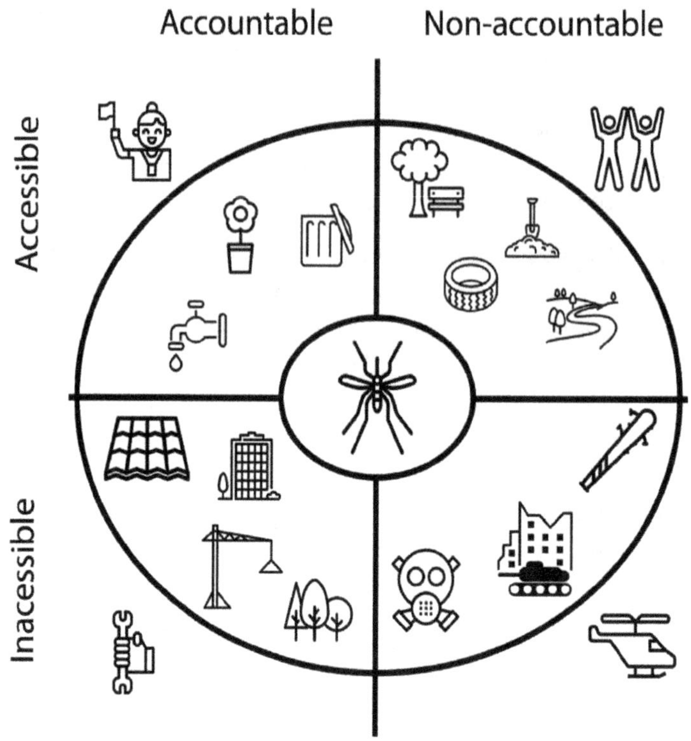

Figure 1. Strategy of societal organization of interventions against *Aedes* species based on the physical and legal accessibility of the space where the mosquito can be eliminated. The concentric rings contain: (i) the threat (*Aedes* mosquitoes), (ii) putative breeding and resting places (PBRP) of *Aedes* mosquitoes based on ownership accountability and physical accessibility, (iii) intervention that would be needed (clockwise, starting from upper-left: Individual citizens, community involvement, governmental direct action, professional assistance) (icon sources: Icons made by Becris, mynamepong, Smashicons, Good Ware, Revicon, Zlatko Najdenovski, Nikita Golubev and Freepik from www.flaticon.com).

proposed in **Figure 1** distinguishes societal actors (individuals, communities, government) who can be engaged in and held responsible for *Aedes* management. This classification, detailed below, enables both the identification of optimal allocation of private and public responsibilities in each case, but also defines the most suitable set of strategies:

(A) Easily accessible & accountable PBRPs. In areas that are both easily accessed and under accountable stewardship, for example, occupied private dwellings, or public facilities under effective management, we propose that the private individuals within the premises are engaged and mobilized. Plates under potted plants, water tanks, garden fountains, birdbaths, water bowls for pets, laundry tubs, toys, swimming pools, cisterns, ponds, etc. can be directly managed by individuals either by draining out the water or filling with sand to prevent adults laying eggs. Current WHO recommendations [17, 18] already charge private individuals with management of PBRPs within 100 m of their homes, which is likely to capture the majority of *Aedes aegypti* PBRPs [19, 20], and places of public congregation. However we would suggest this be expanded to all owners of accessible spaces with the active encouragement and support of government agencies (an interesting example is the "domestic trap strategy"; **Box 1**). Such activities are likely to be regular, for example putting out garbage, or infrequent, for example putting lids on water containers, but are seldom labor intensive, assuming changes in routine behavior. Ironically, some urban areas may be more accountable to individuals than municipal authorities as facilities (such as piped water or sewerage) fail to keep pace with urban spread [21, 22].

BOX 1. Domestic traps: Crowdsourcing Aedes elimination.
Controlling domestic pests like cockroaches, fleas, flies or ants depends on denying them basic resources (e.g., exposed food and breeding places). However, more radical measures are often needed, and traps are a popular choice, not only due to their effectiveness, but also because they (as opposed to chemical sprays) present less danger to humans and pets. The use of mosquito traps domestically is, however, not simple. For example, blood-feeding traps are not practical, as they can hardly compete with mosquitoes' attraction towards human bodies. Similarly, nectar-feeding based traps have no specificity, and would kill many insects (including bees and butterflies). Breeding traps, although potentially effective, are perceived as dangerous if not well implemented or supervised could promote the multiplication of mosquitoes.

Domestic breeding traps that eliminate the aquatic stages of mosquitoes hold great potential if their hazardous implementation can be eliminated. One way to attempt to bias oviposition to more manageable sites is the use of domestic traps that can be readily managed through regular reminders, once a week, for volunteer households and public facility managers who are charged with cleaning out the water in containers functioning as PBRPs [23–25].

The domestic trap strategy (which would be greatly beneficial to the *Mosquito Drain;* **Box 2**) is gaining impetus with the invention of an ingenious house-made trap made with widely available and affordable components (**Figure 2**, an empty PET bottle, adhesive tape and few square centimeters of mesh fabric source). When the eggs hatch in the cone, the larvae migrate to the bottom of the trap through the mesh, but this same mesh prevents adult mosquitoes from leaving the trap. The "mosquitérica," as it is known, presents several advantages over other domestic trap methods. First, it eliminates the concern about occasional negligence in the periodic need to cleaning up and/or adding larvicide to breeding traps. Second, it is unlikely that mosquitoes would develop resistance to this sort of trap –as opposed to chemical spray or even traps that use larvicide (as in the latter case mosquitoes could avoid surfaces or breeding places based on the odors of those substances). And third, it has been shown that egg-laying females are most attracted to sites containing other immature *Ae. aegypti* [9] – something this trap offers, since only the hatching adults are killed (by entrapment). Instructions for building such traps went viral in social networks, and it is having wide acceptance among the population.

This crowdsourcing method of mosquito elimination could be promoted by governments through, for instance, calls for co-ordinated action on a fixed date (e.g. mosquito eradication day [26]). Setting a weekly reminder during the epidemic season would be epidemiologically sound, as it is more frequent than the time of larval development (approximately 8–10 days), hence ideal for cleaning plant pots, water fountains, etc. Concerted action propelled by an official reminder (mainly in TV and social media) could create a collective drive and a positive sense of societal engagement–a study of community-based *Aedes* control showed, the most prominent benefit was the satisfaction created by 'working together' [27].

(B) Difficult to access, but accountable PBRP sites. Despite the best efforts of conscientious individuals, it can be difficult to eliminate all breeding places that can be hidden in corners of the urban landscape such as building cracks, roof gutters, crevices in the high trees canopy and slabs [1]. Both private and public agents who find such situations should be encouraged to request professional assistance. Legislation can also be used to improve building practices to

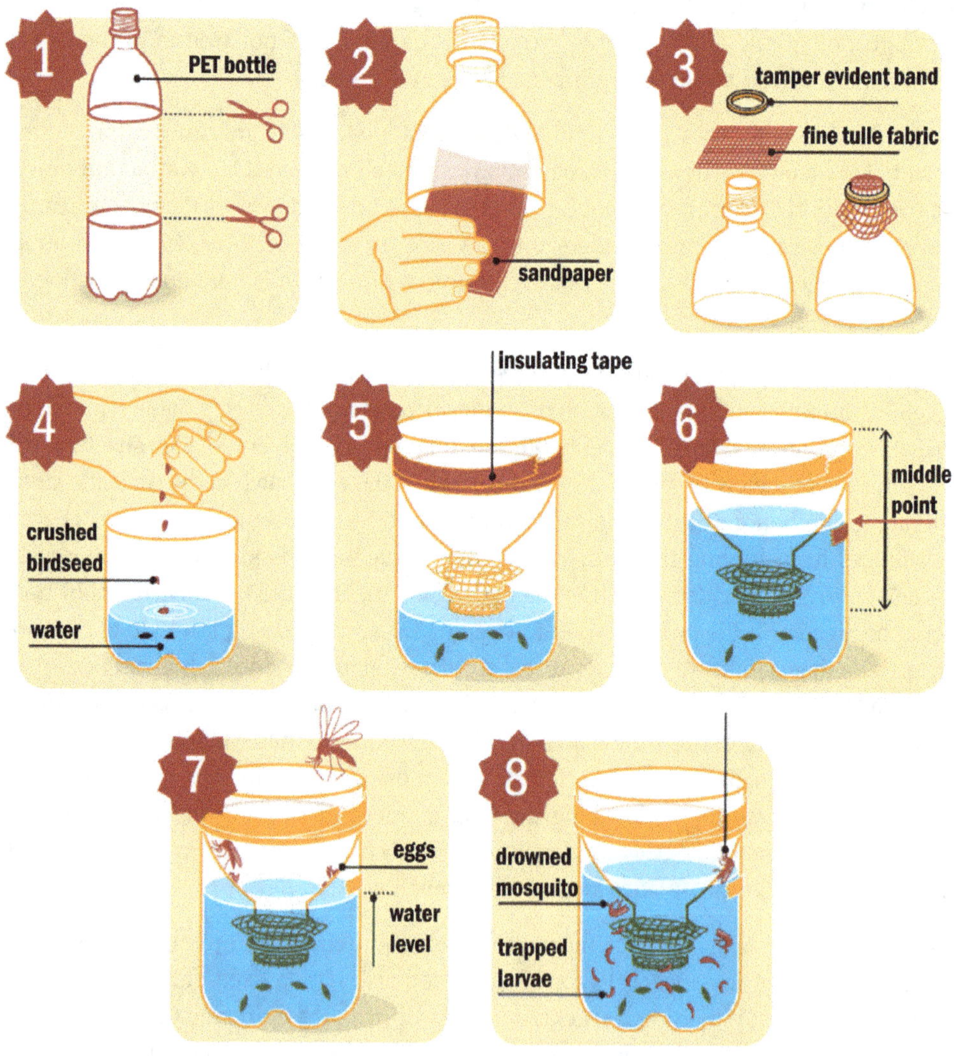

Figure 2. The mosquitérica, a simple larval trap that can be fashioned from common household products (reproduced and translated with permission from UOL, Brazil).

reduce PBRPs with difficult access [28], for example, encouraging architects to eliminate open gutters that are hard to access [29]. However, the inevitable existence of those PBRPs almost ubiquitously demand interventions that are applied in a "diffuse way", such as "peri-focal" interventions with residual insecticides [1], release of sterile adult mosquitoes or strategies involving multiple traps ("Mosquito Drain"; **Box 2**).

Box 2. Mosquito drain.

The *Mosquito Drain* is based on the idea of attracting females to ubiquitous oviposition places where larvae can be eliminated (e.g. domestic breeding traps, see **Box 1**) rather than natural, but inaccessible sites thereby eliminating the next generation of mosquitoes.

In an urban environment, some breeding and resting sites are likely to be inaccessible for cleaning and control (e.g., roofs, crevices, tree holes, etc.; **Figure 1**). However, not all potential breeding places are equally attractive to laying mosquitoes and "compete" for females' preference. Removal of accessible breeding sites would have the following effects on female mosquitoes in search for oviposition sites:

1. impel females to search for alternative potential breeding places;
2. impel females to over-disperse [30, 31] (so infected mosquitoes will cover an area quicker)
3. reduce the quality of potential breeding places sought by females (potential reduction -but not elimination- of viable broods).

Because "egg-laying females were most attracted to sites containing other immature *Aedes*, rather than to sites containing the most food" [9], home traps could become especially attractive to gravid females, and therefore be disproportionally important in reducing the mosquito population. Alternatively, attractants can be added to encourage mosquitoes to preferentially use lethal ovitraps that can be managed or left to biodegrade rather than inaccessible natural PBRPs [32–34]. The *Mosquito Drain* posits that it is not necessary to eliminate all breeding sites to cause the population to crash, which would not be practicable anyway, but that by (i) removing manageable breeding sites (e.g. putting lids on water containers), (ii) providing alternative attractive breeding sites that are easily managed (e.g. 'lure' breeding adults with a suitable trap) and that (iii) kill future generations of mosquitoes (e.g. adding larvicide to ovitraps) would eliminate sufficient reproductive capability of the mosquito population as to drive the population to extinction or at least pushing the biting population below levels at which virus circulation is sustained.

This is a societal effort that depends on collaboration between (many) individuals and government agencies: individuals would be in charge of eliminating any larvae, pupae and/or eggs that could have been accumulated in domestic breeding places (like plant pots and fountains) whilst governments should broadcast a reminder and coordinate that effort. Government agencies would then be freed to tackle hard to access and public spaces.

(C) Accessible, but non-accountable PBRP sites. Neglected public spaces with rubble, trash (tires, cups, cans, plastic bags and discarded containers) and facilities in neglected public spaces and vacant lands or empty lots are accessible to individuals without special knowledge or expertise. Volunteers from the neighborhood (e.g. coordinated by the community), could engaged, and perhaps incentivized, by government or emerging from social media networks in clean-up campaigns where, periodically, debris is removed, trash cleaned, ditches on the ground sealed, and other sensible interventions that destroy and negate breeding sites for *Aedes* performed. A survey in Singapore found that vacant properties and construction sites (the latter more appropriately belonging to accountable sites) had a four to seven times higher premises index than landed premises (which were three and a half times higher than apartments) [19, 35].

(D) Difficult to access and non-accountable sites. A comprehensive strategy that accounts for the whole gamut of access for mosquito control measures cannot ignore that there are patches where the capability of the government to influence behavior, enforce the law, or simply access places can provide major challenges - for example due to violent conflict. In those circumstances, top-down interventions (fogging, aerial fumigation, biological control and release of biologically modified Aedes males [7, 11, 36]) may be the only strategies that can promote vector control. We need to be caution about these approaches though, as these specialized and expensive activities offer diffuse control efforts that target adult mosquitoes rather than destroy PBRPs have a long history of use, but little recent evidence for effectiveness in reducing disease burden [37]. Restricting their use to epidemics is recommended because of cost and environmental impact [17].

3. A comprehensive approach for engaging society

Mosquito control depends on human actions, yet those actions are often at the mercy of legal and physical constraints. Dissecting the legal and physical complexity of contemporary urban ecosystems results in a categorization that can assist the effective implementation of interventions. These categories – based on the diversity of putative oviposition and resting sites – can be easily integrated into existing habitat management behaviors, and can be readily integrated into GIS mapping technologies to generate actionable information to tackle endemic infestations and unfolding outbreaks [29, 38].

One principle reason for successful control in the past century was the implementation of aggressive top-down measures [8, 12, 39]. The erosion of governmental capabilities to interfere with individual liberties does not necessarily impede mosquito control, as that "loss" may be compensated by an increasingly technologically-savvy, knowledge-avid and social media linked population can be mobilized to combat mosquito populations [40–42]. The proposed framework assumes that it is possible to effectively engage the local population [7], not only by suppressing areas of infection where they can easily act (e.g. their properties), but also by collaborating in a forcing a "Mosquito Drain" (**Box 2**) to reach beyond their immediate domain of direct impact.

Prioritizing citizens' actions has several potential benefits: (a) reduced strain on limited public resources that are stretched during public health crises (e.g. epidemics); (b) individuals can act on more targeted and sustained activities [43]; (c) reduction of harmful interventions (e.g. use of fogging in urban spaces that can be practically managed by community initiatives). The local population is also most likely to recognize hotspots of mosquitoes [41, 44, 45] and appreciate local conditions of epidemiological importance [18]. Although evidence for effectiveness of individual community-based interventions is sparse [37], it appears that integrating community participation into schemes reduces costs and increases effectiveness [46–48].

Engaging populations need not be costly (in time or money) given new communication technologies [40] (**Figure 3**) and, by stimulating and coordinating positive bottom-up initiatives, health agencies can co-opt allies in collective health emergencies [49]. In contrast, top-down approaches to combat Aedes risk treating citizens like irresponsible actors (for example threatening fines [35, 39]) fail to realize the emergent benefits of community participation. Emphasizing the power of bottom-up initiatives is not meant to marginalize the role of top-down activities [7, 8, 12]: as shown in our categorization (**Figure 1**), even the most engaged community will not be able to manage all putative mosquitoes breeding sites. Public authorities have an immense role to play, but are perhaps more efficient exercising their mandate in the expensive activities of avoiding a state of neglect in public spaces that risks them becoming the foci of urban pests and then efficiently using a smaller budget to encourage and support societal initiatives (e.g. nudging behavioral change [52]) to address readily accessible environments that would otherwise rapidly drain central resources.

The challenge is also to effectively manage activities, whether top-down or bottom-up that risk being popular, but ill conceived. The WHO emphasizes detailed planning to achieve successful behavioral change and recommend a series of steps to capitalize on public engagement to avoid what they consider the two greatest barriers of doing nothing or, perhaps worse, doing the wrong thing (hence putting people off further interventions if their efforts fail) [50]. In addition to combating lack of knowledge or misinformation, governmental activities need to manage social engagement campaigns beyond planning and into co-ordination since such campaigns to change behaviors have been most successful when combined with feedback

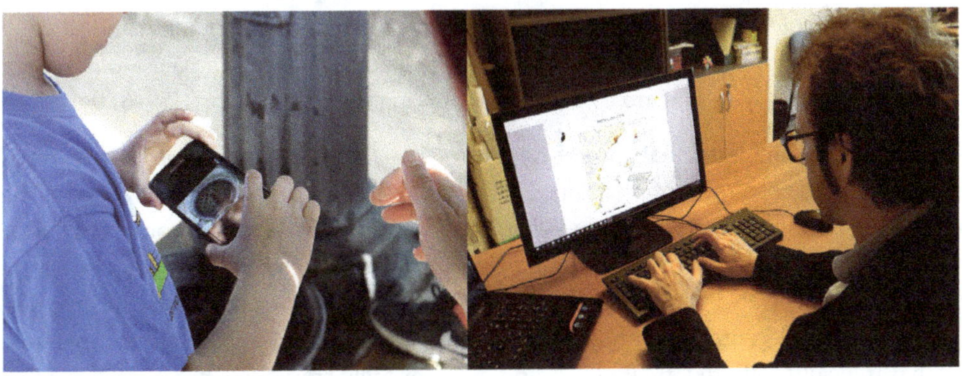

Figure 3. Interface from a citizen-science mosquito identification and reporting application used in Spain to assist in the surveillance efforts. Provided by mosquito alert CC-BY [41].

and regular reminders [39, 51]–for example to clean out water containers, mosquito traps or remove refuse each week [17]. Over reliance on past success risks mosquito populations rebounding, for example because surveillance priorities shift and vigilance suffers [35].

The key challenge in community participation is sustaining interest. As an example of citizen engagement in action, in two Cuban cities house blocks were randomly enrolled in a trial to control PBRPs (2000–2002), resulting in 75% reduction in *Aedes* populations through adding lids to water containers (*i.e.* monitoring accessible and accountable), repairing drains and transforming areas of garbage into (maintained) flowerbeds (*i.e.* accessible but not necessarily accountable) [53]. Importantly, these neighborhood task forces were still in operation 5 years later when there was an outbreak of dengue and proved cost and health effective [43, 47, 48]. However this sustainability may be unusual with evidence from other studies suggest that success may lead to changes in focus that risk lapses in effort [35], volunteers lose enthusiasm [22] and that adherence to control measures diminishes over time (though still out-perform no activity) [54, 55], more so if initiatives (and official cajoling) end [21]. Evidence of citizen science mosquito surveillance suggests good initial participation that rapidly decreased [41], and the few studies that evaluate the effectiveness of community interventions, whilst generally positive for vector control, lasted a year of less [55, 56]. Encouraging appropriate community participation in control measures is likely to be easier in the midst of epidemics when the benefits are visible, but it remains unclear whether this is sustainable in the longer-term in between episodes of, for example, dengue. That is why it is so important that control measures are "cross-cutting" within the context of a community, as we will see below.

4. Transforming cities in a large mosquito trap while improving their livability

Aedes-transmitted diseases are, largely, diseases emanating from neglected private and social spaces [57]. In backyards, buildings, vacant lands and empty lots, trash and untended structures provide perfect breeding places not only for *Aedes* mosquitoes, but also for many other urban and domestic pests. These neglected places have a negative impact on the environment and quality of life of the community, as well as on their economic development and safety [58]. Therefore, a campaign to remove mosquito breeding places is also a campaign to reinvigorate depressed or unplanned urban areas, thereby improving living conditions [59–61].

It is important to highlight that mosquito control has to be integrated into "cross-cutting" solutions for public health, turning societal vulnerabilities into resilience [61, 62] – i.e. what is good for elimination of *Aedes*, should also be beneficial on other societal fronts. For instance, environmental management of *Aedes* might discourage traditional *ad hoc* water storage practices such as private water-storage systems [16, 28]. But resilience to crises and catastrophes are enhanced through decentralized and resource-autonomous societies [63], for example potable water that is locally collected, treated [64] and appropriately stored (so that it is inaccessible to mosquitoes) would still be available even if the water supply from a centralized provider is unavailable, disrupted or fails.

5. Conclusion

The impact of *Aedes* mosquitoes on human health and the prospect of losing the battle against this species requires urgent and scientifically sound strategies [6, 7]. Here, we propose an adaptation to existing recommendations to rationalize, catalyze and coordinate the capabilities of modern society. More responsible societal co-ordination and allocation of limited resources based on existing accountability and physical accessibility can more effectively eliminate these deadly foes, but as a fortuitous by-product presents an opportunity to additionally improve the quality of life by improving the livability, cleanliness and beauty of shared social spaces.

Acknowledgements

We are grateful to the support of the Fogarty International Center and the helpful comments of Drs. Paul Reiter, Oliver Brady, Ellis Mackenzie, Joshua Rosenthal, Gerardo Ulibarri, Yifen Liu and Prof. Chwan-Chuen King. The findings and conclusions in this report are those of the authors and do not necessarily represent the official position of the U.S. National Institutes of Health, Department of Health and Human Services, Department of Genetics and Evolutionary Biology or University of São Paulo.

Author details

Wladimir J. Alonso[1]* and Benjamin J.J. McCormick[2]

*Address all correspondence to: wladimir.j.alonso@wolfson.oxon.org

1 Laboratory for Human Evolutionary and Ecological Studies, Department of Genetics and Evolutionary Biology, University of São Paulo, Brazil

2 Fogarty International Center, National Institutes of Health, Bethesda, MD, USA

References

[1] Reiter P. Control of urban Zika vectors: Should we return to the successful PAHO/WHO strategy? PLoS Neglected Tropical Diseases. 2016;**10**:e0004769. DOI: 10.1371/journal.pntd.0004769

[2] Gubler DJ. Prevention and control of Aedes aegypti-borne diseases: Lesson learned from past successes and failures. Asia-Pacific Journal of Molecular Biology and Biotechnology. 19th ed. 2011:111-114

[3] Reiner RC Jr, Achee N, Barrera R, Burkot TR, Chadee DD, Devine GJ, et al. Quantifying the epidemiological impact of vector control on dengue. PLoS Neglected Tropical Diseases. 2016;**10**:e0004588. DOI: 10.1371/journal.pntd.0004588

[4] Bhatt S, Gething PW, Brady OJ, Messina JP, Farlow AW, Moyes CL, et al. The global distribution and burden of dengue. Nature. 2013;**496**:504-507. DOI: 10.1038/nature12060

[5] Paixão ES, Teixeira MG, Rodrigues LC. Zika, chikungunya and dengue: The causes and threats of new and re-emerging arboviral diseases. BMJ Global Health. 2018;**3**:e000530. http://dx.doi.org/10.1136/bmjgh-2017-000530

[6] Achee NL, Gould F, Perkins TA, RCR J, Morrison AC, Ritchie SA, et al. A critical assessment of vector control for dengue prevention. PLoS Neglected Tropical Diseases. 2015;**9**: e0003655. DOI: 10.1371/journal.pntd.0003655

[7] Erlanger TE, Keiser J, Utzinger J. Effect of dengue vector control interventions on entomological parameters in developing countries: A systematic review and meta-analysis. Medical and Veterinary Entomology. 2008;**22**:203-221. DOI: 10.1111/j.1365-2915.2008.00740.x

[8] Morrison AC, Zielinski-Gutierrez E, Scott TW, Rosenberg R. Defining challenges and proposing solutions for control of the virus vector *Aedes aegypti*. PLoS Medicine. 2008;**5**: e68. DOI: 10.1371/journal.pmed.0050068

[9] Wong J, Stoddard ST, Astete H, Morrison AC, Scott TW. Oviposition site selection by the dengue vector Aedes aegypti and its implications for dengue control. PLoS Neglected Tropical Diseases. 2011;**5**:e1015. DOI: 10.1371/journal.pntd.0001015

[10] PAHO. Dengue and Dengue Hemorrhagic Fever in the Americas: Guidelines for Prevention and Control. Washington, DC: Pan American health Organization; 1994. Available from: http://apps.who.int/bookorders/anglais/detart1.jsp?codlan=1&codcol=61&codcch=548

[11] WHO. Mosquito control: Can it stop Zika at source? [cited 28 Sep 2016]. Available from: http://www.who.int/emergencies/zika-virus/articles/mosquito-control/en/

[12] Gubler DJ. Aedes aegypti and Aedes aegypti-borne disease control in the 1990s: Top down or bottom up. Charles Franklin Craig lecture. The American Journal of Tropical Medicine and Hygiene. 1989;**40**:571-578

[13] Nguyen TH, Nguyen HL, Nguyen TY, Vu SN, Tran ND, Le TN, et al. Field evaluation of the establishment potential of wMelPop wolbachia in Australia and Vietnam for dengue control. Parasites & Vectors. 2015;**8**:563. DOI: 10.1186/s13071-015-1174-x

[14] Ritchie SA, Johnson BJ. Advances in vector control science: Rear-and-release strategies show promise… but don't forget the basics. The Journal of Infectious Diseases. 2017;**215**: S103-S108. DOI: 10.1093/infdis/jiw575

[15] Lindsay SW, Wilson A, Golding N, Scott TW, Takken W. Improving the built environment in urban areas to control Aedes aegypti-borne diseases. Bulletin of the World Health Organization. 2017;**95**:607-608. DOI: 10.2471/BLT.16.189688

[16] Arunachalam N, Tana S, Espino F, Kittayapong P, Abeyewickreme W, Wai KT, et al. Eco-bio-social determinants of dengue vector breeding: A multicountry study in urban and periurban Asia. Bulletin of the World Health Organization. 2010;**88**:173-184. DOI: 10.2471/BLT.09.067892

[17] World Health Organization. Special programme for research and training in tropical diseases (TDR). In: Dengue Guidelines for Diagnosis, Treatment, Prevention and Control: New Edition [Internet]. Geneva, Switzerland: World health Organization; 2009 Available from: http://www.who.int/rpc/guidelines/9789241547871/en/

[18] UNICEF. World Health Organization, Pan American Health Organization, International Federation of Red Cross and Red Crescent Societies (IFRC). Risk Communication and Community Engagement for Zika Virus Prevention and Control [Internet]. New York, USA: UNICEF. 2016 Available from: http://www.who.int/csr/resources/publications/zika/community-engagement/en/

[19] Chan KL, Ho BC, Chan YC. *Aedes aegypti* (L.) and *Aedes albopictus* (Skuse) in Singapore City. 2. Larval habitats. Bulletin of the World Health Organization. 1971;**44**:629-633

[20] Maciel-de-Freitas R, Avendanho FC, Santos R, Sylvestre G, Araújo SC, Lima JBP, et al. Undesirable consequences of insecticide resistance following *Aedes aegypti* control activities due to a dengue outbreak. PLoS One. 2014;**9**:e92424. DOI: 10.1371/journal.pone.0092424

[21] Crabtree SA, Wong CM, Mas'ud F. Community participatory approaches to dengue prevention in Sarawak, Malaysia. Human Organization. 2001;**60**:281-287. DOI: 10.17730/humo.60.3.3767huwef8fdtv5c

[22] Chan KL, Chang MS, Laird M, Phanthumachinda B. Control of Aedes mosquitoes by the community. In: Curtis CF, editor. Appropriate Technology in Vector Control. Boca Raton, FL: CRC press; 1990. pp. 103-119 Available from: https://www.cabdirect.org/cabdirect/abstract/19900500195

[23] Alonso WJ. Epidemiology and ethology in the study of the infectious agents: A desirable mutual contamination. In: Research Gate. 2002 Available from: https://www.researchgate.net/publication/215677443_Epidemiology_and_ethology_in_the_study_of_the_infectious_agents_a_desirable_mutual_contamination

[24] dothnews.com.br. Ajudar Aedes a botar ovos é melhor tática, diz doutor [cited 28 Sep 2016]. Available from: http://www.diariodigital.com.br/geral/dengue-tirar-agua-do--potinho-nao-dianta-nada/140130/

[25] United Nations. UN news-Zika: UN agriculture agency provides expertise to help curb spread of virus. 2016 [cited 28 Sep 2016]. Available from: http://www.un.org/apps/news/story.asp?NewsID=53198#.V-t9FjI-Ku7

[26] Ribeiro Montiani HC, Gutemberg Lima Silva C. Social Mobilization of City Residents in Dengue Control. Best Practices for Dengue Prevention and Control in the Americas. Washington, DC: USAID; 2003. pp. 43-50

[27] Arunachalam N, Tyagi BK, Samuel M, Krishnamoorthi R, Manavalan R, Tewari SC, et al. Community-based control of *Aedes aegypti* by adoption of eco-health methods in Chennai City, India. Pathogens and Global Health. 2012;**106**:488-496. DOI: 10.1179/2047773212Y.0000000056

[28] WHO. Environmental management. [cited 28 Sep 2016]. Available from: http://www.who.int/denguecontrol/control_strategies/environmental_management/en/

[29] Teng TB. New Initiatives in Dengue Control in Singapore; 2001. Available from: http://www.who.int/iris/handle/10665/163695

[30] Reiter P, Amador MA, Anderson RA, Clark GG. Short report: Dispersal of *Aedes aegypti* in an urban area after blood feeding as demonstrated by rubidium-marked eggs. The American Journal of Tropical Medicine and Hygiene. 1995;**52**:177-179

[31] Edman JD, Scott TW, Costero A, Morrison AC, Harrington LC, Clark GG. *Aedes aegypti* (Diptera: Culicidae) movement influenced by availability of oviposition sites. Journal of Medical Entomology. 1998;**35**:578-583

[32] Ritchie SA, Long SA, McCaffrey N, Key C, Lonergan G, Williams CR. A biodegradable lethal Ovitrap for control of container-breeding Aedes. Journal of the American Mosquito Control Association. 2008;**24**:47-53. DOI: 10.2987/5658.1

[33] Williams CR, Ritchie SA, Russell RC, Zborowski P. Development and application of "lure and kill" strategies for the dengue vector Aedes aegypti in Australia. Arbovirus Research in Australia. 2005;**9**:397-402

[34] Ulibarri G, Betanzos A, BetanzosM, Rojas JJ. Preliminary results on the control of Aedes spp. in a remote Guatemalan community vulnerable to dengue, chikungunya and Zika virus: Community participation and use of low-cost ecological ovillantas for mosquito control [version 3; referees: 1 approved, 3 approved with reservations]. F1000 Research. 2017;**5**:598 DOI: 10.12688/f1000research.8461.3

[35] Ooi E-E, Goh K-T, Gubler DJ. Dengue prevention and 35 years of vector control in Singapore. Emerging Infectious Diseases. 2006;**12**:887-893. DOI: 10.3201/10.3201/eid1206.051210

[36] Alphey L. Genetic control of mosquitoes. Annual Review of Entomology. 2014;**59**:205-224. DOI: 10.1146/annurev-ento-011613-162002

[37] Bowman LR, Donegan S, McCall PJ. Is dengue vector control deficient in effectiveness or evidence?: Systematic review and meta-analysis. PLoS Neglected Tropical Diseases. 2016;**10**:e0004551. DOI: 10.1371/journal.pntd.0004551

[38] Chang AY, Parrales ME, Jimenez J, Sobieszczyk ME, Hammer SM, Copenhaver DJ, et al. Combining Google Earth and GIS mapping technologies in a dengue surveillance system for developing countries. International Journal of Health Geographics. 2009;**8**:49. DOI: 10.1186/1476-072X-8-49

[39] Trewin BJ, Darbro JM, Jansen CC, Schellhorn NA, Zalucki MP, Hurst TP, et al. The elimination of the dengue vector, Aedes aegypti, from Brisbane, Australia: The role of surveillance, larval habitat removal and policy. PLoS Neglected Tropical Diseases. 2017;**11**:e0005848. DOI: 10.1371/journal.pntd.0005848

[40] Lwin MO, Vijaykumar S, Fernando ONN, Cheong SA, Rathnayake VS, Lim G, et al. A 21st century approach to tackling dengue: Crowdsourced surveillance, predictive mapping and tailored communication. Acta Tropica. 2014;**130**:100-107. DOI: 10.1016/j.actatropica.2013.09.021

[41] Palmer JRB, Oltra A, Collantes F, Delgado JA, Lucientes J, Delacour S, et al. Citizen science provides a reliable and scalable tool to track disease-carrying mosquitoes. Nature Communications. 2017;**8**:916. DOI: 10.1038/s41467-017-00914-9

[42] Ledogar RJ, Arosteguí J, Hernández-Alvarez C, Morales-Perez A, Nava-Aguilera E, Legorreta-Soberanis J, et al. Mobilising communities for *Aedes aegypti* control: The SEPA approach. BMC Public Health. 2017;**17**:403. DOI: 10.1186/s12889-017-4298-4

[43] Toledo ME, Rodriguez A, Valdés L, Carrión R, Cabrera G, Banderas D, et al. Evidence on impact of community-based environmental management on dengue transmission in Santiago de Cuba. Tropical Medicine & International Health: TM & IH. 2011;**16**:744-747. DOI: 10.1111/j.1365-3156.2011.02762.x

[44] Ranard BL, Ha YP, Meisel ZF, Asch DA, Hill SS, Becker LB, et al. Crowdsourcing—Harnessing the masses to advance health and medicine, a systematic review. Journal of General Internal Medicine. 2013;**29**:187-203. DOI: 10.1007/s11606-013-2536-8

[45] Hay SI, George DB, Moyes CL, Brownstein JS. Big data opportunities for global infectious disease surveillance. PLoS Medicine. 2013;**10**:e1001413. DOI: 10.1371/journal.pmed.1001413

[46] Alvarado-Castro V, Paredes-Solís S, Nava-Aguilera E, Morales-Pérez A, Alarcón-Morales L, Balderas-Vargas NA, et al. Assessing the effects of interventions for *Aedes aegypti* control: Systematic review and meta-analysis of cluster randomised controlled trials. BMC Public Health. 2017;**17**:384. DOI: 10.1186/s12889-017-4290-z

[47] Baly A, Toledo ME, Boelaert M, Reyes A, Vanlerberghe V, Ceballos E, et al. Cost effectiveness of Aedes aegypti control programmes: Participatory versus vertical. Transactions of the Royal Society of Tropical Medicine and Hygiene. 2007;**101**:578-586. DOI: 10.1016/j.trstmh.2007.01.002

[48] Baly A, Toledo ME, Vanlerberghe V, Ceballos E, Reyes A, Sanchez I, et al. Cost-effectiveness of a community-based approach intertwined with a vertical Aedes control program. The American Journal of Tropical Medicine and Hygiene. 2009;**81**:88-93

[49] Alonso WJ, Schuck-Paim C. Public preparedness guidance for a severe influenza pandemic in different countries: A qualitative assessment and critical overview. PLOS Currents Influenza. 2010 Apr 15. Edition 1. DOI: 10.1371/currents.RRN1128

[50] Parks W, Lloyd L, Diseases UBSP for R and T in T. Planning social mobilization and communication for dengue fever prevention and control: A step-by-step guide. Planificación de la movilización y comunicación social para la prevención y el control del dengue: guía paso a paso; 2004. Available from: http://www.who.int/iris/handle/10665/42832

[51] Webb TL, Joseph J, Yardley L, Michie S. Using the internet to promote health behavior change: A systematic review and meta-analysis of the impact of theoretical basis, use of behavior change techniques, and mode of delivery on efficacy. Journal of Medical Internet Research. 2010;**12**:e4. DOI: 10.2196/jmir.1376

[52] Marteau TM, Ogilvie D, Roland M, Suhrcke M, Kelly MP. Judging nudging: Can nudging improve population health? BMJ. 2011;**342**:d228. DOI: 10.1136/bmj.d228

[53] Toledo ME, Vanlerberghe V, Baly A, Ceballos E, Valdes L, Searret M, et al. Towards active community participation in dengue vector control: Results from action research in Santiago de Cuba, Cuba. Transactions of the Royal Society of Tropical Medicine and Hygiene. 2007;**101**:56-63. DOI: 10.1016/j.trstmh.2006.03.006

[54] Kay BH, Tuyet Hanh TT, Le NH QTM, Nam VS, PVD H, et al. Sustainability and cost of a community-based strategy against Aedes aegypti in northern and Central Vietnam. The American Journal of Tropical Medicine and Hygiene. 2010;**82**:822-830. DOI: 10.4269/ajtmh.2010.09-0503

[55] Tapia-Conyer R, Méndez-Galván J, Burciaga-Zúñiga P. Community participation in the prevention and control of dengue: The patio Limpio strategy in Mexico. Paediatrics and International Child Health. 2012;**32**(Suppl 1):10-13. DOI: 10.1179/2046904712Z.00000000047

[56] Heintze C, Garrido MV, Kroeger A. What do community-based dengue control programmes achieve? A systematic review of published evaluations. Transactions of the Royal Society of Tropical Medicine and Hygiene. 2007;**101**:317-325. DOI: 10.1016/j.trstmh.2006.08.007

[57] Gubler DJ. Dengue, urbanization and globalization: The unholy trinity of the 21st century. Tropical Medicine and Health. 2011;**39**:3-11. DOI: 10.2149/tmh.2011-S05

[58] Srinivasan S, O'Fallon LR, Dearry A. Creating healthy communities, healthy homes, healthy people: Initiating a research agenda on the built environment and public health. American Journal of Public Health. 2003;**93**:1446-1450

[59] Wallace R, Wallace D. Origins of public health collapse in new york city: The dynamics of planned shrinkage, contagious urban decay and social disintegration. Bulletin of the New York Academy of Medicine. 1990;**66**:391-434

[60] MacGregor C. Urban regeneration as a public health intervention. The Journal of Social Intervention: Theory and Practice. 2010;**19**:38. DOI: 10.18352/jsi.225

[61] Harpham T, Molyneux C. Urban health in developing countries: A review. Progress in Development Studies. 2001;**1**:113-137. DOI: 10.1177/146499340100100202

[62] Alonso WJ, McCormick BJ, Miller MA, Schuck-Paim C, Asrar GR. Beyond crystal balls: Crosscutting solutions in global health to prepare for an unpredictable future. BMC Public Health. 2015;**15**:955. https://doi.org/10.1186/s12889-015-2285-1

[63] Taleb NN. Antifragile: Things that Gain from Disorder. New York: Random House, Penguin; 2012

[64] Sobsey MD. Managing Water in the Home : Accelerated Health Gains from Improved Water Supply. Geneva, Switzerland: World Health Organization; 2002

10

Mathematical Model as a Tool for the Control of Vector-Borne Diseases: *Wolbachia* Example

Meksianis Z. Ndii, Eti D. Wiraningsih,
Nursanti Anggriani and Asep K. Supriatna

Abstract

Dengue is a vector-borne disease that risks two-thirds of the world's population particularly in tropical and subtropical regions. Strategies have been implemented, but they are only effective in the short term. A new innovative and promising strategy against dengue is by the use of *Wolbachia* bacterium. This requires that *Wolbachia*-carrying mosquitoes should persist in the population. To assess the persistence of *Wolbachia*-carrying mosquitoes and its effects on dengue, a number of mathematical models have been formulated and analysed. In this chapter, we review the existing mathematical models of *Wolbachia*-carrying mosquito population dynamics and dengue with *Wolbachia* intervention and provide examples of the mathematical models. Simulations of the models are presented to illustrate the model's solutions.

Keywords: Wolbachia, dengue, mathematical model

1. Introduction

Dengue is a vector-borne disease caused by four distinct serotypes (DEN1–DEN4), and is endemic in most countries particularly in tropical and subtropical areas [1]. It is estimated that around 390 million cases happen each year [2]. Individuals obtain lifelong immunity to the serotype that they are infected with, but have a higher chance to get the most severe form of dengue in the subsequent infection [1]. It is estimated that around 500,000 individuals get severe dengue and require hospitalisation. Of these, about 2.5% die [3]. Without a proper treatment, the fatality rate can reach 20% [3]. Dengue is also a substantial public health and economic burden [4].

A number of strategies have been implemented, but they are generally effective in the short term. Although some progresses have been made for dengue antiviral treatment, dengue control strategies still depend on vector control [5]. One of the strategies against dengue is by the use of *Wolbachia* bacterium. There are two *Wolbachia* strains used in the experiments: *WMelPop* and *WMel*. *WMelPop* strain can reduce the mosquito lifespan of more than 50% and almost 20% reduction in fecundity [6]. *WMel* strain reduces the lifespan of around 10% and only small reduction in fecundity [6]. *Wolbachia* can reduce the level of virus in the salivary glands. *Wolbachia* gives reproductive advantage for *Wolbachia*-carrying female mosquitoes known as cytoplasmic incompatibility (CI). The *Wolbachia*-carrying female mosquitoes can reproduce when mating with both non-*Wolbachia* and *Wolbachia*-carrying male mosquitoes. Non-*Wolbachia* female mosquitoes can reproduce when mating with non-*Wolbachia* males [7]. Field experiments showed that *Wolbachia*-carrying mosquitoes have established and dominated the population [8]. When *Wolbachia*-carrying mosquitoes persist in the field, the *Wolbachia* intervention can be implemented. The question that arises is that to what extend this intervention can reduce dengue transmission? To answer the above question, a number of mathematical models have been formulated and analysed. Mathematical model is a useful tool to understand complex phenomena. This can be used to understand population dynamics [9], disease transmission dynamics [10, 11], and others [12, 13]. A number of mathematical models have been developed to examine the persistence and spread of *Wolbachia*-carrying mosquitoes and its effects on dengue transmission dynamics. In this chapter, we review the existing mathematical models of *Wolbachia*-carrying mosquito population dynamics and dengue with *Wolbachia* intervention, give examples of the mathematical models, and show several numerical simulations to illustrate the model's solutions.

2. Mathematical modelling

This section presents background on mathematical modelling of infectious diseases. Mathematical modelling is a useful tool to understand complex phenomena including disease transmission dynamics and their control strategies. There are several types of modelling that are generally used: deterministic, stochastic, statistical, agent-based modelling, and the others. A deterministic model is mostly used because it is easily solved and can include many parameters or variables. The model is in the form of system of differential equations.

Many mathematical models have been developed to investigate disease transmission dynamics including vector-borne diseases [14]. The model is based on a standard SIR model where the human population is divided into susceptible (S), infected (I), and recovered (R) [15]. The susceptible individuals become exposed after being contacted with infected individuals at a rate β. They then recover at a rate γ. The model is written in the following system of differential equations:

$$\frac{dS}{dt} = -\beta\frac{SI}{N}, \quad \frac{dI}{dt} = \beta\frac{SI}{N} - \gamma I, \quad \frac{dR}{dt} = \gamma I. \tag{1}$$

The model can then be extended to include other compartments and parameters depending on the characteristics of diseases. For example, if the disease has long incubation period, we can add exposed compartment. If the disease is transmitted via vector, we can add another system of equations describing vector dynamics. When one aims to investigate the effects of vaccination, vaccinated compartment can be included. The important principles in modelling are to know characteristics of studied phenomena and the purpose of the research. The principles have been applied when we formulate mathematical models for *Wolbachia*-carrying mosquito population dynamics and dengue with *Wolbachia*.

3. Overview of mathematical models of *Wolbachia* and dengue

In this section, we review existing mathematical model of *Wolbachia*-carrying mosquito population dynamics and dengue with *Wolbachia* intervention.

Many (spatial and non-spatial) mathematical models have been formulated to analyse the persistence and spread or dispersal of *Wolbachia*-carrying mosquitoes in the populations [9, 16–29]. The general aim is to understand the underlying factors required for the persistence and spread of *Wolbachia*-carrying mosquitoes.

A number of nonspatial mathematical model for *Wolbachia*-carrying mosquito population dynamics have been developed. Ndii et al. [19] developed a mathematical model for *Wolbachia*-carrying mosquito population dynamics and assessed the persistence of *Wolbachia*-carrying mosquito populations. They found that *Wolbachia*-carrying mosquitoes persist in the population given that the death rate is not too high. Zhang et al. [30] formulated a mathematical model to assess the best strategies for releasing *Wolbachia*-carrying mosquitoes. They found that initial quantities of non-*Wolbachia* and *Wolbachia*-carrying mosquitoes and augmentation methods (timing, quantity, and order of frequency) determine the success of the *Wolbachia* intervention. They also formulated birth-pulse model with different density dependent death rate functions. They found that for condition with a strong density dependent death rate, the initial ratio of non-*Wolbachia* and *Wolbachia*-carrying mosquitoes should exceed a critical threshold for *Wolbachia*-carrying mosquitoes to dominate the population.

The spatial mathematical models have been developed to assess the *Wolbachia*-carrying mosquitoes' dispersal. Chan and Kim [9] used reaction diffusion approach and incorporated slow and fast dispersal mode to assess the dynamics of the *Wolbachia* spread. They found that temperature affects the wavespeed of the *Wolbachia*-carrying *Aedes aegypti*, that is, *Wolbachia* invasion for *Aedes aegypti* increases when the temperature decreases within the optimal temperature rate for mosquito survival. Hancock et al. [17] developed a metapopulation model to assess the spatial dynamics of *Wolbachia*. They found that spatial variation in the density-dependent competition experienced by juvenile host insects can influence the spread of *Wolbachia* into population. In their other paper [16], they found a new expression for the threshold which takes into account the main aspects of insects' life history. They showed that constant or pulsed immigrations affect the spread of *Wolbachia*-carrying mosquitoes.

Mathematical models for *Wolbachia*-carrying mosquitoes' populations consider several important aspects. They are cytoplasmic incompatibility (CI), the maternal transmission, *Wolbachia*-carrying mosquito death rate, release strategies of *Wolbachia*-carrying mosquitoes [9, 16–29, 31, 32]. These are expressed in the parameters, variables, or simulations.

A number of mathematical models have been developed to understand dengue transmission mathematical models [33, 34]. However, little mathematical models have been developed to investigate the efficacy of *Wolbachia*-intervention [35–40] in reducing dengue transmission. Hancock et al. [39] developed a mathematical model and investigated the strategies for releasing *Wolbachia*-carrying mosquitoes and its effects on dengue transmission dynamics. They found that male-biased releases can substantially reduce the dengue transmission. Furthermore, male-biased release can be an effective strategy that results in the persistence of *Wolbachia*-carrying mosquitoes. Ndii et al. [36, 41, 42] formulated single and two serotype dengue mathematical models to investigate the *Wolbachia* effectiveness in reducing dengue transmission. They found that *Wolbachia* can reduce primary and secondary dengue infections with higher reduction in secondary infections. Hughes and Britton [35] found that *Wolbachia* can reduce dengue transmission in areas where the basic reproduction number is not too high. This implies that *Wolbachia* can reduce dengue transmission in areas with low to moderate transmission settings, which is similar to that found Ndii et al. [36] and Ferguson et al. [37]. Supriatna et al. [40] showed that *Wolbachia* can reduce the value of basic reproduction number. In their other paper, they showed that the predatory and *Wolbachia* can reduce primary and secondary infections [43]. Furthermore, Supriatna et al. [44] investigated the use of vaccine and *Wolbachia* on dengue transmission dynamics [44] and showed that the optimal dengue control is determined by the epidemiological parameters and economic factors. Furthermore, they found that introducing too many *Wolbachia*-carrying mosquitoes would be counter-productive.

4. Examples and numerical simulations of mathematical models

In this section, we present examples of mathematical models of *Wolbachia*-carrying mosquito population dynamics and dengue with *Wolbachia* intervention and their numerical simulations.

4.1. Mathematical model of *Wolbachia*-carrying mosquito population dynamics and numerical simulations

4.1.1. Mathematical model of Wolbachia*-carrying mosquito population dynamics*

Here, we present an example of the mathematical model of the *Wolbachia*-carrying mosquito population dynamics. We present the model by Ndii et al. [19, 45] and show several numerical simulations. The mosquito population is divided into aquatic (A_N and A_W), male (M_N and M_W) and female (F_N and F_W) mosquitoes. Note that the aquatic compartment consists of eggs, larvae and pupae, which are grouped into one compartment. Furthermore, the subscripts M and W denote non-*Wolbachia* and *Wolbachia*-carrying mosquito population.

The effect of CI is captured by the following expression. The non-*Wolbachia* female mosquitoes reproduce when mating with non-*Wolbachia* males, which is governed by the following equations:

$$\rho_N \frac{M_N F_N}{M_N + F_N + M_W + F_W} \tag{2}$$

and the *Wolbachia*-carrying females reproduce when mating with non-*Wolbachia* and *Wolbachia*-carrying males, which is governed by the following equations:

$$\rho_W \frac{F_W(M_N + M_W)}{M_N + F_N + M_W + F_W} \tag{3}$$

Note that the population growth is limited by carrying capacity *K*. The maternal transmission is not perfect [46]. This means that not all *Wolbachia*-carrying aquatic mature to be *Wolbachia*-carrying adult. There is a proportion of $(1-\alpha)$ that mature to be non-*Wolbachia* adults that is $\epsilon_{NW}(1-\alpha)$. Note that the ratio of male and female mosquitoes is denoted by ϵ $(\epsilon_N, \epsilon_W, \epsilon_{NW})$. The model is governed by the following systems of differential equations:

$$\begin{aligned}
\frac{dA_N}{dt} &= \rho_N \frac{M_N F_N}{P}\left(1 - \frac{(A_N + A_W)}{K}\right) - \mu_{NA} A_N - \gamma_N A_N, \\
\frac{dM_N}{dt} &= \epsilon_N \gamma_N A_N - \mu_N M_N + \epsilon_{NW}(1-\alpha_W)\gamma_W A_W, \\
\frac{dF_N}{dt} &= (1-\epsilon_N)\gamma_N A_N - \mu_N F_N + (1-\epsilon_{NW})(1-\alpha_W)\gamma_W A_W, \\
\frac{dA_W}{dt} &= \rho_W \frac{F_W(M_W + M_N)}{P}\left(1 - \frac{(A_N + A_W)}{K}\right) - \mu_{WA} A_W - \gamma_W A_W, \\
\frac{dM_W}{dt} &= \epsilon_W \alpha_W \gamma_W A_W - \mu_W M_W, \\
\frac{dF_W}{dt} &= (1-\epsilon_W)\alpha_W \gamma_W A_W - \mu_W F_W.
\end{aligned} \tag{4}$$

where $P = M_N + F_N + M_W + F_W$ is the total population.

4.1.2. Numerical simulations

In this section, numerical simulations are conducted to illustrate the solutions of the model. The parameter values used are given in **Table 1**. The initial conditions are $A_{N0} = 0$, $F_{N0} = M_{N0} = 7253$, $A_{W0} = 0$, and $M_{W0} = F_{W0} = 14200$.

Figure 1 shows the numerical solutions of the model using the parameter values given in **Table 1**, but the *Wolbachia* adult mosquito death rate is $2 \times \mu_N$. This reflects the *WMelPop Wolbachia* strain which reduces the mosquito lifespan by a half. **Figure 1** shows that the non-*Wolbachia* mosquitoes dominate the population. This means that this strain cannot be used as a strategy to reduce dengue transmission. **Figure 2** shows the numerical solutions of the model

Symbol	Description	Value	Unit	Source
ρ_N	Non-*Wolbachia* reproductive rate	1.25	day^{-1}	[19]
μ_{NA}	Non-*Wolbachia* aquatic death rate	1/7.78	day^{-1}	[47]
γ_N	Non-*Wolbachia* maturation rate	1/6.67	day^{-1}	[48]
ϵ_N	The proportion of non-*Wolbachia* adult male offspring	0.5	Proportion	[49]
μ_N	Non-*Wolbachia* adult death rate	1/14	day^{-1}	[47]
μ_{WA}	*Wolbachia* aquatic death rate	1/7.78	day^{-1}	[47]
μ_W	*Wolbachia* adult death rate	1/7	day^{-1}	[46]
ρ_W	*Wolbachia* reproductive rate	$0.95\rho_N$	day^{-1}	[19]
γ_W	*Wolbachia* maturation rate	1/6.67	day^{-1}	[46]
ϵ_W	The proportion of *Wolbachia*-infected male adults	0.5	N/A	Assumed
ϵ_{NW}	The rate of uninfected males hatched from a *Wolbachia*-infected mother	0.5	N/A	Assumed
α_W	The proportion of *Wolbachia*-infected offspring from a *Wolbachia*-infected mother	0.9	N/A	[7, 46, 50, 51]
K	Carrying capacity	300,000		[48]

Table 1. Parameters, description, values and sources for the model of *Wolbachia*-carrying mosquitoes.

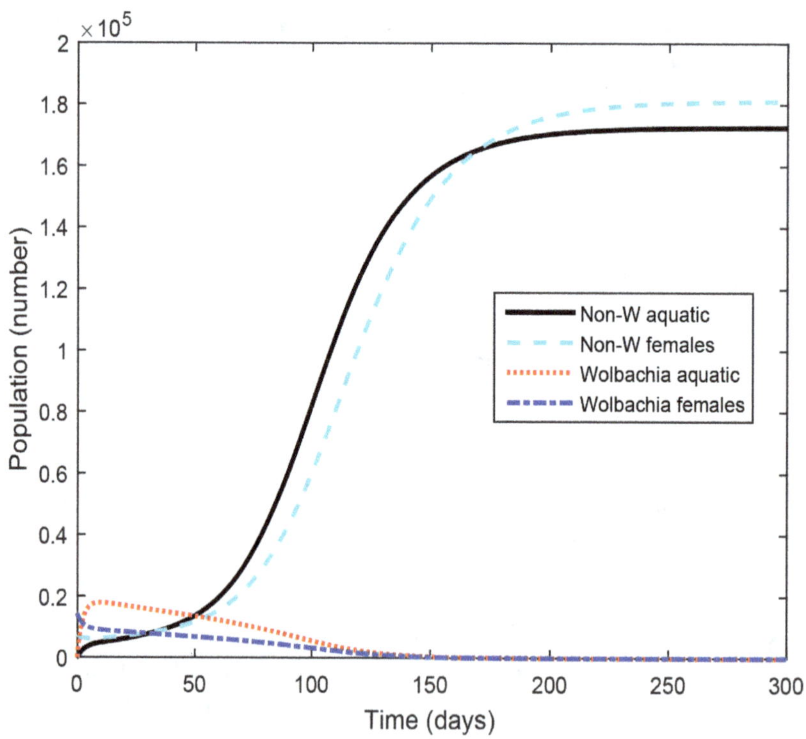

Figure 1. Numerical simulations of the Model (4). The parameter values used are given in **Table 1**, but the parameter μ_W is $2 \times \mu_N$ to reflect the *WMelPop Wolbachia* strain.

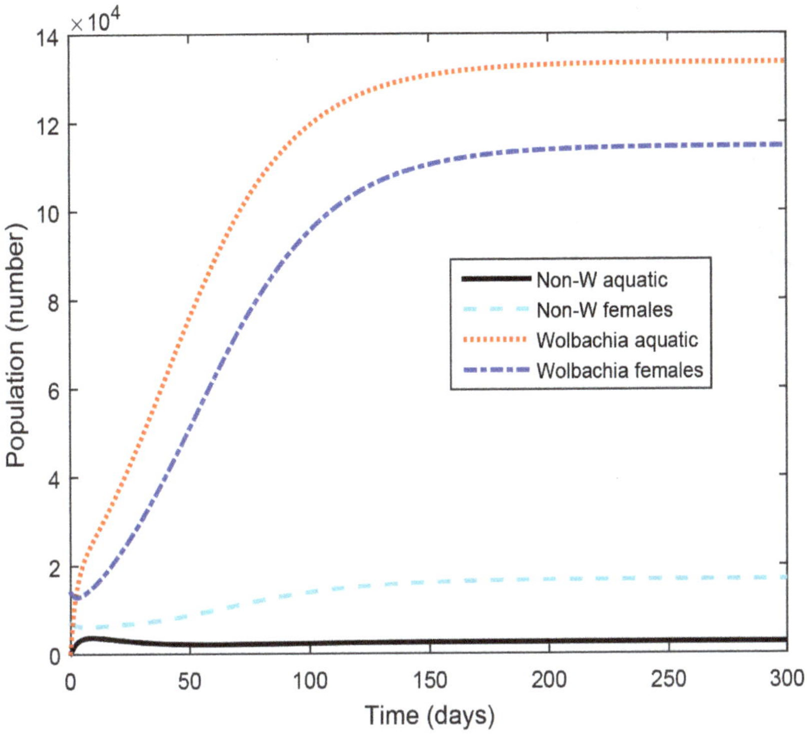

Figure 2. Numerical simulations of the Model (4). The parameter values used are given in **Table 1**. The parameter values reflect the *WMel Wolbachia* strain.

using the parameter values given in **Table 1**. The *Wolbachia* mosquito death rate is $1.1 \times \mu_N$ which reflects the *WMel Wolbachia* strain. This strain reduces the mosquito lifespan by around 10%. It shows that the *Wolbachia*-carrying mosquitoes dominate the population. This means that *WMel* strain can be used in the *Wolbachia* intervention. **Figure 3** shows the simulation results using *WMel* parameter values with initial conditions of $A_{N0} = 0$, $F_{N0} = M_{N0} = 7253$, $A_{W0} = 0$, and $M_{W0} = F_{W0} = 145$. It shows that the non-*Wolbachia* mosquitoes dominate the populations. It implies that the initial conditions also affects the persistence of *Wolbachia*-carrying mosquitoes.

4.2. Dengue mathematical model and numerical simulations

4.2.1. *Dengue mathematical model in the presence of* Wolbachia

In this section, we give example of two-serotype dengue mathematical model. We present the model by Ndii et al. [42]. The model consists of human, non-*Wolbachia* and *Wolbachia*-carrying mosquito population. The human population is divided into susceptible (S_H), exposed to serotype i (E_H^i), infected to serotype i (I_H^i), temporary immunity to the serotype i (X_H^i), recovered class (R_H), susceptible, exposed and infected to j strain ($S_H^{ji}, E_H^{ji}, I_H^{ji}$, respectively). The superscript ji means individuals that were previously infected by serotype i and currently infected by serotype j. The mosquito population is divided into susceptible (S_N and S_W),

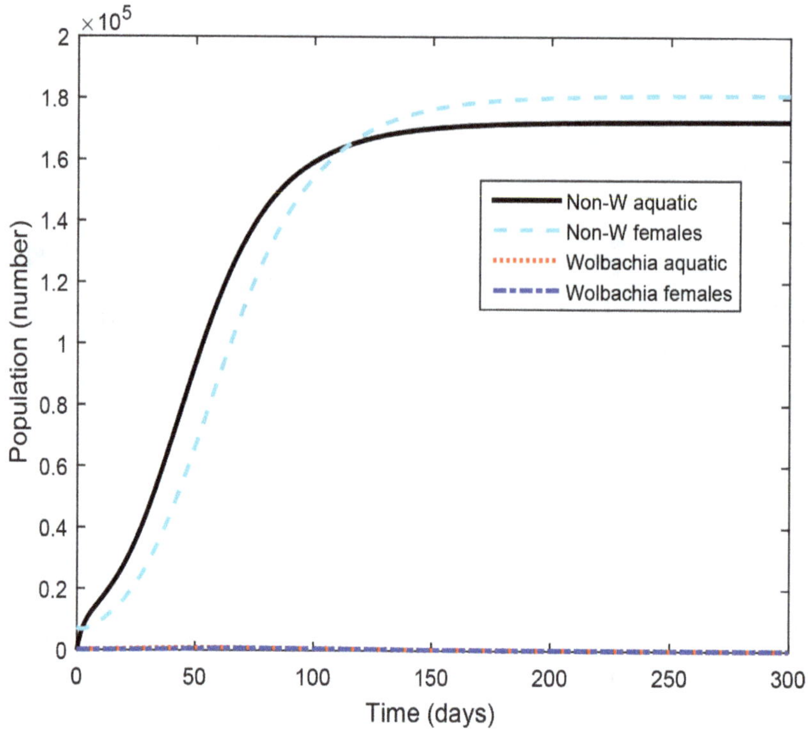

Figure 3. Numerical simulations of the Model (4). The parameter values used are given in **Table 1**. The parameter values reflect the *WMel Wolbachia* strain but different initial conditions. The initial conditions are $A_{N0} = 0$, $F_{N0} = M_{N0} = 7253$, $A_{W0} = 0$, and $M_{W0} = F_{W0} = 145$.

exposed to serotype i (E_N^i and E_W^i) and infected to serotype i (I_N^i and I_W^i). The subscript N and W is for non-*Wolbachia* and *Wolbachia*-carrying mosquitoes.

The model is governed by the following system of differential equations:

$$\frac{dS_H}{dt} = BN_H - \sum_{i=1}^{2} \lambda_H^i S_H - \mu_H S_H, \tag{5}$$

$$\frac{dE_H^i}{dt} = \lambda_H^i S_H - \gamma_H E_H^i - \mu_H E_H^i, \tag{6}$$

$$\frac{dI_H^i}{dt} = \gamma_H E_H^i - \sigma I_H^i - \mu_H I_H^i, \tag{7}$$

$$\frac{dX_H^i}{dt} = \sigma I_H^i - \theta^i X_H^i - \mu_H X_H^i, \tag{8}$$

$$\frac{dS_H^{ji}}{dt} = \lambda_H^j S_H^{ji} - \mu_H S_H^{ji}, \tag{9}$$

$$\frac{dE_H^{ji}}{dt} = \lambda_H^j S_H^{ji} - \gamma_H E_H^{ji} - \mu_H E_H^{ji}, \tag{10}$$

$$\frac{dI_H^{ji}}{dt} = \gamma_H E_H^{ji} - \sigma I_H^{ji} - (\mu_H + d) I_H^{ji}, \tag{11}$$

$$\frac{dR_H}{dt} = \sum_{j=1, j\neq i}^{2} \sigma I_H^{ji} - \mu_H R_H, \tag{12}$$

Model for non-*Wolbachia* mosquito population

$$\frac{dA_N}{dt} = \frac{\rho_N F_N^2}{2(F_N + F_W)}\left(1 - \frac{A_N + A_W}{K}\right) - \tau_N A_N - \mu_{NA} A_N, \tag{13}$$

$$\frac{dS_N}{dt} = \frac{\tau_N A_N}{2} + \frac{(1-\alpha)\tau_W A_W}{2} - \sum_{i=1}^{2} \lambda_N^i S_N - \mu_N S_N, \tag{14}$$

$$\frac{dE_N^i}{dt} = \lambda_N^i S_N - \gamma_N E_N^i - \mu_N E_N^i, \tag{15}$$

$$\frac{dI_N^i}{dt} = \gamma_N E_N^i - \mu_N I_N^i. \tag{16}$$

Model for *Wolbachia*-carrying mosquito population

$$\frac{dA_W}{dt} = \frac{\rho_W F_W}{2}\left(1 - \frac{A_N + A_W}{K}\right) - \tau_W A_W - \mu_{WA} A_W, \tag{17}$$

$$\frac{dS_W}{dt} = \frac{\alpha \tau_W A_W}{2} - \sum_{i=1}^{2} \lambda_W^i S_W - \mu_W S_W, \tag{18}$$

$$\frac{dE_W^i}{dt} = \lambda_W^i S_W - \gamma_W E_W^i - \mu_W E_W^i, \tag{19}$$

$$\frac{dI_W}{dt} = \gamma_W E_W^i - \mu_W I_W^i, \tag{20}$$

where the force of infections are

$$\lambda_H^i = \frac{b_N T^i I_N^i}{N_H} + \frac{b_W T_{HW}^i I_W^i}{N_H}, \tag{21}$$

$$\lambda_N^i = \frac{b_N T^i I_H^i}{N_H} + \phi_i \frac{b_N T^i I_H^{ij}}{N_H}, \tag{22}$$

$$\lambda_W^i = \frac{b_W T^i I_H^i}{N_H} + \phi_i \frac{b_W T^i I_H^{ij}}{N_H}, \tag{23}$$

where ϕ_i is the antibody-dependent enhancement factor for serotype i. Note that the susceptible human becomes exposed to dengue after being bitten by non-*Wolbachia* and *Wolbachia*-infected

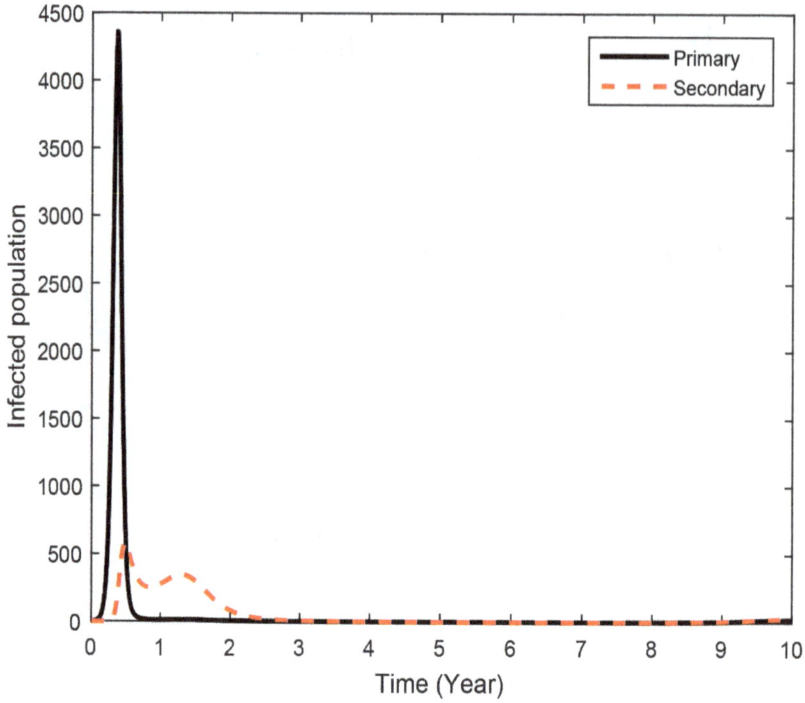

Figure 4. Numerical simulations of primary and secondary infections in the absence of *Wolbachia*-carrying mosquitoes. The parameters values used are given in **Table 2**. Initial conditions are $I_H^1(0) = I_H^2(0) = 1$ and $N_H = 10^5$. $A_N(0) = S_N(0) = 3 \times N_H$.

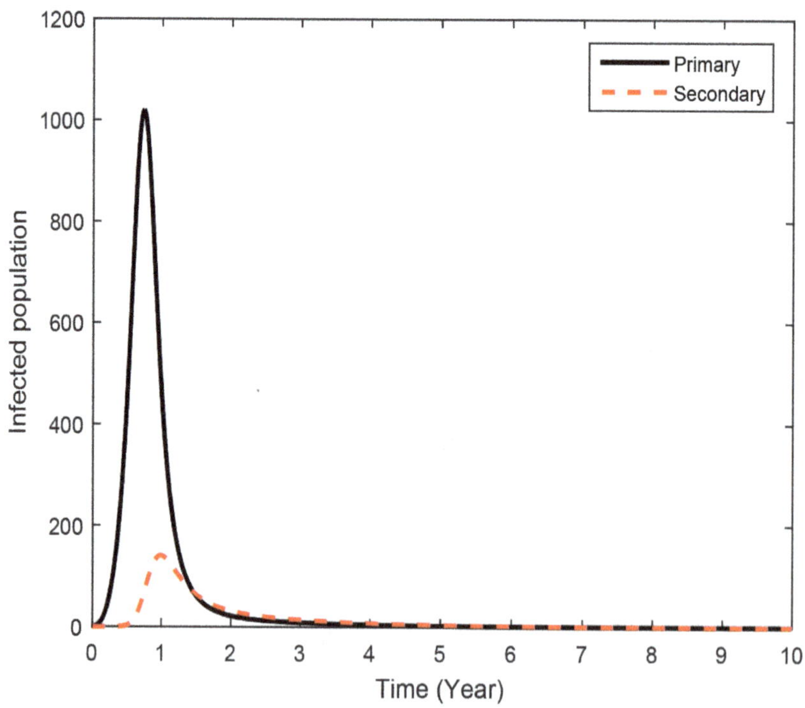

Figure 5. Numerical simulations of primary and secondary infections in the presence of *Wolbachia*-carrying mosquitoes. The parameters values used are given in **Table 2**. Initial conditions are $I_H^1(0) = I_H^2(0) = 1$ and $N_H = 10^5$. $A_N(0) = S_N(0) = A_W(0) = S_W(0) = 1.5 \times N_H$.

mosquitoes, which then becomes infected and have temporary immunity. After a certain period in temporary immunity class, they become susceptible to the other dengue serotype. They will have secondary infection after being bitten by infected mosquitoes carrying different dengue serotype to that they are previously infected.

4.2.2. Numerical simulations

This section presents numerical simulations of the model. **Figures 4** and **5** show the numerical simulations of primary and secondary infections in the absence and presence of *Wolbachia*, respectively.

Figures 4 and **5** show that *Wolbachia* can reduce dengue transmission. The number of infections in the presence of *Wolbachia*-carrying mosquitoes (see **Figure 5**) is smaller than that in the absence of *Wolbachia*-carrying mosquitoes (see **Figure 4**). This means that the *Wolbachia* can

Symbol	Description	Value	Unit	Source
α	Maternal transmission	0.9	N/A	[19, 46, 52]
B	Human birth rate	$1/(70 \times 365)$	day^{-1}	[3]
b_N	Biting rate of non-W mosquitoes	0.63	day^{-1}	[53]
b_W	Biting rate of W mosquitoes	$0.95\ b_N$	day^{-1}	[54]
γ_H	Progression rate from exposed to infectious	1/5.5	day^{-1}	[1]
γ_N	Progression from exposed to infectious class of non-W mosquitoes	1/10	day^{-1}	[55]
γ_W	Progression from exposed to infectious class of W mosquitoes	1/10	day^{-1}	[55]
K	Carrying capacity	$3 \times N_H$	N/A	[55]
λ	Force of infection	Eqs. (21)–(23)		
μ_N	Adult mosquito death rate (non-W)	1/14	day^{-1}	[47]
μ_H	Human death rate	$1/(70 \times 365)$	day^{-1}	[3]
μ_{NA}	Death rate of aquatic non-W mosquitoes	1/14	day^{-1}	[47]
μ_W	Adult aquatic death rate	$1.1\mu_N$	day^{-1}	[46, 51]
μ_{WA}	Death rate of W mosquitoes	1/14	day^{-1}	[47]
ϕ	ADE	1.1	N/A	[56]
ρ_N	Reproductive rate of non-W mosquitoes	1.25	day^{-1}	[19]
ρ_W	Reproductive rate of W-mosquitoes	$0.95\rho_N$	day^{-1}	[46]
σ	Recovery rate	1/5	day^{-1}	[1]
T_N	Transmission probability from non-W mosquitoes to human	0.5	N/A	[36]
T_{HW}	Transmission probability from W mosquitoes to human	$0.5T_N$	N/A	[36, 57]
θ	Progression rate from temporary immunity class to susceptible class	$1/(0.5 \times 365)$	day^{-1}	[58]
τ_N	Maturation rate of non-W mosquitoes	1/10	day^{-1}	[47]
τ_W	Maturation rate of W mosquitoes	1/10	day^{-1}	[47]

Table 2. Parameter descriptions, values, and sources. Note that W and N are used to indicate Wolbachia-carrying and non-Wolbachia mosquitoes in the parameter descriptions, respectively. $N_H = 10^5$.

potentially be used to break the cycle of dengue transmission. Note that the parameter values are largely uncertain. Therefore, large data set is needed to validate the model against data.

5. Discussion and conclusions

The use of *Wolbachia* bacterium has been proposed as a new innovative strategy against dengue. A lot of research have been conducted to look at the persistence of *Wolbachia*-carrying mosquitoes and the potential reduction in the number of dengue cases by the use of *Wolbachia* bacterium. One of the approaches is by the use of mathematical model. It can be seen that mathematical model can provide insights into the persistence and the effectiveness of the *Wolbachia* in reducing dengue transmission dynamics.

One of the important steps in modelling is model's validation. The model can be validated against the real data. Although several parameters can be obtained from literature, it is important to estimate the influential parameters such as transmission rate against the real data. Ferguson et al. [37] validated their model against the real data. Furthermore, most parameters are strongly uncertain, which indicate that sensitivity analysis is strongly required. This aims to find the most important parameters which can guide us in collecting appropriate data to be estimated.

Models presented in this work do not take into account the environmental factors such as temperature and rainfall. These may affect the dynamics of mosquito population and hence dengue transmission dynamics. Furthermore, in our work, the ratio of male and female mosquitoes is equal, which possibly affects the mosquito's population dynamics. It is important to consider sex-biased ratio to determine its effects on the persistence of *Wolbachia*-carrying mosquitoes and dengue reduction.

In this paper, we review existing mathematical models of *Wolbachia*-carrying mosquitoes' population dynamics and dengue with *Wolbachia*. Examples of the mathematical models are given. It shows that *Wolbachia*-carrying mosquitoes can persist in the population depending on the *Wolbachia* strains. Furthermore, the initial conditions also affect the persistence of *Wolbachia*-carrying mosquito populations. It is shown that *Wolbachia* can potentially reduce the primary and secondary infections with higher reduction in secondary infections. Results suggest that using *Wolbachia* can potentially reduce the transmission of dengue and hence minimise the public health and economic burden.

The results showed that the *Wolbachia* can persist in the population. When mosquitoes are infected with the *WMel* strain of *Wolbachia*. For dengue mathematical models with *Wolbachia*, it shows that the *Wolbachia* can potentially reduce the primary and secondary infections. This means that using *Wolbachia* can be an alternative strategy against dengue.

Acknowledgements

MZN acknowledges funding from Ministry of Research, Technology and Higher Education of Indonesia through Penelitian Pascadoctor scheme 2018 (Grant No: 70/UN15.19/LT/2018). EDW received funding from Ministry of Research, Technology and Higher Education of Indonesia (Grant No: 3/E/KPT/2018). NA received Academic Leadership Grant from Padjadjaran University (Grant No: 2297 /UN6.D/KS/2018) and Penelitian Dasar Unggulan Perguruan Tinggi (Grant No: 1126/UN6.D/LT/2018).

Author details

Meksianis Z. Ndii[1]*, Eti D. Wiraningsih[2], Nursanti Anggriani[3] and Asep K. Supriatna[3]

*Address all correspondence to: meksianis.ndii@staf.undana.ac.id

1 Department of Mathematics, Faculty of Sciences and Engineering, University of Nusa Cendana, Kupang NTT, Indonesia

2 Department of Mathematics, Faculty of Mathematics and Natural Sciences, State University of Jakarta, Jakarta DKI, Indonesia

3 Department of Mathematics, Faculty of Mathematics and Natural Sciences, Padjadjaran University, Jawa Barat, Indonesia

References

[1] Gubler DJ. Dengue and dengue hemorrhagic fever. Clinical Microbiology Reviews. 1998; **11**:480-496

[2] Bhatt S, Gething PW, Brady OJ, Messina JP, Farlow AW, et al. The global distribution and burden of dengue. Nature. 2013;**496**:1476-4687

[3] World Health Organisation. Dengue and Severe Dengue, Fact Sheet No. 117 [Online]. February 2018. Available from: http://www.who.int/news-room/fact-sheets/detail/dengue-and-severe-dengue [Accessed: June 1, 2018]

[4] Shepard DS, Undurraga EA, Halasa YA, Stanaway JD. The global economic burden of dengue: A systematic analysis. The Lancet Infectious Diseases. 2016;**16**(8):935-941

[5] Dorigatti I, McCormack C, Nedjati-Gilani G, Ferguson NM. Using *Wolbachia* for dengue control: Insights from modelling. Trends in Parasitology. 2018;**34**(2):102-113

[6] McMeniman CJ, Lane RV, Cass BN, Fong AWC, Sidhu M, Wang Y-F, O'Neill SL. Stable introduction of a life-shortening *Wolbachia* infection into the mosquito *Aedes aegypti*. Science. 2009;**323**(5910):141-144

[7] Sinkins SP. *Wolbachia* and cytoplasmic incompatibility in mosquitoes. Insect Biochemistry and Molecular Biology. 2004;**34**(7):723-729

[8] Hoffmann AA, Iturbe-Ormaetxe I, Callahan AG, Phillips BL, Billington K, Axford JK, Montgomery B, Turley AP, O'Neill SL. Stability of the *WMel Wolbachia* infection following invasion into *Aedes aegypti* populations. PLoS Neglected Tropical Diseases. 2014;**8**:e3115

[9] Chan MHT, Kim PS. Modelling a *Wolbachia* invasion using a slow–fast dispersal reaction–diffusion approach. Bulletin of Mathematical Biology. 2013;**75**(9):1501-1523

[10] Ndii MZ, Supriatna AK. Stochastic mathematical models in epidemiology. Information. 2017;**20**:6185-6196

[11] Ndii MZ, Amarti Z, Wiraningsih ED, Supriatna AK. Rabies epidemic model with uncertainty in parameters: Crisp and fuzzy approaches. IOP Conference Series: Materials Science and Engineering. 2018;**332**(1):012031

[12] Ndii MZ, Carnia E, Supriatna AK. Mathematical models for the spread of rumors: A review. In: Gaol FL, Hutagalung F, Chew FP, editors. Issues and Trends in Interdisciplinary Behavior and Social Science. USA: CRC Press; 2018. pp. 266-290

[13] Tambaru D, Djahi BS, Ndii MZ. The effects of hard water consumption on kidney function: Insights from mathematical modelling. AIP Conference Proceedings. 2018;**1937**(1): 020020

[14] Reiner RC, Perkins T, Barker CM, et al. A systematic review of mathematical models of mosquito-borne pathogen transmission: 1970–2010. Journal of the Royal Society Interface. 2013;**10**(81):20120921

[15] Keeling MJ, Rohani P. Modeling Infectious Diseases in Humans and Animals. USA: Princeton University Press; 2008

[16] Hancock PA, Sinkins SP, Godfray HCJ. Population dynamic models of the spread of *Wolbachia*. The American Naturalist. 2011;**177**(3):323-333

[17] Hancock PA, Godfray HCJ. Modelling the spread of *Wolbachia* in spatially heterogeneous environments. Journal of Royal Society Interface. 2012;**9**(76):3045-3054

[18] Hancock PA, White VL, Callahan AG, Godfray CHJ, Hoffmann AA, Ritchie SA. Density dependent population dynamics in *Aedes aegypti* slow the spread of *wMel Wolbachia*. Journal of Applied Ecology. 2016;**53**(3):785-793

[19] Ndii MZ, Hickson RI, Mercer GN. Modelling the introduction of *Wolbachia* into *Aedes aegypti* to reduce dengue transmission. The ANZIAM Journal. 2012;**53**:213-227

[20] Li Y, Liu X. An impulsive model for *Wolbachia* infection control of mosquito-borne diseases with general birth and death rate functions. Nonlinear Analysis: Real World Applications. 2017;**37**:412-432

[21] Turelli M, Barton NH. Deploying dengue-suppressing *Wolbachia*: Robust models predict slow but effective spatial spread in *Aedes aegypti*. Theoretical Population Biology. 2017;**115**:45-60

[22] Xue L, Manore CA, Thongsripong P, Hyman JM. Two-sex mosquito model for the persistence of *Wolbachia*. Journal of Biological Dynamics. 2017;**11**(Suppl. 1):216-237

[23] Zhang X, Tang S, Liu Q, Cheke RA, Zhu H. Models to assess the effects of non-identical sex ratio augmentations of *Wolbachia*-carrying mosquitoes on the control of dengue disease. Mathematical Biosciences. 2018;**299**:58-72

[24] Guevara-Souza M, Vallejo EE. A computer simulation model of *Wolbachia* invasion for disease vector population modification. BMC Bioinformatics. 2015;**16**(1):317

[25] Strau JF, Telschow A. Modeling the indirect effect of *Wolbachia* on the infection dynamics of horizontally transmitted viruses. Frontiers in Microbiology. 2015;**6**:378

[26] Bliman PA, Aronna MS, Coelho FC, Moacyr A, da Silva HB. Ensuring successful introduction of *Wolbachia* in natural populations of *Aedes aegypti* by means of feedback control. Journal of Mathematical Biology. 2018;**76**(5):1269-1300

[27] Li Y, Liu X. A sex-structured model with birth pulse and release strategy for the spread of *Wolbachia* in mosquito population. Journal of Theoretical Biology. 2018;**448**:53-65

[28] Huang M, Luo J, Hu L, Zheng B, Yu J. Assessing the efficiency of *Wolbachia* driven aedes mosquito suppression by delay differential equations. Journal of Theoretical Biology. 2018;**440**:1-11

[29] Zheng B, Guo W, Hu L, Huang M, Yu J. Complex *Wolbachia* infection dynamics in mosquitoes with imperfect maternal transmission. Mathematical Biosciences and Engineering. 2018;**15**:523-541

[30] Zhang X, Tang S, Cheke RA. Models to assess how best to replace dengue virus vectors with *Wolbachia*-infected mosquito populations. Mathematical Biosciences. 2015;**269**:164-177

[31] Keeling MJ, Jiggins FM, Read JM. The invasion and coexistence of competing *Wolbachia* strains. Heredity. 2003;**91**:382-388

[32] Rasgon JL. Using Predictive Models to Optimize *Wolbachia*-Based Strategies for Vector-Borne Disease Control. New York, NY: Springer New York; 2008. pp. 114-125

[33] Supriatna AK, Soewono E, van Gils SA. A two-age-classes dengue transmission model. Mathematical Biosciences. 2008;**216**(1):114-121

[34] Anggriani N, Supriatna AK, Soewono E. A critical protection level derived from dengue infection mathematical model considering asymptomatic and symptomatic classes. Journal of Physics: Conference Series. 2013;**423**(1):012056

[35] Hughes H, Britton NF. Modelling the use of *Wolbachia* to control dengue fever transmission. Bulletin of Mathematical Biology. 2013;**75**(5):796-818

[36] Ndii MZ, Hickson RI, Allingham D, Mercer GN. Modelling the transmission dynamics of dengue in the presence of *Wolbachia*. Mathematical Biosciences. 2015;**262**:157-166

[37] Ferguson NM, Kien DTH, Clapham H, Aguas R, Trung VT, Chau TNB, Popovici J, Ryan PA, O'Neill SL, McGraw EA, Long VT, Dui LT, Nguyen HL, Van Vinh Chau N, Wills B, Simmons CP. Modeling the impact on virus transmission of *Wolbachia*-mediated blocking of dengue virus infection of *Aedes aegypti*. Science Translational Medicine. 2015;**7**(279):279ra37

[38] Qu Z, Xue L, Hyman JM. Modeling the transmission of *Wolbachia* in mosquitoes for controlling mosquito-borne diseases. SIAM Journal on Applied Mathematics. 2018;**78**(2): 826-852

[39] Hancock PA, Sinkins SP, Godfray HCJ. Strategies for introducing *Wolbachia* to reduce transmission of mosquito-borne diseases. PLoS Neglected Tropical Diseases. 2011;**5**(4):1-10

[40] Supriatna AK, Anggriani N. System dynamics model of *Wolbachia* infection in dengue transmission. Procedia Engineering. 2012;**50**:12-18

[41] Ndii MZ, Allingham D, Hickson RI, Glass K. The effect of *Wolbachia* on dengue outbreaks when dengue is repeatedly introduced. Theoretical Population Biology. 2016;**111**:9-15

[42] Ndii MZ, Allingham D, Hickson RI, Glass K. The effect of *Wolbachia* on dengue dynamics in the presence of two serotypes of dengue: Symmetric and asymmetric epidemiological characteristics. Epidemiology and Infection. 2016;**144**(13):2874-2882

[43] Anggriani N, Supriatna AK. The effect of *Wolbachia* introduction and predatory in dengue disease transmission. Advanced Science, Engineering and Medicine. 2015;**7**(10):864-868

[44] Supriatna AK, Anggriani N, Nurulputri L, Wulantini R, Aldila D. The optimal release strategy of *Wolbachia* infected mosquitoes to control dengue disease. Advanced Science, Engineering and Medicine. 2014;**6**(8):831-837

[45] Ndii MZ. Analysis of a *Wolbachia* intervention to reduce dengue spread [Master's thesis]. The Australian National University; 2011

[46] Walker T, Johnson PH, Moreira LA, Iturbe-Ormaetxe I, Frentiu FD, et al. The *WMel Wolbachia* strain blocks dengue and invades caged *Aedes aegypti* populations. Nature. 2011; **476**:450-453

[47] Yang HM, Macoris MLG, Galvani KC, Andrighetti MTM, Wanderley DMV. Assessing the effects of temperature on the population of *Aedes aegypti*, the vector of dengue. Epidemiology and Infection. 2009;**137**(8):1188-1202

[48] Maidana NA, Yang HM. Describing the geographic spread of dengue disease by traveling waves. Mathematical Biosciences. 2008;**215**(1):64-77

[49] Ruang-areerate T, Kittayapong P. *Wolbachia* transinfection in aedes aegypti: A potential gene driver of dengue vectors. Proceedings of the National Academy of Sciences. 2006; **103**(33):12534-12539

[50] Xi Z, Khoo CCH, Dobson SL. *Wolbachia* establishment and invasion in an *Aedes aegypti* laboratory population. Science. 2005;**310**:326-328

[51] Yeap HL, Mee P, Walker T, Weeks AR, O'Neill SL, et al. Dynamics of the "Popcorn" *Wolbachia* infection in outbred *Aedes aegypti* informs prospects for mosquito vector control. Genetics. 2011;**187**:583-595

[52] Hoffmann AA, Turelli M, Harshman LG. Factors affecting the distribution of cytoplasmic incompatibility in *Drosophila simulans*. Genetics. 1990;**126**:933-948

[53] Scott TW, Amerasinghe PH, Morrison AC, Lorenz LH, Clark GG, Strickman D, Kittayapong P, Edman JD. Longitudinal studies of *Aedes aegypti* (Diptera: Culicidae) in Thailand and Puerto Rico: Blood feeding frequency. Journal of Medical Entomology. 2000;**37**:89-101

[54] Turley AP, Moreira LA, O'Neill SL, McGraw EA. *Wolbachia* infection reduces blood–feeding success in the dengue fever mosquito, *Aedes aegypti*. PLoS Neglected Tropical Diseases. 2009; **3**:e516

[55] Chowel G, Diaz-Duenas P, Miller JC, Velazco AA, Hyman JM, Fenimore PW, Castillo-Chaves C. Estimation of the reproduction number of dengue fever from spatial epidemic data. Mathematical Biosciences. 2007;**208**:571-589

[56] Hu K, Thoens C, Bianco S, Edlund S, Davis M, Douglas J, Kaufman JH. The effect of antibody-dependent enhancement, cross immunity, and vector population on the dynamics of dengue fever. Journal of Theoretical Biology. 2013;**319**:62-74

[57] Bian G, Xu Y, Lu P, Xie Y, Xi Z. The endosymbiotic bacterium *Wolbachia* induces resistance to dengue virus in *Aedes aegypti*. PLoS Pathogen. 2010;**6**:e1000833

[58] Wearing HJ, Rohani P. Ecological and immunological determinants of dengue epidemics. Proceedings of the National Academy of Sciences. 2006;**103**:11802-11807

11

Current Status of Vaccines against Dengue Virus

Jhon Carlos Castaño-Osorio,
Alejandra María Giraldo-Garcia and
Maria Isabel Giraldo

Abstract

Dengue is a disease caused by the dengue virus (DENV), being the most important arbovirus in the world. About 3.97 billion people live in countries at risk and 400 million infections occur each year, of which 500,000 suffer from the most severe form of the disease and 25,000 of these die. The clinical spectrum of Dengue ranges from asymptomatic infection to severe Dengue characterized by increased vascular permeability, bleeding disorders, shock, and death. The increase in global cases of this disease is due in part to the absence of effective public intervention measures and lack of a specific treatment and vaccines licensed for human use. Therefore, in this review, we will present the different strategies known to date for the development of vaccines for this disease, as well as the results and limitations obtained in the different clinical studies.

Keywords: dengue, vaccine, tetravalent, immunopathogenesis

1. Introduction

Dengue is a mosquito-borne viral disease caused by four types of dengue viruses, which, in the recent years, has rapidly become widespread worldwide. Dengue virus transmission is attributed to female mosquitoes of the species *Aedes aegypti*, in the majority of cases, as well as *Ae. albopictus* to a lesser extent. Other diseases that are transmitted by this mosquito include chikungunya, yellow fever, and Zika infection [1]. Dengue is a very rapidly growing public health problem being currently faced by approximately 40% of the global population living in more than a hundred tropical and subtropical countries [2]. Dengue is widespread throughout the tropics, with local variations in risk influenced by rainfall, temperature as consequence of climate change, unplanned rapid urbanization, unprecedented population growth, increasing movement of people (and consequently viruses), international travel and breakdown in public health infrastructure, and vector control programs. The actual numbers of dengue cases are underreported and many cases are misclassified. The prevalence of dengue is estimated at 3.9 billion people who are at risk of infection in 128 tropical and subtropical countries, mainly southeast and south Asia, Central and South America, and the Caribbean. A recent estimate indicates 390 million dengue infections per year (95% credible interval 284–528 million), of which 96 million (67–136 million) manifest clinically (with any severity of disease), with an estimated 500,000 cases each year of life-threatening disease in the form of severe dengue—including dengue hemorrhagic fever and dengue shock syndrome mostly in the pediatric population, with about 20,000 succumbing to it, and is the leading cause of childhood death in many countries [1–3]. Dengue is associated with considerable social, economic, and political consequences caused by urban epidemics, such as those seen in Delhi (1996), Cuba (1977–1979 and 1997), Taiwan (2002), and Brazil (2008). Furthermore, Dengue is currently also a major cause of morbidity in American and European travelers and military personnel [4]. This disease places a high economic burden on both governments and individuals; for instance, in America, Dengue illness costs US$2.1 billion per year on average, excluding vector control, exceeding costs of other viral illnesses. In addition, in Southeast Asia, there is an estimate of 2.9 million dengue episodes and 5906 deaths annually, with an annual economic burden of $950 million [3].

2. Natural clinical evolution

Dengue virus infections encompass a range of well-described clinical illnesses ranging from an asymptomatic infection to a self-limiting febrile illness, dengue fever, to severe dengue (shock and death), a clinical syndrome that typically presents with capillary permeability and can lead to dengue shock syndrome and dengue hemorrhagic fever. Among less common presentations of severe dengue are encephalitis, hepatitis, and renal dysfunction [4]. Infection by any dengue virus requires a 4- to 8-day incubation period and can produce a wide spectrum of illnesses, the majority of these being asymptomatic or subclinical. Although most patients are able to recover after a self-limiting (yet debilitating) illness, a small proportion develops a severe form of the disease, which is mainly characterized by plasma leakage with or without bleeding [3]. The acute illness is usually benign and self-limiting. Moreover, a secondary infection, corresponding to a subsequent infection with a different serotype is also characterized by acute fever and several other nonspecific signs and symptoms, usually indistinguishable from a range of other illnesses. However, in 2–3% of secondary infections with another serotype there is a higher risk of increased disease severity, causing life-threatening Dengue with Warning Signs (DWS+) and Severe dengue (SD), according to the revised WHO dengue case classification (DENCO) [2, 5]. Serotype-cross-reactive antibodies facilitate DENV infection in Fc-receptor-bearing cells by promoting virus entry via Fcγ receptors (FcγR), a process known as antibody-dependent enhancement (ADE) [6, 7]. Dengue without Warning Signs (DWS−) is more often observed in adults and adolescents and can manifest with only a mild fever only or a more disabling disease. This latter form is characterized by symptoms occurring mainly in the early febrile stage, such as the sudden onset of high fever, severe headache, retro-orbital pain, myalgia, arthralgia, and rash. In the critical phase, the skin is flushed with the appearance of a petechial rash, occurring predominantly around the time of defervescence, when an increase in capillary permeability accompanied by increased hematocrit can occur, leading to hypovolemic shock that can result in organ impairment, metabolic acidosis, disseminated intravascular coagulation, and severe hemorrhage. If untreated, mortality can be as high as 20%, whereas appropriate case management and intravenous rehydration can reduce mortality to less than 1% [3]. SD usually affects children younger than 15 years of age, although it can occur in adults. SD is characterized by a transient increase in vascular permeability resulting in plasma leakage with high fever, bleeding, thrombocytopenia, and hemoconcentration, which can lead to shock [5]. Two factors, namely, antibody-dependent-enhancement (ADE) and inherent virulence of the DEN viruses, appear to contribute the most to disease pathogenesis [2].

3. Pathogenesis of Dengue virus infection

The pathophysiological basis for severe dengue is multifactorial, resulting from a complex interaction between the virus, the host, and, at least in part, immune-mediated mechanisms. Individuals with primary Dengue virus infection induce a lifelong protective immunity to the infecting serotype, accompanied by a short-term cross-immunity against other serotypes and development only leads to self-limited dengue fever characterized by high fever and debilitating joint pain, recovery from infection by one provides lifelong immunity against that serotype. However, subsequent infection with a different dengue serotype is more likely to cause DWS+/SD, and cross-immunity to the other serotypes after recovery is only partial and temporary. Epidemiological data suggest an increased risk of DWS+/SD in people with preexisting heterotypic dengue virus antibodies, and this has led to research in dengue pathogenesis focusing on the subsequent infections by other serotypes and an increased risk of developing severe dengue. Accordingly, antibodies against a given serotype can cross-react with, but not cross-protect against, the remaining three virus serotypes [4] during secondary infections. Immunopathological mechanisms have been proposed, such as the immune system improvement phenomenon (immunopotentiation), which contribute to the increased risk of DWS+ or SD. It is widely accepted that these cross-reactive antibodies can promote enhanced uptake of the heterologous virus into host cells, precipitating a hyperimmune reaction resulting in blood vessel leakage and potentially fatal hypovolemic shock [1, 2]. This increase occurs when nonneutralizing antibodies resulting from the primary infection favor the invasion of the second virus with a different serotype into the target cells, a phenomenon known as antibody-dependent amplification or antibody-dependent enhancement (ADE) [8, 9]. Subsequent infection with a different dengue serotype is more likely to cause DWS+/SD [8, 9]. According to the ADE hypothesis, a primary infection with DENV produces an insufficient concentration of antibodies or avidity to neutralize a secondary infection by DENV of a different serotype that differs in its amino acid sequence by 30–35%; and these sub-neutralizing antibody concentrations can promote infection in such cells by facilitating Fc-receptor-mediated entry [10]. These concentrations could be enough to opsonize the secondary virus and target it for Fc-receptor-mediated endocytosis into myeloid cells such as monocytes and macrophages (which constitute the main site of DENV replication) and in this manner promote higher viral loads. ADE can be observed *in vitro* and has also been proven to drive higher viral loads of DENV in animal models [11]. The following findings support the hypothesis of the antibody-dependent enhancement (ADE): undiluted sera obtained early from patients with secondary infection was shown to enhance dengue virus infection *in vitro,* infants born from dengue-immune mothers displayed a higher viral burden than infants born to dengue nonimmune mothers and further demonstrated immune activation associated with disease severity, and lethal antibody-dependent enhancement has been shown in dengue mouse models, and virus-antibody complexes bind to Fcγ receptor-bearing cells, resulting in increased infected cell mass and a rise in viremia. The cardinal feature of DWS+ is plasma leakage believed to arise from pro-inflammatory cytokine-inflicted damage to the vascular endothelium. Although the cause of severe form of dengue infection is not clear, it has been revealed that secondary infection with a different serotype of DENV, or even a homotypic reinfection, are major risk factors for SD probably due to antibody-dependent enhancement. The phenomena of original antigenic sin, as well as immune evasion that inhibits interferon (IFN)-α and IFN-β signaling by suppressing Jak-Stat activation, a cytokine storm, and autoimmune responses are thought to contribute to the pathogenesis of severe form of dengue disease [12, 13], see **Figure 1**. Dengue virus (DENV) can inhibit both type I IFN production and signaling in susceptible human cells, including dendritic cells (DCs). The proteolytic activity of the NS2B3 protease complex of DENV allows it to function as an antagonist of type I IFN production. Other DENV proteins that antagonize type I IFN signaling include NS2A, NS4A, NS4B, and NS5 by targeting different components of this signaling pathway, such as STATs [15]. During a primary infection, serotype-specific as well as cross-reactive memory T-cell responses are produced. On the other hand, during a secondary dengue virus infection, viral epitopes expressed on infected cells trigger activation of serotype-cross-reactive memory T-cells, with the production of pro-inflammatory cytokines. The latter ultimately lead to plasma leakage in the vascular endothelium. The specific cellular

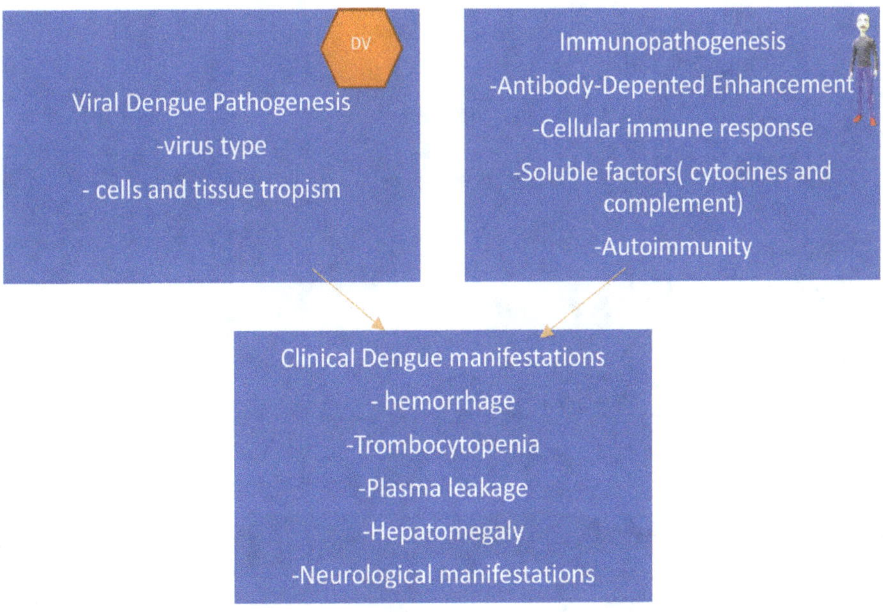

Figure 1. A hypothetical model of dengue pathogenesis. Viral and immunological factors contribute to clinical manifestations, including severe hemorrhage, thrombocytopenia, plasma leakage, hepatomegaly, and neurological compromise. DV: dengue virus. Adapted from Wan et al. [14].

response against DENV begins with the activation of CD4+ T-cell during viremia and subsequently the activation of CD8+ T-cell. In individuals with DHF or DWS+ due to secondary infections, the presence of CD4+/CD8+ memory T-cell and cytotoxic CD4+/CD8+ T-cell has been demonstrated [16], and the activation of T-cell and the production of cytokines are important factors in the pathogenesis of DWS+ [17]. Likewise, the cellular immune response, in the case of DWS+, exacerbates the activation and release of cytokines, which is related to the greater severity of the clinical picture. The activation of the complement system has also been demonstrated in DHF, and high concentrations of C3 and C1q proteins can be detected in severe cases. It is suggested that complex virus-circular antibodies could activate the cascade reaction of the complement [18], see **Figure 2**. Regulatory immune pattern in homologous versus a pro-inflammatory pattern in heterologous dengue virus secondary infection has been reported. Several soluble factors produced by T cells, monocytes, macrophages, and mast cells have been proposed to increase vascular permeability in primary endothelial cells. These factors include TNFα, interleukin 6, interleukin 8, interleukin 10, interleukin 12, macrophage migration inhibitory factor, HMGB1, MCP-1, and matrix metalloproteinases. Endothelial permeability can also be influenced by the maturation state of NS4B, which modulates the cytokine response in monocytic cell lines. In addition, secreted NS1 protein, along with anti-NS1 antibodies and complement activation, might be involved in dengue virus-induced vascular leakage. Moreover, around defervescence, when plasma leakage is apparent, high levels of complement activation products C3a and C5a are detected in plasma, followed by accelerated consumption and large reduction of complement components in patients with dengue shock syndrome. Activation of the complement system can stimulate the production of inflammatory cytokines associated with DWS+/SD, and trigger local and systemic effects implicated

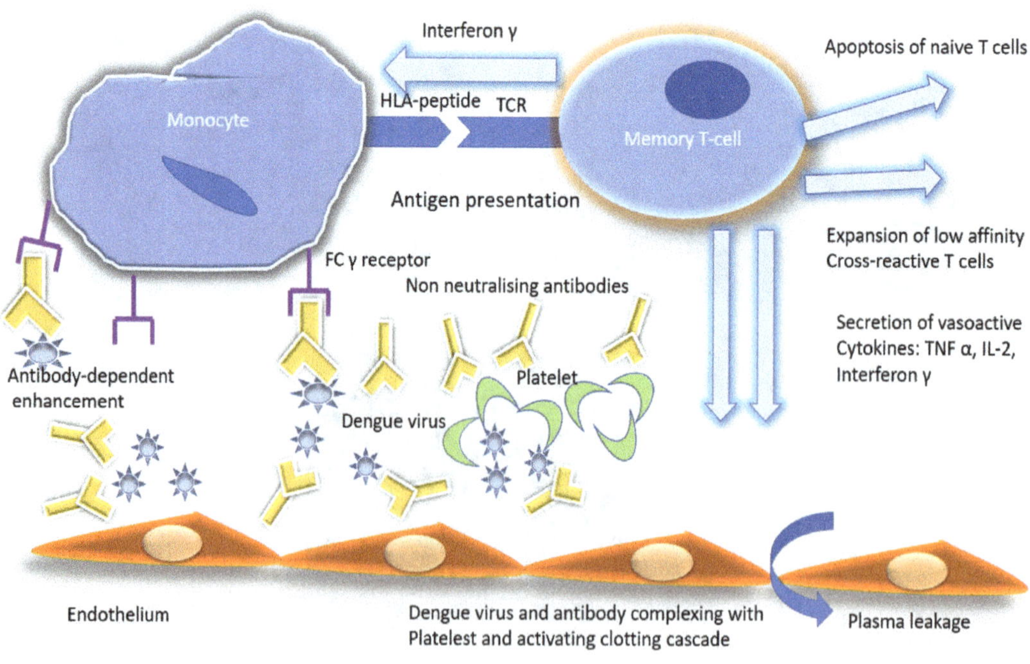

Figure 2. Schematic representation of the immunopathogenesis of severe dengue disease. Adapted from Webster et al. [4].

in intravascular coagulation. Finally, although controversial, the role of autoimmunity in the pathogenesis of dengue is mentioned, as autoantibodies resulting in platelet and endothelial cell dysfunction might be involved in severe dengue pathogenesis. Not all cases of DWS+ occur in people who experience a secondary infection, since in some cases the virus' own virulence, added to the characteristics of the host, leads to the complication of the disease [19], which may be due to the presence of antibodies against viral proteins that have cross-reactivity with platelets and coagulation factors [18]. Certain nonstructural proteins such as NS1, NS2, and NS3 appear to have a certain structural homology with coagulation factors, platelets, integrins, and adhesins of human endothelial cells, allowing the activation of autoreactive T lymphocytes that participate in the pathology of dengue [16, 20]. Anti-NS1 antibodies correlate with disease severity, and cross-reaction of anti-NS1 antibodies with liver and endothelial cells are also implicated in affecting the integrity of the vascular endothelium and platelets has been proposed to trigger these cells to express nitric oxide and undergo apoptosis [2, 3, 14]. Certain antibodies to some E protein epitopes can bind to human plasminogen and inhibit plasmin activity (see **Figure 3**). Recently, it has been reported that Tropomyosin (TPM)-1 may play an important role in the pathogenesis of SD. It is plausible that the elevation of TPM-1 in the plasma of SD patients can be due to excessive cell death, thereby releasing TPM into the circulation as DAMPs, and leading to mast cell activation. Moreover, the insulin pathway may play a role in the pathogenesis of SD, hence, regulating the insulin

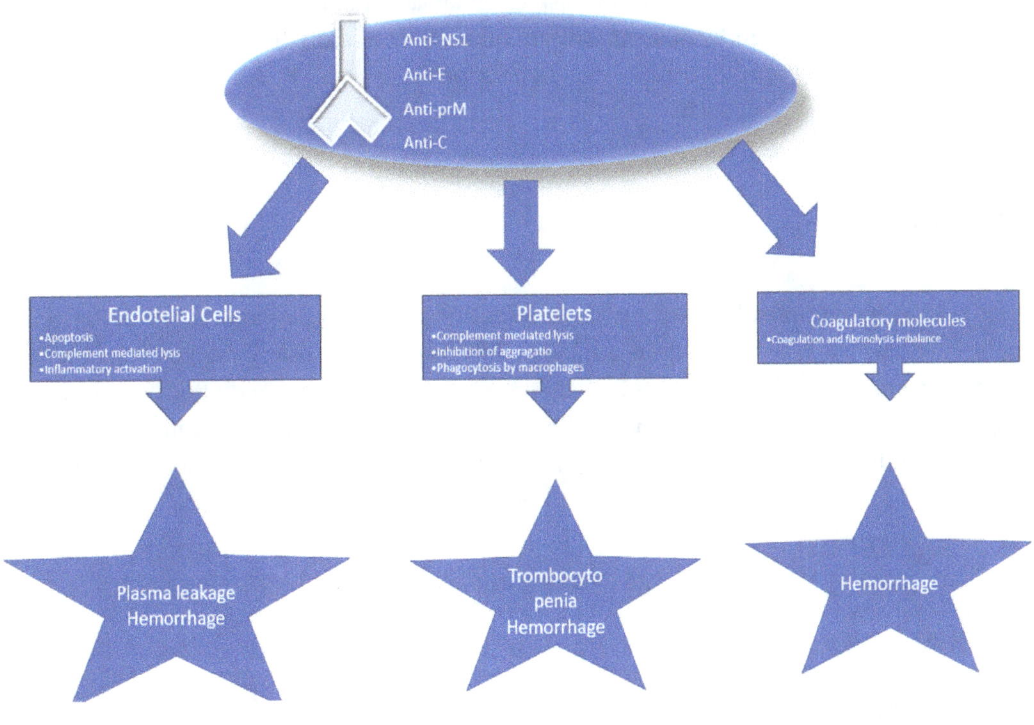

Figure 3. A schematic model of autoantibody-mediated immunopathogenesis in DENV infection. Molecular mimicry between platelets, endothelial cells, and coagulatory molecules with NS1, prM, E, and C proteins underlies the cross-reactivity of anti-NS1, anti-prM, anti-E, and anti-C Abs, respectively, to host proteins. Abs Z antibodies; C Z capsid protein; DENV Z dengue virus; E Z envelope protein; NS Z nonstructural protein; prM Z precursor membrane protein. Adapted from Wan et al. [14].

signaling pathway may be a key intervention to reduce plasma leakage in patients with SD [12], see **Figures 1–3**.

A protective versus pathological outcome depends on the balance between the host's genetic and immunological background and viral factors. Vaccine development has been slowed by fears that immunization might predispose individuals to the severe form of dengue infection [3, 4]. There are four distinct, but closely related, serotypes of the virus that cause dengue (DEN-1, DEN-2, DEN-3, and DEN-4).

No DENV-specific therapies are available, while a DENV vaccine that elicits protection in people with prior DENV exposure but not in naive individuals and that is not equally protective against all four serotypes has recently begun to be licensed on a country-by-country basis. This is mostly due to an incomplete understanding of the interplay between viral and host factors that contribute to DENV pathogenesis. On the virus side, some DENV lineages are more virologically and epidemiologically fit than others and are thus associated with DWS+/SD manifestations. On the host side, DENV infection history is the primary determinant associated with the development of more severe dengue disease, with potential contributions from other factors such as genetic variation, age, and sex.

Several studies have demonstrated that DENV-specific antibodies can protect against infection and, under certain conditions, enhance infection and disease severity, whereas the role of T cells remains unclear. Thus, to avoid the risk of enhancement, a safe vaccine against dengue virus will need to confer protective immunity against all four serotypes [10]. Consequently, the adaptive immune response to dengue can be both protective and pathogenic, which complicates vaccine development, as discussed in this chapter.

4. Dengue vaccines

Dengue virus is widespread throughout the tropics, representing an important, rapidly growing public health problem with an estimated 2.5–3.9 billion people at risk of dengue fever and the life-threatening severe dengue disease. Therefore, the need for a safe and effective vaccine for dengue is immediate. Vaccine development has been slowed by fears that immunization might predispose individuals to the severe form of dengue infection [4]. The characteristics and challenges that the ideal vaccine for the dengue virus must have are described in the following.

4.1. Characteristics of an ideal dengue vaccine and challenges to its development

4.1.1. Characteristics

- Safe in children and adults [3, 4]
- Avoids ADE (antibody-dependent enhancement) and pathogenesis
- Rapid immunization regime requiring a single vaccine or two that fit in with established vaccine programs

- Induces a balance between reactogenicity and immunogenicity
- Suitable for use in target age groups
- Genetically stable
- Stimulates neutralizing antibodies and Th1 cell-mediated immunity
- Induces long-lasting immunity, safety, and protection
- Generates neutralizing immunity to all four serotypes
- Does not contribute to immunopathogenesis (vaccine-induced enhancement)
- Easy storage and transportation
- Affordable and cost effective

4.1.2. Challenges

- Existing possibility of triggering ADE
- Vaccine must be tetravalent
- Dengue virus serotypes do not induce long-lasting heterotypic immunity
- No suitable or ideal animal model exists for immunization studies
- No well-established viral virulence markers are available
- Correlates of protection are not well defined
- Subsequent infection (especially, after a long-time interval) may lead to severe dengue
- Vaccine candidates should be evaluated in geographic areas with different transmission patterns [3].

To date, there are several DENV vaccines under development, with some in phase 3 safety and efficacy testing. These include inactivated, live attenuated, recombinant subunit, viral vectored, and DNA vaccines. Dengue vaccine development has aimed to elicit a neutralizing antibody response, as T cells are assumed to contribute a minor or secondary role in dengue vaccine-mediated protection. Next, we will describe each of these vaccines.

4.2. Vaccine types

4.2.1. Live-attenuated virus (LAV)

The fundamental aim of vaccination is to promote protective immunity while avoiding disease from the vaccine itself. The first generation of viral vaccines was based on empirical attenuation by repeated passage in cultured cells. Several LAVs are eligible vaccines as they meet the following criteria; they elicit a strong and protective immune response with a low risk of disease from the vaccine itself. In the present regulatory environment, the use of LAVs has also been limited by safety concerns, including reversion to wild-type virulence. Because LAVs are shed from vaccines, they sometimes present a risk to unvaccinated individuals with impaired immunity. Although LAV vaccines have been developed for many RNA viruses, the mutability of these pathogens presents unique challenges for vaccine design [21].

4.2.2. Purified inactivated virus (PIV)

It is widely believed that inactivated dengue virus vaccines are impractical given the difficulty in obtaining sufficiently high titers of the virus in a suitable cell substrate. However, this was challenged when dengue type-2 (dengue-2) virus was adapted to replicate to high titers in certified Vero and fetal rhesus lung (FRhL-2) cell cultures and used to make prototype purified, inactivated virus (PIV) vaccines. In addition, in formulation with an aluminum hydroxide adjuvant, these vaccines elicit virus-neutralizing antibodies in mice and rhesus macaques and provide at least partial protection against virus challenge [22].

4.2.3. Recombinant subunits

Recombinant subunit-based vaccines may prove to be significantly advantageous compared to other approaches currently being implemented for development of a dengue vaccine. First of all, the lack of a replicating virus helps to ensure the safety of the product by avoiding the possibility for inadequate attenuation or reversion in the context of live virus approaches, or inadequate inactivation in the context of killed virus vaccines. Furthermore, under a tetravalent formulation, the ability to induce a balanced immune response may be more easily manipulated through dose adjustments using recombinant subunits compared to four replicating viruses. Finally, in terms of yield and cost effectiveness, and since the dengue vaccine mainly targets developing areas, a high yielding, highly immunogenic, recombinant subunit could prove to be an attractive alternative to vaccines based on virus replication, (live attenuated or killed) where yields may be lower than required [23].

Recombinant subunit vaccines stand as one of the safest alternatives, as a means to bypass the issue of viral interference, offering the possibility to administer a tetravalent formulation on an accelerated schedule. An advantage of an accelerated schedule is that full protective immunity could be induced more quickly, thus avoiding the potential of exacerbated disease due to partial immunity during an extended immunization course. Among other advantages of an accelerated schedule are better general compliance, more suitability for travelers and military personnel, easier integration into existing immunization schedules, and the potential for use in an outbreak setting. A balanced tetravalent immune response may also be more readily accomplished through simple dose adjustments for each of the four recombinant proteins, in comparison to live virus vaccines where the interactions between viruses can be complex and unpredictable [24].

4.2.4. Virus-like particles (VLPs)

VLP vaccines are virus-like particles that do not contain replicative genetic material, but permit presentation of antigen in a repetitive, ordered array similar to the virion structure, which is thought to increase immunogenicity [25]. Thus, the safety concerns of virus vaccines regarding reversion mutants and immunocompromised individuals are obviated. The recombinant of

VLP allows these vaccines to be usually manufactured large-scale in a cost-effective manner, following current good manufacturing practices. They induce quick and fulminant humoral immune responses by displaying antigens in an ordered and repetitive way. Their particulate nature and dimensions allows an efficient assimilation by dendritic cells (DCs) and transportation to lymph nodes, followed by presentation and induction of optimal immune responses. VLPs are renowned for inducing rapid and strong antibody responses. This trait is attributed to their dense, highly repetitive, quasi-crystalline structures [26], see Dengue vaccine candidates in **Table 1**.

Candidate name/ identifier	Antigen	Vaccination	Developer	Preclinical	Phase I	Phase II	Phase III
CYD Live recombinant based on a yellow fever vaccine 17D backbone	DENV-1-4 prM/E	3 doses (0/6/12 months)	Sanofi Pasteur	X	X	X	X
TV003/TV005 Tetravalent live, attenuated/ recombinant (whole virus DENV1–3 and recombinant DENV2 in DENV4 backbone)	DENV-1,3,4 whole genome, DENV-2 prM/E	1 dose	US National Institutes of Health and Butantan (with licenses to other manufacturers)	X	X	X	X
DENVax Tetravalent live, attenuated/ recombinant (whole virus DENV2 and recombinant DENV1/ 3/4 in DENV2 backbone)	DENV-2 whole genome, DENV-1, -3, -4 prM/E	2 doses (0/ 90 days)	Takeda	X	X	X	
DPIV Tetravalent purified inactivated vaccine	DENV-1–4 whole genome	2 doses (0/ 28 days)	GSK/US WRAIR/ Fiocruz	X	X		
DEN-80ETetravalent E protein subunit vaccine	Soluble DEN 1/2/ 3/4 prM/E protein	3 doses (0/1/ 2 months)	Merck	X	X		
TVDVTetravalent "shuffled" prM/E expressed from plasmid vector DNA vaccine	Plasmid DNA expressing DENV 1/2/3/4 prM-E	3 doses (0/1/ 3 months)	US Naval Medical Research Center	X	X		
TLAV-TPIV Heterologous prime-boost with live-attenuated tetravalent, live-attenuated vaccine and tetravalent alum-adjuvanted purified inactivated vaccine	Purified inactivated DENV or plasmid vector expressing prM/E (prime) and live-attenuated DENV (boost)		US WRAIR	X	X		

Dengue vaccine candidates; adapted from Kirsten et al. [27].

Table 1. Dengue vaccine candidates.

4.3. Vaccines under clinical trials

4.3.1. CYD-TDV Dengvaxia

Sanofi Pasteur's CYD vaccine is a live-attenuated tetravalent chimeric vaccine. In this vaccine, the premembrane and envelope proteins from a wild-type dengue virus corresponding to each of the four serotypes are substituted into the yellow fever (YF) 17D vaccine backbone. A strong neutralizing antibody response to DENV2 was elicited in the first CYD clinical trial in healthy adults, which evaluated only the serotype 2 vaccine strain. Participants previously given YF vaccine seroconverted to all four dengue serotypes [28]. The first licensed dengue vaccine, a live, attenuated, tetravalent dengue vaccine (CYD-TDV; Dengvaxia), has recently been registered in 15 countries as a three-dose immunization schedule administered subcutaneously at 6-month intervals [29]. In the case of Dengvaxia, vaccination of children with no previous infection (seronegative) may mimic an initial infection during the first step in the development of ADE. Because vaccine protection is incomplete and unequal against the four serotypes, a natural infection later in life can complete the sequence of events, causing ADE and severe, life-threatening dengue fever [30].

Following CYD-TDV introduction, it should be administered as a three-dose series given on a 0-/6-/12-month schedule. However, additional evidence is required in order to determine whether equivalent or better protection may be obtained through simplified schedules. In response to a delay in a vaccine dose for any reason, the vaccine course should be resumed (not restarted), maintaining the 6-month interval between subsequent doses. Given the 12-month duration of the immunization schedule and to enable better vaccine monitoring, countries should have vaccine tracking systems implemented. CYD-TDV is not recommended for use in children under 9 years of age, consistent with current labeling, in view of the association of CYD-TDV with increased risk of hospitalized and severe dengue illness in the 2- to 5-year age group. The target age for routine vaccination should be defined by each country, intended to maximize the vaccination impact and programmatic feasibility of targeting specific age groups. For instance, some countries may present the highest incidence of dengue illness among the adult age population and may consider vaccinating people up to 45 years of age in routine programs. The implementation of a routine CYD-TDV vaccination program at 9 years of age in settings meeting the criteria mentioned above is expected to contribute to a 10–30% reduction in symptomatic and hospitalized dengue illness over 30 years [31], see **Table 2**. This vaccine will be reviewed further in a separate section since, differently to other vaccines in this section, Dengvaxia has already been registered.

4.3.2. TV003 and TV005 Dengue vaccine

The Laboratory of Infectious Diseases at the U.S National Institutes of Health has evaluated numerous monovalent and tetravalent dengue candidate vaccines to identify candidates with the most acceptable safety, infectivity, and immunogenicity profile. Among these, TV003 is an admixture of four live-attenuated recombinant dengue vaccine candidate viruses (rDEN1D30, rDEN2/4D30, rDEN3D30/31, and rDEN4D30) [36]. Various monovalent candidates were initially tested in Phase 1 trials in order to optimize each of the four vaccine virus strains. Vaccine virus serotypes 1, 3, and 4 are based on complete viruses, while serotype 2 is a recombinant

Reference	Lead author /year	Conclusion
Four-year safety follow-up of the tetravalent dengue vaccine efficacy randomized controlled trials in Asia and Latin America,	Arredondo-García et al. 2018 [32]	Data from the clinical trials for up to year 4 after first vaccination indicate a positive benefit–risk profile for the CYD-TDV vaccine for the population aged 9 years old.
A multi-country study of dengue vaccination strategies with Dengvaxia and a future vaccine candidate in three dengue-endemic countries: Vietnam, Thailand, and Colombia.	Lee et al. 2018 [33]	Given the absence of efficacy and half-life data for any of the second-generation vaccine candidates, it was assumed that NVC is 80% efficacious with a half- life of 8 years.
Dengue vaccination during pregnancy—an overview of clinical trials data.	Skipetrova et al. [34]	In the small dataset assessed, no evidence of increased adverse pregnancy outcomes has been identified from inadvertent immunization of women in early pregnancy with CYD-TDV compared with the control group. The conclusions are limited to vaccination in CYD-TDV in the first trimester, since no data are available on pregnancy outcome for administration of this vaccine in the second or third trimester. The data described here, and those continuing to emerge from the on-going clinical development and post-marketing of CYD-TDV, provide a valuable contribution to the currently limited available information on the use of the dengue vaccine in pregnant women.
Live-attenuated, tetravalent dengue vaccine in children, adolescents and adults in a dengue-endemic country: Randomized controlled phase I trial in the Philippines.	Capeding et al. 2011 [35]	The safety profile of TDV in a flavivirus endemic population was consistent with previous reports from flavivirus-naïve populations. A vaccine regimen of either three TDV vaccinations administered over a year or two TDV vaccinations given more than 8 months apart resulted in a balanced antibody response to all four dengue serotypes in this flavivirus-exposed population, including children.

Table 2. Some CYD-TDV Dengue vaccine safety and immunogenicity studies in different populations.

virus based on the serotype 4 vaccine strain with the structural proteins replaced by those of serotype 2. A single dose of TV005 elicits seroconversion rates above 90% against each serotype, and 90% of flavivirus-naive recipients displayed a tetravalent response. TV003 or TV005 has been licensed to several manufacturers, including Butantan, VaBiotech, and Merck. Phase 2 studies are underway in Brazil and Thailand, and a Phase 3 trial led by Butantan began in February, 2016, in Brazil [27], see **Table 3**.

4.3.3. *DENVax*

Takeda's live tetravalent dengue vaccine (TDV) candidate is based on a molecularly characterized attenuated serotype 2 strain (TDV-2). The DENV-2 PDK-53 virus was initially obtained through 53 serial passages of the wild-type (wt) DENV-2 16681 in primary dog kidney (PDK)

Reference	Lead author /year	Conclusion
In a randomized trial, the live-attenuated tetravalent dengue vaccine TV003 is well- tolerated and highly immunogenic in subjects with flavivirus exposure prior to vaccination	Whitehead et al. 2017 [37]	In summary, the authors demonstrated that the NIH tetravalent dengue vaccine TV003 is well-tolerated in flavivirus-experienced individuals and elicits robust post-vaccination neutralizing antibody titers.
The live-attenuated dengue vaccine TV003 elicits complete protection against dengue in a human challenge model	Kirkpatrick et al. 2016 [36]	TV003 induced complete protection against challenge with rDEN2Δ30 administered 6 months after vaccination. TV003 will be further evaluated in dengue-endemic areas.

Table 3. Some TV003 vaccine safety and immunogenicity studies.

cells. The DENV-2 PDK-53 virus has proved to be safe, well-tolerated, immunogenic, and elicits long-term humoral and cellular immune responses to DENV-2, based on clinical trials conducted in the United States and Thailand [38]. Three chimeric strains (TDV-1, TDV-3, and TDV-4) were engineered by substituting the premembrane (prM) and envelope (E) structural genes of the respective DENV strains into the attenuated TDV-2 backbone [39]. TDV is designed to promote humoral and cellular protective immune responses against all four dengue serotypes, as it contains the premembrane and envelope proteins unique to each serotype. These specific proteins are needed to induce neutralizing antibodies. The use of DENV-2 as a backbone for TDV may confer additional protection against dengue. In particular, TDV contains the genes encoding the conserved nonstructural (NS) proteins within the dengue backbone; and these proteins have been shown to be important in generating T-cell-mediated responses to dengue infection. Furthermore, anti-NS1 antibodies have been associated with cross-protective humoral immune responses [40]. **Table 4** shows some of the studies conducted to determine the effectiveness of this vaccine.

4.3.4. DPIV tetravalent purified inactivated vaccine

The Walter Reed Army Institute of Research (WRAIR) in collaboration with GlaxoSmithKline Vaccines (GSK) developed a live-attenuated tetravalent dengue virus vaccine candidate comprised of four live virus strains representing each of the four DENV types. These strains were attenuated by serial passage in primary dog kidney (PDK) cells [44]. The US Navy Naval Medical Research Center (NMRC) has developed a tetravalent DNA vaccine (TVDV), formulated with Vical's Vaxfectin adjuvant, containing genes encoding the premembrane (prM) and envelope (E) proteins for all four serotypes of dengue virus. Both Vaxfectin-formulated and unformulated vaccines are currently being evaluated in Phase I human testing [45].

Inactivated vaccines are assumed to provide acceptable safety profiles across a wide age range as well as in immunocompromised hosts. In addition, these can be co-administered with other vaccines. Shortened vaccination schedules and rapid immunization are also feasible using this type of vaccines. For these reasons, a safe and efficacious tetravalent DENV PIV could be suitable for national immunization programs across broad age ranges and baseline health status, as well as an active immunization option for travelers and military personnel, and a potential tool for outbreak response [46]. **Table 5** shows several DPIV vaccine safety and immunogenicity studies.

Reference	Lead author /year	Conclusion
Safety and immunogenicity of a live-attenuated tetravalent dengue vaccine candidate in flavivirus-naive adults: a randomized, double-blinded Phase 1 clinical trial	George et al. 2015 [41]	TDV was generally well-tolerated, induced trivalent or broader neutralizing antibodies to DENV in most flavivirus-naive vaccines, and is undergoing further development.
Safety and immunogenicity of a recombinant live-attenuated tetravalent dengue vaccine (DENVax) in flavivirus-naive healthy adults in Colombia: a randomized, placebo-controlled, phase 1 study	Osorio et al. 2014 [42]	The authors emphasize the acceptable tolerability and immunogenicity of the tetravalent DENVax formulations in healthy, flavivirus-naive adults. Further clinical testing of DENVax in different age groups and in dengue-endemic areas is warranted.
Development of DENVax: A chimeric dengue-2 PDK-53-based tetravalent vaccine for protection against dengue fever	Osorio et al. 2011 [43]	The DENVax vaccine is considerably different from previously tested tetravalent vaccines in that all four strains contain the same attenuating mutations as the DEN-2 PDK-53 strain, a strain that has been shown to be both safe and immunogenic in humans. Such vaccine is critically needed to protect people from the threat of dengue infection and improve public health worldwide.

Table 4. Some TDV(DENVax) vaccine safety and immunogenicity studies.

Reference	Lead author /year	Conclusion
Phase I randomized study of a tetravalent dengue purified inactivated vaccine in healthy adults from Puerto Rico.	Diaz et al. 2018 [47]	Results from this first phase I study of a new vaccine candidate with inactivated DENV in a dengue-primed population showed that all four DPIV vaccine formulations were well-tolerated and immunogenic. This new investigational DPIV vaccine had an acceptable safety profile in a small number of flavivirus-primed healthy adult subjects and all formulations boosted neutralizing antibodies (Nab) responses, with complex adjuvants increasing immunogenicity versus alum adjuvantation. Nab titers remained high (and above baseline titers) through M13. These results encourage continuation of DPIV clinical development.
Phase 1 randomized study of a tetravalent dengue purified inactivated vaccine in healthy adults in the United States	Lepine et al. 2017 [48]	All DPIV formulations were well-tolerated. No vaccine-related serious adverse events were observed through 12 months after the second vaccine dose. In all DPIV groups, geometric mean antibody titers peaked at Day 56, waned through 6 months after the second vaccine dose, and then stabilized. In the nine subjects where boosting was evaluated, a strong anamnestic response was observed. These results support continuation of the clinical development of this dengue vaccine candidate.

Table 5. Some DPIV vaccine safety and immunogenicity studies.

4.3.5. DEN 80E vaccine

This vaccine (developed by Hawaii Biotech and now licensed to Merck) is composed of a recombinant truncated protein corresponding to 80% of the N-terminal DENV E protein (DEN-80E). The C-terminal truncation of the E protein at amino acid 395 removes the membrane anchor sequence of the protein, resulting in a recombinant E protein with improved secretion, purification and immunogenicity. The DEN-80E protein for each of the four dengue serotypes has been expressed in the Drosophila S2 expression system to produce a tetravalent vaccine [49], which induces a high level expression of proteins of interest. Specifically, the system was chosen to express a plasmid containing the prM and N-terminal 80% of the E gene sequence of DENV-2. The resulting polyprotein undergoes cleavage by endogenous proteases and the 80E protein with a native-like N terminus is released. Two doses of the DENV-2 subunit 80E protein were administered to rhesus macaques in combination with one of seven different adjuvants at a 3-month dosing interval. Following this administration, animals were challenged with wild-type DENV-2 2 months after the last dose of vaccine. Neutralizing antibodies were detected in all study animals after the first dose and this response was boosted by the second dose. The highest neutralizing antibody titers were produced by the r80E protein formulated with the adjuvants AS05 or AS08, and protection against viremia was correlated with a higher neutralizing antibody titer at challenge. The same system was employed to generate recombinant subunit E proteins (80E) of the other DENV serotypes. A tetravalent formulation of the recombinant 80E proteins was evaluated in mice and nonhuman primate experiments. In some instances, the NS1 protein of DENV-2 was included in the formulation to potentially enhance the immune response to the vaccine. Macaques were immunized with the tetravalent formulation four times (day 0, 28, 67, and 102) and were challenged 5 months after the last dose. Due to the limited number of monkeys in each group, monkeys were only challenged with DENV-2 or DENV-4. Monkeys developed a robust neutralizing antibody response to all four DENV serotypes and were completely protected from DENV-2 challenge [50]. **Table 6** shows some of the studies conducted to determine the effectiveness of this vaccine.

4.3.6. TVDV tetravalent "shuffled" prM/E expressed from a plasmid vector DNA vaccine

The U.S. Naval Medical Research Center (NMRC) developed a tetravalent plasmid DNA vaccine candidate using prM and E protein genes expressed in a plasmid vector. A DENV-1 monovalent candidate of this vaccine was evaluated for safety and immunogenicity through a phase I clinical trial on healthy flavivirus-naïve adults using a three-dose schedule at 0/1/5 months. The results showed poor immunogenicity. Although it is possible that TVDV may have a role as a travel vaccine in the future, the available data is currently insufficient to anticipate its potential use as a travel vaccine [52].

The TVDV is a mixture of equal amounts of four monovalent double-stranded plasmid DNA vaccines produced under current Good Manufacturing Practices conditions in the United States. Each monovalent plasmid contains the prM and E genes of dengue 1, 2, 3, or 4 viruses cloned into the backbone plasmid VR1012 (Vical Incorporated, San Diego, CA) [53]. **Table 7** shows some of the studies conducted to determine the effectiveness of this vaccine.

Reference	Lead author/ year	Conclusion
Preclinical development of a dengue tetravalent recombinant subunit vaccine: Immunogenicity and protective efficacy in nonhuman primates	Govindarajan et al. 2015 [51]	Overall, the subunit vaccine was demonstrated to induce strong neutralization titers resulting in protection against viremia following challenge even 8–12 months after the last vaccine dose.
The development of recombinant subunit envelope-based vaccines to protect against dengue virus induced disease	Coller et al. 2011 [24]	The DEN-80E recombinant subunit proteins for all four dengue virus types are expressed at high levels and have been shown to maintain native-like conformation. When formulated with a variety of adjuvants the antigens are potent immunogens and induce high titer virus-neutralizing antibody responses. Furthermore, the antigens have been shown to protect against viral challenge in both mouse and nonhuman primate models. Tetravalent vaccine formulations have also been evaluated in preclinical models with no evidence of immune interference or competition between the four DEN-80E antigens being observed. These proofs of concept preclinical studies led to the advancement of a monovalent DEN1-80E vaccine candidate into clinical testing.
Development of a recombinant tetravalent dengue virus vaccine: immunogenicity and efficacy studies in mice and monkeys	Clements et al. 2010 [23]	The production of recombinant dengue 80E proteins in Drosophila S2 cells that are capable of eliciting potent immune responses in mice and nonhuman primates represents a major achievement in the effort to develop a recombinant dengue vaccine. The S2 cell expression system efficiently produces 80E from all four dengue serotypes. Our data show that co-administration of the subunits from the four serotypes results in a balanced immune response, equivalent to that observed when the four individual components are administered separately. Furthermore this response can be induced in a relatively short period of time (2–3 months).

Table 6. Some DEN 80E Vaccine safety and immunogenicity studies.

4.4. Vaccine candidates under preclinical assays

There are numerous vaccine candidates that are being studied in preclinical trials, as can be seen in **Table 8**.

4.4.1. EDIII-p64k fusion proteins and EDIII-capsid fusion proteins expressed in E. coli

Te Pedro Kourí Tropical Medicine Institute (IPK) in collaboration with the Center for Genetic Engineering and Biotechnology (CIGB) in Cuba have led the development of various recombinant subunit vaccine candidates. One approach is based on fusion of DENV EDIII to the carrier protein p64k of *Neisseria meningitidis,* and this EDIII-p64k fusion protein is then expressed in *E. coli*. Evaluations in mice showed that monovalent vaccine candidates for all

Reference	Lead author/ year	Conclusion
Safety and immunogenicity of a tetravalent dengue DNA vaccine administered with a cationic lipid-based adjuvant in a Phase 1 clinical trial	Thomas et al. 2018 [53]	TVDV-Vaxfectin was safe and well-tolerated in this early Phase 1 human clinical trial. Whereas anti-dengue IFNγ T-cell responses occurred in most of the study subjects, anti-dengue neutralizing antibody responses were poor. Utilization of alternative delivery methods as well as examining prime-boost approaches may result in a more robust and long-lasting humoral immune response.
A dengue DNA vaccine formulated with Vaxfectin® is well-tolerated, and elicits strong neutralizing antibody responses to all four dengue serotypes in New Zealand white rabbits	Raviprakash et al. 2012 [54]	The formulated vaccine and the adjuvant were tested for safety and/or immunogenicity in New Zealand white rabbits using a repeat dose toxicology study. The formulated vaccine and the adjuvant were found to be well-tolerated by the animals. Animals injected with formulated vaccine produced strong neutralizing antibody response to all four dengue serotypes.

Table 7. Some TVDV vaccine safety and immunogenicity studies.

DENV serotypes were able to induce neutralizing antibodies and protect against viral challenge. DENV-1 and DENV-2 monovalent candidates have also been evaluated in NHPs. Monkeys were immunized subcutaneously with four doses of the monovalent vaccine (50–100 g protein per dose, formulated in Freund's adjuvant), which proved to be immunogenic and provided protection against viral challenge. Adjuvants suitable for human use are under evaluation, including *N. meningitidis* serogroup A capsular polysaccharide (CPSA) adsorbed on aluminum hydroxide [25].

5. Final thoughts

Finally, we want to reflect on the implications of the co-circulation of the dengue virus and the Zika virus, as well as on the new indications for the use of the Dengvaxia vaccine.

First, we will analyze the fact that the appearance of the infection by the Zika virus (another flavivirus) in zones of high prevalence for dengue constitutes an interesting challenge for the development of the ideal vaccine for both viruses.

5.1. Zika virus infection means new challenges in dengue vaccine development

Among pathogenic human flaviviruses, DENV and ZIKV are most closely related to each other, with 55.1–56.3% amino acid sequence identity. Zika virus is closer to dengue virus than to any of the other flaviviruses and indeed is almost close enough to think of it as a fifth serotype [10]. Accordingly, emerging literature indicates many similarities between these two viruses in terms of interactions between the virus and host immune system. For both viruses, the interferon system is the central mediator of host defense and target of a viral counterattack,

Techonological approach	Antigen	Vaccine developer	Valency under evaluation or evaluated in NHP
Recombinant subunit vaccines	EDIII-p64k fusion proteins and EDIII-capsid fusion proteins expressed in *E. coli*	IPK/CIGB	Monovalent
	Bivalent 80E-STF2 fusion proteins expressed in baculovirus/insect cells	VaxInnate	Tetravalent
	Tetravalent consensus EDIII protein expressed in *E. coli.*	NHRI	Tetravalent
DNA vaccine	prM/E expressed from plasmid vector DNA vaccine	US CDC	Tetravalent
VLP Vaccines	EDIII-HBsAg VLPs or ectoE-based VLPs expressed in *P. pastoris*	ICGEB	Tetravalent
Virus-vectored vaccines	Tetravalent EDIII and DENV-1 ectoM expressed from live-attenuated measles virus vector	Themis Bioscience/Institut X Pasteur	Tetravalent
	E85 expressed from single-cycle VEE virus vector	Global Vaccines	Tetravalent
Purified inactivated virus vaccine	Psoralen-inactivated DENV	US NMRC	Monovalent
Purified inactivated DENV	Purified inactivated DENV	WRAIR/GSK/FIOCRUZ	Tetravalent
	Inactivated virus (+VEE-particle adjuvant)	Global Vaccines	Tetravalent
Live-attenuated virus vaccines	DEN/DEN chimeric viruses, live, attenuated	Chiang Mai University/ Mahidol X University/ NSTDA/BioNet-Asia	Monovalent
	DEN host range mutations	Arbovax	Tetravalent

Table 8. Active dengue vaccine candidates in preclinical development that have been evaluated in NHP models.

whereas complex interplays between antibody and T cell responses likely determine the outcome of infection in flavivirus immune settings [55]. Dejnirattisai et al. found that most mAbs to DENV also bound to ZIKV, yet the antibodies targeting the major linear fusion-loop epitope (FLE) did not neutralize ZIKV, whereas they showed neutralizing activity against DENV. ZIKV virus infection was found to be potently enhanced by DENV-immune plasma and mAbs to DENV, suggesting the possibility that preexisting immunity to DENV might increase ZIKV replication; thus, this data indicate that immunity to DENV might drive greater ZIKV replication and have clear implications for disease pathogenesis and future vaccine programs for ZIKV and DENV [11]. There have been safety concerns related to Dengvaxia resulting from long-term vaccine trials. In patient groups under 9 years of age, hospitalization from DENV infection was greater for vaccinated children than for the nonvaccinated control group. These findings suggest ADE of infection in DENV naive children at the start of the study trial and who had been primed by but not protected by the vaccine. Consequently, the vaccine is not licensed for use in children under 9 years of age and, furthermore, it is recommended for use only in populations with a seroprevalence of 70% or greater of prior DENV exposure in the age group to be vaccinated [56].

Currently, there is a high pressure to produce a vaccine against ZIKV, and in this context, the extensive serological cross-reaction between DENV and ZIKV must be considered. It is likely necessary that the vaccine be used in areas with high seroprevalence for DENV and raising de novo ZIKV-neutralizing responses in such a setting might be challenging. It is likewise possible that vaccination of DENV-naive subjects against ZIKV might promote ADE of DENV infection and, conversely, that vaccination against DENV might promote ADE of ZIKV infection. In summary, cross-reaction of antibodies to DENV with ZIKV and promotion of ADE of infection can occur due to the existing similarities between the two viruses, even though ZIKV differs in sequence identity from DENV by around 41–46% (in the sequence of the envelope protein). In this context, ZIKV could be considered a fifth member of the DENV serocomplex, a factor that must be considered in vaccine approaches to these two viruses [11]. The results of Barba-Spaeth group suggest that the epitope targeted by the EDE1 bnAbs is more adequate for developing an epitope-focused vaccine for viruses of the ZIKV/DENV super serogroup than is the FLE, which induces poorly neutralizing and strongly infection-enhancing antibodies [57].

5.2. The Dengvaxia future

Dengvaxia is the only vaccine licensed to date for use in humans, which is why epidemiologists, health professionals, clinical physicians, and basic researchers (virologists, immunologists, molecular biologists, etc.) should be concerned about the future of this vaccine, which has had a reverse according to the latest publications of its results, so we will end this chapter with the following reflection based on the publications from 2016 to date.

Since April 2016, Dengvaxia has been licensed for use in 19 countries, and was recommended by the WHO Strategic Advisory Group of Experts (SAGE) on immunization to be used in regions with high endemicity, as defined by a prevalence of dengue antibodies of more than 50% in the targeted age group of people aged 9–45 years. Nevertheless, Guiar's mathematical model finds that a significant reduction of hospitalizations can be only achieved when the vaccine is directed exclusively to seropositive individuals [58]. Along this same line, this group of researchers in 2017 predicted a significant reduction in dengue virus infection-related hospital admissions resulting from the administration of Dengvaxia only to dengue seropositive individuals, based on the analysis of an age-structured model using the available vaccine trial data. Moreover, the researchers predicted a significant increase in the number of dengue-related admissions, over a 5-year period, if the vaccine is to be administered without previous population screening for serostatus. The take-home message is that individual serostatus is the most important feature when implementing this vaccine and that only individuals of any age who have experienced at least one dengue virus infection will benefit from vaccination [59, 60]. New data by Sanofi in November 2017 showed that Dengvaxia could increase the risk of severe dengue in people who had not been previously exposed to the virus. For any countries considering vaccination as part of their dengue control program, the WHO recommends a "prevaccination screening strategy," in which only dengue seropositive people are vaccinated. The prescreening process could be achieved by conventional serological testing for dengue virus to identify people who have had previous dengue infections. As Sanofi stated, "We are confident in Dengvaxia's safety and its proven potential to reduce dengue disease burden in endemic countries. We will continue to work with the international public health community and endemic countries, to ensure the best usage of the vaccine to increase protection for populations at risk of subsequent dengue infections [that are] potentially more debilitating" [61].

Author details

Jhon Carlos Castaño-Osorio[1]*, Alejandra María Giraldo-Garcia[1] and Maria Isabel Giraldo[2]

*Address all correspondence to: jhoncarlos@uniquindio.edu.co

1 Quindio University, Armenia, Quindio, Colombia

2 Department of Microbiology and Immunology, University of Texas Medical Branch, Galveston, TX, USA

References

[1] Who. Dengue and Severe Dengue. WHO Fact Sheet [Internet]. 2012. pp. 1-4. Available from: www.who.int/mediacentre/factsheets/fs117/en/index.html

[2] Swaminathan S, Khanna N. Dengue: Recent advances in biology and current status of translational research. Current Molecular Medicine [Internet]. 2009;**9**(2):152-173. Available from: http://www.eurekaselect.com/openurl/content.php?genre=article&issn=1566-5240&volume=9&issue=2&spage=152

[3] Guzman MG, Harris E. Dengue. Lancet (London, England) [Internet]. 2015;**385**(9966):453-465. Available from: http://griffith.summon.serialssolutions.com/2.0.0/link/0/eLvHCXMwnV07T8MwED5BQQgJ8ShQAgV1hCGt49iJM_GuWJgAic3yky0Npf3_2Hn0BWJgyZBYUXJn3333-e4MEOM-CldsQoKlDzSIRJIJRLRmSapUZnTq4mlcttZbZDJuGqag0nZjJEvLrUfKk-YDh_OziDgPxa6Lz9AfI-W3W-szNdZhA_tG5W6Cp-93vxVKljnv85

[4] Webster DP, Farrar J, Rowland-Jones S. Progress towards a dengue vaccine. The Lancet Infectious Diseases. 2009;**9**(11):678-687

[5] Hadinegoro SRS. The revised WHO dengue case classification: Does the system need to be modified? Paediatrics and International Child Health. 2012;**32**(supp 1):33-38

[6] Silveira GF, Wowk PF, Cataneo AHD, Dos Santos PF, Delgobo M, Stimamiglio MA, Lo Sarzi M, et al. Human T lymphocytes are permissive for dengue virus replication. Journal of Virology [Print 15 May 2018]. 2018;**92**(10):e02181-17. DOI: 10.1128/JVI.02181-17

[7] Wang M, Yang F, Huang D, Huang Y, Zhang X, Wang C, et al. Anti-idiotypic antibodies specific to prM monoantibody prevent antibody dependent enhancement of dengue virus

infection. Frontiers in Cellular and Infection Microbiology. 2017;**7**:157. DOI: 10.3389/fcimb.2017.00157

[8] Morens DM. Antibody-dependent enhancement of infection and the pathogenesis of viral disease. Clinical Infectious Diseases. 1994;**19**(3):500-512

[9] Morens DM, Halstead SB. Measurement of antibody-dependent infection enhancement of four dengue virus serotypes by monoclonal and polyclonal antibodies. The Journal of General Virology. 1990;**71**:2909-2914

[10] Harrison SC. Immunogenic cross-talk between dengue and Zika viruses. Nature Immunology [Internet]. 2016 Sep 19;**17**(9):1010-1012. Available from: http://dx.doi.org/10.1038/ni.3539

[11] Dejnirattisai W, Supasa P, Wongwiwat W, Rouvinski A, Barba-Spaeth G, Duangchinda T, et al. Dengue virus sero-cross-reactivity drives antibody-dependent enhancement of infection with zika virus. Nature Immunology [Internet]. 2016 Jun 23;**17**:1102. Available from: http://dx.doi.org/10.1038/ni.3515

[12] Soe HJ, Yong YK, Al-Obaidi MMJ, Raju CS, Gudimella R, Manikam R, et al. Identifying protein biomarkers in predicting disease severity of dengue virus infection using immune-related protein microarray. Khan NA, ed. Medicine. 2018;**97**(5):e9713. DOI: 10.1097/MD.0000000000009713

[13] Rothman AL. Immunity to dengue virus: A tale of original antigenic sin and tropical cytokine storms. Nature Reviews. Immunology. 2011;**11**(8):532-543

[14] Wan S-W, Lin C-F, Yeh T-M, Liu C-C, Liu H-S, Wang S, et al. Autoimmunity in dengue pathogenesis. Journal of the Formosan Medical Association [Internet]. 2013 Jan;**112**(1):3-11. Available from: http://linkinghub.elsevier.com/retrieve/pii/S0929664612005281

[15] Morrison J, Aguirre S, Fernandez-Sesma A. Innate immunity evasion by dengue virus. Viruses. 2012;**4**(3):397-413

[16] Zivny J, DeFronzo M, Jarry W, Jameson J, Cruz J, Ennis F, et al. Partial agonist effect influences the CTL Response to a heterologous dengue virus serotype. Journal of Immunology. 1999;**163**:2754-2760

[17] Hober D, Poli L, Roblin B, Gestas P, Chungue E, Granic G, et al. Serum levels of tumor necrosis factor-alpha (TNF-alpha), interleukin-6 (IL-6), and interleukin-1 beta (IL-1 beta) in dengue-infected patients. The American Journal of Tropical Medicine and Hygiene. 1993;**48**(3):324-331

[18] Lei HY, Yeh TM, Liu HS, Lin YS, Chen SH, Liu CC. Immunopathogenesis of dengue virus infection. Journal of Biomedical Science. Sep 2001;**8**(5):377-388

[19] Bravo JR, Guzmán MG, Kouri GP. Why dengue haemorrhagic fever in Cuba? 1. Individual risk factors for dengue haemorrhagic fever/dengue shock syndrome (DHF/DSS). Transactions of the Royal Society of Tropical Medicine and Hygiene. 1987;**81**(5):816-820

[20] Markoff LJ, Innis BLHRH. Development of cross-reactive antibodies to plasminogen during the immune response to dengue virus infection. The Journal of Infectious Diseases. 1991;**164**(2):294-301

[21] Lauring AS, Jones JO, Andino R. Rationalizing the development of live attenuated virus vaccines. Nature Biotechnology. 2010;**28**(6):573-579

[22] Putnak JR, Coller BA, Voss G, Vaughn DW, Clements D, Peters I, et al. An evaluation of dengue type-2 inactivated, recombinant subunit, and live-attenuated vaccine candidates in the rhesus macaque model. Vaccine. 2005;**23**(35):4442-4452

[23] Clements DE, Coller BAG, Lieberman MM, Ogata S, Wang G, Harada KE, et al. Development of a recombinant tetravalent dengue virus vaccine: Immunogenicity and efficacy studies in mice and monkeys. Vaccine. 2010;**28**(15):2705-2715

[24] Coller BAG, Clements DE, Bett AJ, Sagar SL, Ter Meulen JH. The development of recombinant subunit envelope-based vaccines to protect against dengue virus induced disease. Vaccine. 2011;**29**(42):7267-7275

[25] Schmitz J, Roehrig J, Barrett A, Hombach J. Next generation dengue vaccines: A review of candidates in preclinical development. Vaccine [Internet]. 2011 Sep;**29**(42):7276-7284. Available from: http://linkinghub.elsevier.com/retrieve/pii/S0264410X11010383

[26] Jennings GT, Bachmann MF. The coming of age of virus-like particle vaccines. Biological Chemistry. 2008;**389**(5):521-536

[27] Vannice KS, Durbin A, Hombach J. Status of vaccine research and development of vaccines for dengue. Vaccine [Internet]. 2016 Jun;**34**(26):2934-2938. Available from: http://linkinghub.elsevier.com/retrieve/pii/S0264410X16002930

[28] Schwartz LM, Halloran ME, Durbin AP, Longini IM. The dengue vaccine pipeline: Implications for the future of dengue control. Vaccine. 2015;**33**(29):3293-3298

[29] Ravel G, Mantel N, Silvano J, Rogue A, Guy B, Jackson N, et al. Biodistribution and safety of a live attenuated tetravalent dengue vaccine in the cynomolgus monkey. Vaccine. 2017;**35**(43):5918-5923

[30] Dans AL, Dans LF, Lansang MAD, Silvestre MAA, Guyatt GH. Controversy and debate on dengue vaccine series—paper 1: Review of a licensed dengue vaccine: Inappropriate subgroup analyses and selective reporting may cause harm in mass vaccination programs. Journal of Clinical Epidemiology. 2018;**95**:137-139

[31] World Health Organization. Dengue vaccine: WHO position paper, July 2016 – recommendations. Vaccine [Internet]. 2017 Mar;**35**(9):1200-1201. Available from: http://linkinghub.elsevier.com/retrieve/pii/S0264410X16310192

[32] Arredondo-García J, Hadinegoro S, Reynales H, Chua M, Rivera Medina D, et al. Clinical Microbiology and Infection. 2018;**24**(7):755-763

[33] Lee SH, Hosseindoust AR, Kim JS, Cho YH, Lee JH, Kwon IK, et al. Bacteriophages as a promising anti-pathogenic option in creep-feed for suckling piglets: Targeted to control *Clostridium* spp. and coliforms faecal shedding. Livestock Science. 2016;**191**:161-164

[34] Skipetrova A, Wartel TA, Gailhardou S. Dengue vaccination during pregnancy—An overview of clinical trials data. Vaccine [Internet]. 2018 May;**36**(23):3345-3350. Available from: http://linkinghub.elsevier.com/retrieve/pii/S0264410X18305474

[35] Capeding RZ, Luna IA, Bomasang E, Lupisan S, Lang J, Forrat R, et al. Live-attenuated, tetravalent dengue vaccine in children, adolescents and adults in a dengue endemic country: Randomized controlled phase I trial in the Philippines. Vaccine [Internet]. 2011 May;**29**(22):3863-3872. Available from: http://linkinghub.elsevier.com/retrieve/pii/S0264410X11004397

[36] Kirkpatrick BD, Whitehead SS, Pierce KK, Tibery CM, Grier PL, Hynes NA, et al. The live attenuated dengue vaccine TV003 elicits complete protection against dengue in a human challenge model. Science Translational Medicine [Epub 16 Mar 2016]. 16 Mar 2016;**8**(330): 330ra36. DOI: 10.1126/scitranslmed.aaf1517

[37] Whitehead SS, Durbin AP, Pierce KK, Elwood D, McElvany BD, Fraser EA, et al. In a randomized trial, the live attenuated tetravalent dengue vaccine TV003 is well-tolerated and highly immunogenic in subjects with flavivirus exposure prior to vaccination. Messer WB, editor. PLOS Neglected Tropical Diseases [Internet]. 2017 May 8;**11**(5):e0005584. Available from: http://dx.plos.org/10.1371/journal.pntd.0005584

[38] Brewoo JN, Powell TD, Arguello J, Huang CY-H, Kinney RM, Tary-Lehmann M, et al. Efficacy of a tetravalent chimeric dengue vaccine (DENVax) in cynomolgus macaques. The American Journal of Tropical Medicine and Hygiene [Internet]. 2011 Jun 1;**84**(6):978-987. Available from: http://www.ajtmh.org/content/journals/10.4269/ajtmh.2011.10-0592

[39] Jackson LA, Rupp R, Papadimitriou A, Wallace D, Raanan M, Moss KJ. A phase 1 study of safety and immunogenicity following intradermal administration of a tetravalent dengue vaccine candidate. Vaccine [Epub 19 May 2018]. 2018;**36**(27):3976-3983. DOI: 10.1016/j.vaccine.2018.05.028

[40] Osorio JE, Partidos CD, Wallace D, Stinchcomb DT. Development of a recombinant, chimeric tetravalent dengue vaccine candidate. Vaccine [Internet]. 2015 Dec;**33**(50):7112-7120. Available from: http://linkinghub.elsevier.com/retrieve/pii/S0264410X15016552

[41] George SL, Wong MA, Dube TJT, Boroughs KL, Stovall JL, Luy BE, et al. Safety and immunogenicity of a live attenuated tetravalent dengue vaccine candidate in flavivirus-naive adults: A randomized, double-blinded phase 1 clinical trial. The Journal of Infectious Diseases [Internet]. 2015 Oct 1;**212**(7):1032-1041. Available from: https://academic.oup.com/jid/article-lookup/doi/10.1093/infdis/jiv179

[42] Osorio JE, Velez ID, Thomson C, Lopez L, Jimenez A, Haller AA, et al. Safety and immunogenicity of a recombinant live attenuated tetravalent dengue vaccine (DENVax) in flavivirus-naive healthy adults in Colombia: A randomised, placebo-controlled, phase 1 study. The Lancet Infectious Diseases [Internet]. 2014 Sep;**14**(9):830-838. Available from: http://linkinghub.elsevier.com/retrieve/pii/S1473309914708114

[43] Osorio JE, Huang CY-H, Kinney RM, Stinchcomb DT. Development of DENVax: A chimeric dengue-2 PDK-53-based tetravalent vaccine for protection against dengue fever.

Vaccine [Internet]. 2011 Sep;**29**(42):7251-7260. Available from: http://linkinghub.elsevier.com/retrieve/pii/S0264410X11010413

[44] Eckels KH, Thomas SJ, De La Barrera R, Carletti I, Fernandez S, Dessy F, et al. A phase II, randomized, safety and immunogenicity study of a re-derived, live-attenuated dengue virus vaccine in healthy adults. The American Journal of Tropical Medicine and Hygiene [Internet]. 2013 Jan 9;**88**(1):73-88. Available from: http://www.ajtmh.org/content/journals/10.4269/ajtmh.2012.12-0361

[45] US Navy's Naval Medical Research Center. US Navy Advances Dengue TVDV Using Vaxfectin [Internet]. 2012. Available from: https://www.bmiresearch.com/articles/us-navy-advances-dengue-tvdv-using-vaxfectin

[46] Martinez LJ, Thomas SJ, Teneza-Mora NC, De La Barrera R, Currier JR, Eckels KH, et al. Safety and immunogenicity of a dengue virus serotype-1 purified-inactivated vaccine: Results of a phase 1 clinical trial. The American Journal of Tropical Medicine and Hygiene [Internet]. 2015 Sep 2;**93**(3):454-460. Available from: http://www.ajtmh.org/content/journals/10.4269/ajtmh.14-0819

[47] Thomas SJ, Jarman RG, Febo I, De La Barrera R, Innis BL, Eckels KH, et al. Phase I randomized study of a tetravalent dengue purified inactivated vaccine in healthy adults from Puerto Rico. The American Journal of Tropical Medicine and Hygiene [Internet]. 2018 May 9;**98**(5):1435-1443. Available from: http://www.ajtmh.org/content/journals/10.4269/ajtmh.17-0627

[48] Lepine E, Ruck RC, Thomas SJ, Schmidt AC, Lin L, Paolino KM, et al. Phase 1 randomized study of a tetravalent dengue purified inactivated vaccine in healthy adults in the United States. The American Journal of Tropical Medicine and Hygiene [Internet]. 2017 Jun 7;**96**(6):1325-1337. Available from: http://www.ajtmh.org/content/journals/10.4269/ajtmh.16-0634

[49] Torresi J, Ebert G, Pellegrini M. Vaccines licensed and in clinical trials for the prevention of dengue. Human Vaccines & Immunotherapeutics [Internet]. 2017 May 4;**13**(5):1059-1072. Available from: https://www.tandfonline.com/doi/full/10.1080/21645515.2016.1261770

[50] Durbin AP, Whitehead SS. Next-generation dengue vaccines: Novel strategies currently under development. Viruses. 2011;**3**(10):1800-1814

[51] Govindarajan D, Meschino S, Guan L, Clements DE, ter Meulen JH, Casimiro DR, et al. Preclinical development of a dengue tetravalent recombinant subunit vaccine: Immunogenicity and protective efficacy in nonhuman primates. Vaccine [Internet]. 2015 Aug;**33**(33):4105-4116. Available from: http://linkinghub.elsevier.com/retrieve/pii/S0264410X15008683

[52] Lim S-K, Lee YS, Namkung S, Lim JK, Yoon I-K. Prospects for dengue vaccines for travelers. Clinical and Experimental Vaccine Research [Internet]. 2016;**5**(2):89. Available from: https://synapse.koreamed.org/DOIx.php?id=10.7774/cevr.2016.5.2.89

[53] Thomas SJ, Kochel T, Simmons M, Luke TC, Smith L, Sun P, et al. Safety and immunogenicity of a tetravalent dengue DNA vaccine administered with a cationic lipid-based adjuvant in a phase 1 clinical trial. The American Journal of Tropical Medicine and Hygiene [Internet].

2018 Mar 7;**98**(3):849-856. Available from: http://www.ajtmh.org/content/journals/10.4269/ajtmh.17-0416

[54] Raviprakash K, Luke T, Doukas J, Danko J, Porter K, Burgess T, et al. A dengue DNA vaccine formulated with Vaxfectin® is well tolerated, elicits strong neutralizing antibody responses to all four dengue serotypes in New Zealand white rabbits. Human Vaccines & Immunotherapeutics. 2012;**8**(12):1764-1768

[55] Elong Ngono A, Shresta S. Immune response to dengue and zika. Annual Review of Immunology [Internet]. 2018;**36**(1). Available from: http://www.annualreviews.org/doi/10.1146/annurev-immunol-042617-053142%0Ahttp://www.ncbi.nlm.nih.gov/pubmed/29345964

[56] WHO. World Health Organization (WHO) Strategic Advisory Group of Experts. Dengue Vaccine [Internet]. 2016. Available from: http://www.who.int/immunization/sage/meetings/2016/april/SAGE_April_2016_Meeting_Web_summary.pdf?ua=1

[57] Barba-Spaeth G, Dejnirattisai W, Rouvinski A, Vaney M-C, Medits I, Sharma A, et al. Structural basis of potent Zika–dengue virus antibody cross-neutralization. Nature [Internet]. 2016 Jun 23;**536**:48. Available from: http://dx.doi.org/10.1038/nature18938

[58] Aguiar M, Stollenwerk N, Halstead SB. The risks behind Dengvaxia recommendation. The Lancet Infectious Diseases. 2016;**16**(8):882-883

[59] Aguiar M, Halstead SB, Stollenwerk N. Consider stopping Dengvaxia administration without immunological screening. Expert Review of Vaccines. 2017;**16**(4):301-302

[60] Aguiar M, Stollenwerk N. Dengvaxia: Age as surrogate for serostatus. The Lancet Infectious Diseases [Epub 21 Dec 2017]. 2018;**18**(3):245. DOI: 10.1016/S1473-3099(17)30752-1

[61] Iacobucci G. WHO recommends additional tests for Sanofi's dengue vaccine after safety concerns. BMJ. 2018;**361**:k1765

12

Challenges for the Introduction and Evaluation of the Impact of Innovative *Aedes aegypti* Control Strategies

Héctor Gómez-Dantés, Norma Pavía-Ruz, Fabián Correa-Morales, Abdiel Martín-Park, Gonzalo Vázquez-Prokopec and Pablo Manrique-Saide

Abstract

Innovative control tools for the dengue, chikungunya and Zika vector *Aedes aegypti*, such as genetically modified mosquitoes and biological control and manipulation with the bacteria *Wolbachia*, are now becoming available and their incorporation into institutional vector control programs is imminent. The objective of this chapter is to examine the technical and organizational mechanisms together with the necessary processes for their introduction and implementation, as well as the indispensable indicators to measure their entomological effect on vector populations and their epidemiological impact in the short, medium and long term as part of an integrated vector management approach.

Keywords: dengue, chikungunya, Zika, *Wolbachia*, SIT, RIDL, entomological surveillance, epidemiology

1. Introduction

The tools and strategies that have been implemented in recent decades to control the *Aedes aegypti* mosquito face an efficient vector of various viruses [dengue, chikungunya, Zika and yellow fever, which together are known as *Aedes*-borne diseases (ABD)] that has a great capacity for adaptation to human and urban habitats (domesticated).

Improvements in the quantification and control of this mosquito in urban environments and the transmission of ABD require a reformulation of current control strategies, as well as a stronger focus on reducing vector abundance, preventing human-vector contact and finally, reducing virus transmission [1, 2]. Due to the multiplicity of co-circulating viruses transmitted by the *Aedes* mosquito and the absence of effective treatment or vaccines against these infections, the development of long-term strategies for managing the populations of the *Aedes* mosquito has become a public health priority.

Traditional mosquito control strategies have consisted of nonintegrated vector management of the immature (larvae) mosquito stage and of the use of insecticides that have fairly low—and temporary—mortality rates in adult female mosquitoes. Effective and sustained control by these methods and intervention is impeded by a number of obstacles: effective coverage of all breeding sources, lack of personnel needed, the need of continuous insecticide re-application, the transitory nature of their effects, the false sense of security that they generate and the dependence fomented in both the affected communities and the mosquito management programs.

On February 1, 2016, the World Health Organization (WHO) declared the Zika virus, along with microcephaly and the other associated neurological disorders, a public health emergency of international importance (public health emergency of international concern, PHEIC) [3]. The Zika outbreak rapidly reached across not only the Americas, but also 75 other countries and territories; its control continues to be a long-term challenge to public health even after the declaration of the end of the state of emergency by the WHO Emergency Committee in November of 2016.

Due to this emergency, the scientific community; entrepreneurs and international, regional, and national governmental programs in areas endemic to *Ae. aegypti* and ABD are researching on innovative alternative methods of vector control. WHO has expressed its support for developing and upscaling three novel approaches to controlling the *Ae. aegypti* mosquito: the sterile insect technique (SIT), the release of insects carrying dominant lethal genes (RIDL) and the release of *Wolbachia*-infected mosquitoes.

We find ourselves looking to the possible incorporation of various technological innovations whose application in the field of public health offers positive (theoretical) prospects of success along with new opportunities for enhancing the effectiveness of control programs; however, there are also technical and operational challenges that must be considered before incorporating these innovations into the inventory of mosquito management tools [4].

2. Methods of intervention for *Aedes aegypti* control

Vector control is a complex task. There are a number of options available for different stages (eggs, larvae, pupae and adult) of the mosquito populations; a variety of available tools (physical/mechanical, environmental, biological, chemical and behavioral preventive measures) and different goals for each strategy (covering containers to avoid egg-laying, eliminating breeding sites in order to diminish larval densities, spraying insecticides to kill and reduce adult mosquitoes or installing barriers that diminish vector-human contact). The ultimate goal of each strategy is diminishing transmission. However, experience has shown that there is no "magic bullet" that is effective, lasting, affordable and easy to implement.

The purpose of vector control is to maintain populations at "acceptable" densities, to minimize vector-human contact (to prevent mosquito bites) and to reduce the longevity of female adult mosquitoes, in order to reduce the health problem to a manageable level that does not surpass the capacities of local health systems. The ambitious campaign (1947–1970) promoted by the Pan American Health Organization (PAHO) to eliminate *Ae. aegypti* from the continent was one of the great Latin American public health events due to the extent of its achievements throughout the continent. Eradication is not plausible for *Ae. aegypti*, elimination was a goal pursued in the past, but the desirable goal is now control.

We are challenged by different stages of the vector's life cycle which develop in different environments (air and water) and in different types of breeding sites (natural and artificial), made of a variety of materials (plastic, metal, cement, clay, glass, etc.) and have different productivity, different uses (some may be disposable and others able to be controlled) and can be either permanent or seasonal. This variability in type of vector breeding sites imposes diverse challenges for control—whether it can be sporadic (cleaning campaigns), continuous (use of larvicides or larvivorous fish), or permanent (physical elimination)—and it is not realistic to expect that these differences require a homogenous strategy. The characteristics of the different types of breeding sites require a variety of customized strategies so that the control may be effective and sustainable.

The diversity of available vector control strategies and their implementation in each operation are related to the resources available, the cultural context in which the interventions are performed and the overall capacity for applying them appropriately and with sufficient coverage. These factors can and should be included in the integrated vector management (IVM) approach promoted by the WHO [5, 6]. IVM is based on a spectrum of intervention strategies, frequently utilized in synergy and applied simultaneously, that are selected based off of knowledge of local factors influencing the vector's biology and the disease's transmission and morbidity, with the goal of optimizing resources for vector control.

As dengue spread on the last decades, the idea of vector control replaced that of vector elimination, because the magnitude of the problem surpassed the capacity of institutional responses (vertical programs) and incorporated new approaches such as community participation; biological control of larvae (copepods, *Bacillus thuringiensis* (Bti) and fish); physical control (mosquito nets, curtains, clothing, etc., all impregnated with insecticide); chemical control (repellents, larvicides and novel insecticides); behavior change communication [7] (BCC) and communication for behavioral impact [8, 9] (COMBI); integrated management in the comprehensive control of vectors (EGI-Dengue, 2003) [10] and even the design of multidisciplinary approaches, such as an eco-bio-social emphasis [11]. The incorporation of so many different approaches is a clear sign of the complexity entailed in facing this mosquito.

Despite new vector control strategies being introduced with the goal of diminishing transmission, entomological monitoring indicators were never adapted to the new demands of the programs, and the traditional indices designed to measure the presence and absence of larvae and containers, which were never linked to the risk of transmission, were maintained [12].

The introduction of technological innovations—such as the use of *Wolbachia,* the genetic modification of mosquito (GMM) populations, and/or the use of irradiated mosquitoes—that promise better coverage, impact and sustainability propose to improve the effectiveness and durability of control interventions. Nevertheless, the innovations also present organizational and procedural challenges that must be attended before, during and after their introduction as control measures.

3. Innovations to biological and genetic manipulation of mosquito vectors

The strategies for genetic and biological control/manipulation with *Wolbachia* of mosquito vectors (GMM/BCMW) propose an attack on the mechanisms directly responsible for the proliferation of mosquito populations. Allowing the mosquitoes' reproductive dynamics be the tool for spreading the intervention means that we will allow the modified populations to disperse naturally (through repeated releases) so that little by little the mosquitoes go about occupying the territory of wild populations to the point of reaching our objective by replacing them in their function as vectors or by suppressing them as a species.

The mechanism of dispersion and coverage that is proposed is the male mosquito vector itself; these male mosquitoes will find their female counterparts and transmit the control measure before these females lay their eggs, undiscriminating as to preferred breeding site and location. The progeny (eggs, larvae and adults) will incorporate the intervention naturally and will maintain it in the population that emerges from their lineage (desirable). In essence, the dispersal and upkeep of the intervention will be a product of biological mechanisms rather than human intervention.

Interventions consisting of biological manipulation and genetic control of vectors, furthermore, share many characteristics that again distinguish them from the traditional methods. Among these are as follows: (1) dependence on vertical (maternal) transmission of heritable elements (resistance genes and *Wolbachia*), (2) specificity in regard to affected species, (3) environmental friendliness, (4) harnessing of natural reproductive instincts, (5) noninvasiveness of domestic spaces and (6) large-scale application (indispensable). A common challenge of these innovations and of traditional measures of control is to achieve the coverage necessary to be effective and sustainable.

In general, these innovations to vector manipulation are based on two strategies that can be organized according to the results obtained (population elimination vs. replacement) or to the implantation dynamics (self-sustainable or self-limiting).

Population elimination/suppression: aimed to affect the demographics of the vector population with the goal of eliminating it from the area or reducing it to a low level that will not maintain transmission.

Population substitution/replacement: This strategy seeks to replace wild populations with modified populations that are resistant to the viral infection. One of the most novel mechanisms that produce resistance to infection is transinfection with *Wolbachia*. Other mechanisms are effected through the incorporation of transgenes that—by way of impacting the vectors' survival, physiology (flight, feeding) or susceptibility to the infection—indirectly reduce the mosquito's vectorial competence (interference).

Self-limiting: This strategy implicates the abundant and repeated release of mosquitoes in order to maintain the flux of the genetic change in the target population. It is reversible with the discontinuation of releases.

Self-sustaining: This strategy proposes repeated releases of modified mosquito populations sufficient to establish themselves as the dominant population (replacement), to the end of their persisting in the population even while there may be unforeseen risks.

4. Paradigm shift, focus and objective

One of the most important changes upon incorporating GMM-BCMW into the *Aedes* and ABD control programs is a *paradigm shift* in passing from emphasis on the larval stages to the direct impact on adult populations. These innovations in *Ae. aegypti* control direct efforts to the reproductive capacity or its competence as a vector, rather than the breeding sites. The theoretical assumption is based on the key elements for vector control centered on adult mosquitoes (abundance, survival, incubation periods, biting rate, etc.) [13]. However, directing control toward adult mosquitoes requires information that is not currently produced in traditional control programs.

Traditional programs of control direct their efforts toward larval stages, reducing breeding sites abundance and the density of larvae in houses and containers, while they attack adult mosquitoes with insecticides that have limited coverage, short duration and low mortality at the population level. The focus and objective of integrated vector management (IVM) are directed to the control of mosquito populations through multi-sector interventions with a multidisciplinary and/or eco-bio-social focus based on changes to community practices, achieved by way of educational interventions.

GMM-BCMW are not technologies that can be used in case of emergency (outbreak control). Focus is directed to the reduction, suppression (elimination) or substitution of *Ae. aegypti* populations; but in all cases, they should be visualized within the IVM scheme as complimentary tools. Traditional vector control programs imposed a strong component of entomological surveillance (larval monitoring) not correlated to epidemiological surveillance (incidence of infection and disease); this favored control responses (reactive) before the increase of entomological indicators, without relating them to transmission risk (risk thresholds). This has resulted in reactive interventions based on detection of an increase in breeding sites or of the number of cases that frequently have late entomological effects but no epidemiological effect. With and IVM approach it is expected to use surveillance as a predictor of risk; the identification of priority areas for interventions and to promote actions before, during and after periods of epidemics. In the case of GMM-BCMW, surveillance should be improved so it can be a powerful (proactive) tool that permits entomological, epidemiological and viral surveillance.

5. Challenges to entomological surveillance

Entomological surveillance has been employed to (1) determine changes in the geographical distribution of *Ae. aegypti*, (2) obtain relative measurements of *Ae. aegypti* populations through time and identify areas of "high" infestation or periods of growth in vector populations and (3) evaluate the impact of anti-vector interventions. These indicators cannot be used straightforwardly to estimate the risk of virus transmission in the population at a certain time or location.

Entomological indexes: There are various indicators (indexes) and methods to detect or monitor *Aedes* populations (egg, larval, pupal and adult stages) in relation to their location (containers, home or geographical area). The indicators were initially qualitative (negative/positive breeding sites or houses) and evolved toward being quantitative in order to identify the number of mosquitoes, though without specifying density, productivity or breeding site relevance (cryptic). The indices are not sufficiently exact to identify the risk of transmission [14].

One element of the evolution of control programs has been the slow innovation of entomological monitoring indicators, an area dominated by the traditional *Stegomyia* indexes used in the campaign to eliminate *Ae. aegypti* in the fight against yellow fever: house (HI), container (CI) and Breteau (BI) indexes. These indices were useful in the extent to which they indicated the (qualitative) presence and absence of the vector in a campaign that sought its elimination and attempted to evaluate the endeavors toward physical elimination of breeding sites (positive breeding sites or houses). The focus now turned toward the reduction in density (rather than the elimination) of the vector, and these indicators have lost their usefulness [15, 16].

The need for better indicators led to indices of pupae and oviposition, closer life stages to the ideal measure of adult (female) mosquito populations, which would allow for a better approximation of the estimated risk of transmitting dengue [17, 18]. These indicators of entomological risk did not reduce or eliminate the challenges to evaluate the interventions because the need to relate density and/or the threshold of the different vector stages to risk of transmission still persists [19–21].

The use of "nonentomological" (though associated with infestation and facilitators of vector-human contact and epidemiological risk) indicators has also been proposed and ought to be considered in order to better understand the dynamics of dengue transmission—for example, density and distribution of human populations, socioeconomic conditions, living and public services, climate, etc. [22–27].

The selection of indicators and surveillance methods depends on the objective of surveillance (density reduction, risk detection and outbreak prevention), the levels of infestation and the capacity for implementation. Nevertheless, there is little evidence showing that the control programs employ systematic monitoring of vector populations—in particular, monitoring of adult females—in order to measure infestation and risk of dengue transmission [18, 28, 29]. In the best of cases, programs still employ indices of infested sites/breeding sites [29, 30] in order to establish "areas" of transmission risk without demonstrating the predictive capacity of these indices as indicators of dengue transmission risk in the last 50 years [31].

The limitations of these methods for measuring mosquito populations are the absence of a "gold standard," the fact that all measurements have a range of error (they are not precise) and that only a proportion of the total mosquito population (eggs, larvae or adults) is measured. Furthermore, it must be understood that the risk of transmission can occur in various locations and not necessarily where the measurement and/or intervention is performed and that in the selection of methods of measurement and entomological monitoring, precision is always sacrificed. This is to say that, despite being less precise, easier and cheaper methods are chosen over those (e.g., adult surveys) that require more resources and thus are more expensive [32].

An additional challenge is the combination of strategies (not yet their integration) and the differentiated evaluation of their impact, since while one intervention can modify the physical availability of breeding sites, it does not necessarily result in a decrease of vector density nor control the most stable and productive breeding sites. On the other hand, there is insufficient evidence to support the idea that achieving a lower egg or larval density through a variety of available interventions has an impact on the rate of disease transmission. Nevertheless, the combined use of old strategies and/or the incorporation of new vector control tools imposes various challenges: (1) the use of indicators that measure more specifically the density of mosquitoes in all stages of development in order to more concretely evaluate all available modes of intervention, (2) the definition of risk thresholds and (3) that the programs demonstrate their capacity (in terms of human resources, equipment and finances) to be executed with the coverage and frequency necessary to make them valid [1, 2].

6. Challenges to epidemiological surveillance

The evaluation of interventions to control *Ae. aegypti* faces diverse challenges regarding the potential impact they may have on the risk of transmission not only of dengue but also of other arboviruses recently associated with the region's epidemiological profile: Zika, chikungunya and yellow fever. The first challenge is estimating the impact derived from the disease that may be affected and the second in measuring the direct impact of the interventions on the vector populations in all of their stages and their relation to transmission risk (vectorial competence and capacity).

Systems of epidemiological surveillance now have the task of measuring, in the most precise manner possible, three infections transmitted by *Ae. aegypti*. Now things are complicated because the syndrome of fever and exanthema may be indicative of dengue, Zika and chikungunya. The diseases are also associated with other signs, distinctive symptoms and highly specific clinical complications (hemorrhages with severe dengue, chronic arthralgia with the chikungunya virus and congenital syndromes and neurological complications with Zika).

The estimate of the actual number of dengue cases, and now of Zika and chikungunya, is very difficult to calculate due to *biological problems* inherent to the infection, such as the number asymptomatic infections, or of unspecified fevers, which hinders the correct quantification of the impact of each of these illnesses. Clinical confusion regarding symptomatic fever/exanthema and discriminating diagnosis is reduced when complications are severe and chronic manifestations of each infection are observed. The *operational problems* are evidenced through the low demand of health services—especially during outbreaks—which results in under registration of cases when the person does not demand or lacks access to health services, medicates himself or opts for treatments of symptoms they already recognize through previous exposure to the problem.

Only patients with severe symptoms go to the doctor, and these are the best detected by the surveillance system. An additional operational problem is the lack of sensibility to clinical diagnoses of fever and the limited collection of samples in order to confirm diagnosis—even during an epidemic—now that normative processes restrict the collection of samples to only severe cases or those at the onset of an outbreak. Only those cases confirmed by diagnostic methods available in regional labs (serology and viral isolation) are recorded [33].

These circumstances impact the opportunity for vector control interventions (operational problem) since the presence of asymptomatic cases and unspecified or febrile patients are not registered early, and it is not until the accumulation of many cases that an increase in transmission is detected; it is at this point that control actions are initiated [34]. Among the *cultural problems*, or problems of perception, we find the familiarity with the sickness and its management given prior experience; fever is not considered an important risk to one's health and does not merit a visit to a doctor unless accompanied by more serious symptoms.

The necessity of improving detection, diagnosis and notification: Epidemiological surveillance of arboviruses faces two importance problems that occur in two different spaces: the community and health services. Given the clinical characteristics, an important number of cases do not demand health services due to their asymptomatic status or the unspecified fever that does not merit a visit to a doctor. Even many clinical cases do not consult medical services due to the patient having recognized and identified the case and knowing how to treat it. Due to this situation, we underestimate the number of cases and the detection of the illness and detection for those affected should be improved [35, 36].

In the health services sector, diagnosis and documentation related to cases should be improved by strengthening the capacities of health personnel and local laboratories. To accomplish this, the following are indispensable: (1) counting on clinical guidelines that facilitate the health personnel in the identification and treatment of clinical cases under surveillance (dengue, Zika and chikungunya) and that reduce the identification of false negatives, (2) establishing criteria for the collection of samples and having the supplies necessary for serological and/or viral confirmation of suspected cases, (3) improving the reporting of cases unconfirmed in the laboratory (probable/suspected) following the algorithms of differential diagnosis for the three illnesses, (4) encouraging the reporting of cases by epidemiological association in the case of an outbreak and (5) seeking mechanisms for notification of cases identified by private medical services [37].

7. Operational changes to the programs of control with *Wolbachia* and GMM

Evidence indicates that technological innovations should be viewed as tools complementary to vector control programs—tools whose introduction would be performed in carefully selected sites until the detection of evidence of the sustained impact and the reduction of potential risks of evolution in the manipulated species and introduced genetic or biological marker. It is believed that innovations would be used in places where traditional measures of control have little to no effect and where they may have an important epidemiological impact on transmission dynamics. However, as with any intervention—and especially with innovative interventions—there are some operational changes that will need to be considered for the programs of control with *Wolbachia* and GMM.

Integration of interventions by level of application: A central element is the organization of interventions by level of application. We must keep on with simple practices, such as domestic hygiene (personal level); routine broad procedures such as breeding sites elimination campaigns; technically elaborated entomological sampling and larvicide application (community level); and even specialized, high-cost actions that require equipped, professional personnel, such as insecticide sprays (town level) or programs of medical attention for the correct handling of severe cases (national level). On the other hand, interventions aimed at urban infrastructure (access to potable water, garbage collection and a recycling system) ought to be incorporated bearing in mind that require high-level political commitment and substantial investments (municipal level).

An additional challenge is the integration of abovementioned interventions in order to perform them in a combined and sequential manner and differential intensity in accordance with the epidemiology of each area vulnerable to transmission. Although the available human and financial resources will generally define this, we must pursue on the objective to direct efforts to high-risk areas. The selection of localities in which to introduce these innovations for control should take into account the degree of risk in that area as well as the impact produced by the illnesses.

Program structure: The organization of the control programs has evolved from a vertical centralized structure ("Top-down")—independent of health services and with a "militarized" organization—to a more horizontal and decentralized structure, more tightly linked to services of surveillance and medical care and more participatory ("Bottom-up"). The advances toward a horizontal organization are variable, and in many programs, there exists a combination of both structures, in which the coordination is centralized. The need of coordinating all these processes—including the application of GMM/BCMW-based strategies—implies that programs that adopt these innovations ought to incorporate a centralized perspective, although the host communities ought to participate in the operational unfolding of the new technologies.

Implementation: The traditional control programs have an established procedural routine repeated each year, in the same season, with the same resources (human resources as well as physical, chemical and biological); however, the areas of control must be expanded and the actions intensified due to the increase in at-risk zones. In the case of IVM, it has been proposed that actions implemented should be differential in frequency and intensity in accordance with epidemiological risk.

Human resources and operational infrastructure: The vertical focus of traditional control programs developed a whole line of training for technical vector control personnel totally apart from promotional, preventative and educational health activities. This operational personnel was integrated in brigades separated from other health activities that were not exclusively linked to vector control. This resulted in an independent organization with equipment, vehicles, machinery and supplies (insecticides) that has been growing hand-in-hand with the problem. With IVM, a more rational use of resources is proposed, starting with the multi-sector and multidisciplinary nature (social participation) of the approach, where the social communication component is incorporated as a substantial element of this strategy.

The incorporation of GMM-BCMW into the vector control programs involves the components proposed for IVM, but also requires adaptation of the technology to the local conditions, as well as the development of an infrastructure of basic technology (insectariums and laboratories) to permit mass, sustained production, implementation and appropriate evaluation of the interventions. In this case, a specialized multidisciplinary group—in addition to technical personnel—is needed to achieve the introduction, monitoring and evaluation of new interventional strategies.

Coverage: A problem inherent to the traditional programs of control in urban and suburban areas in countries where ABD are endemic is their limited coverage; not all breeding sites can be protected or removed, and their productive potential cannot be eliminated with biological, chemical or physical agents. It is not possible to protect or control the totality of the most productive and stable breeding sites in urban centers due to their number, seasonal productivity, location and access ("cryptic" breeding sites).

The coverage of a vector control program functions at the level of the individual, the household, the block or neighborhood, but rarely at the town level. With the IVM programs, the target for intensive application of control efforts will be the neighborhood and towns at greatest risk; there are no claims that all affected areas, neighborhoods or towns will be covered. Coverage in the case of GMM-BCMW can include areas, towns, or medium-sized urban centers, since the mass release of treated mosquitoes cannot limit itself to blocks or a neighborhood. Thus, monitoring and maintenance in such broad areas is complicated by the necessity of technical and (specially trained) human resources and not presently contemplated by surveillance programs.

Scale: One of the most important challenges for any vector control intervention is reaching a level of sufficient coverage (breeding sites, houses, people or communities) in order to effectively limit transmission. These technological innovations are proposed as intervention at a scale larger than that established by traditional vector control strategies. However, all of the processes of production, introduction and maintenance must be initially evaluated at an intermediate scale before considering their application at the regional or national level.

Their application for control of mosquitoes that transmit disease is today only viewed within the context of the strategy of integrated vector management (IVM). This implies necessary adaptations in control programs as regard production of biological materials as well as in relation to the operation, which should be designed in accordance with the technical specifications of the modified organisms.

Efficiency in large-scale production: In order to obtain the desired results, it is necessary to release a large quantity of mosquitoes (sterile, genetically manipulated or infected) into the environment in a reasonably short period of time that will allow for reduction and substitution of wild mosquito populations. Production, handling (separation), distribution and release may affect the capacity and competence of freed vectors. Production is easy to evaluate, but the same may not be said for the competence of the generated mosquitoes.

Quality: The performance, or *fitness*, of the vector should be evaluated, and there is not much experience with this sort of evaluation. Some factors to be evaluated are physical distinctions (pupa and/or adult size), survival rate, dispersal, mating capabilities, sperm quality, competition with wild or native species, and so on. Training of technical personnel and a specialized multidisciplinary group is needed.

Social participation: Social and community participation are essential to the acceptance, monitoring and evaluation of GMM strategies. Given the nature of the new GMM methods, communication with the communities is necessary in order to introduce these methods, which are conceptually very different from traditional methods of control.

Sustainability: The re-introduction of an eliminated species is possible if control interventions cease or diminish in intensity and frequency. Invasion or re-introduction from other nontreated areas requires a containment plan with geographical barriers to inhibit vector migration. The concerns are more environmental than health-related. The emptied niche may promote the invasion of a more dangerous, competent and effective species.

Costs: Cost-effectiveness studies of traditional control methods begin to be an important strategy in evaluating their potential and their degree of incorporation, and in defining the conditions that create for their maximum usefulness. The success of an intervention in terms of costs is subject to the context of where it is applied, the scale of implementation, the availability of personnel and appropriate equipment and the scale of the problem (endemic, epidemic, hyperendemic and introduction of new agents). Traditional control programs require resources in response to the growing magnitude and breadth of the problem. The investments associated with IVM increase costs because of the community and multi-sector participation and the necessary social communication, which touch on other relevant community issues. The incorporation of GMM-MBW needs to be accompanied by an important investment in infrastructure, personnel training, equipment and supplies, along with a strong social communication component that ought to be considered within the comprehensive cost of the program.

8. Final considerations

During the last decade, the WHO has been promoting IVM but has been using only those intervention methods traditionally available. Several innovative methods are being developed to complement the current control of *Ae. aegypti* populations and affect the transmission of ABD. Some show great potential, such as the use of GMM-BCMW, but are not yet available as part of institutional prevention and control programs. In addition to the challenges exposed earlier, other limitations include a lack of scientific and technological infrastructure of the quality and capacity necessary for the implementation of novel methods of mosquito control. This extends to laboratories, systems for the mass rearing of mosquitoes and processes such as quality control, transportation, field release, monitoring and evaluation of effectiveness. Both WHO and the Pan American Health Organization (PAHO) are offering their technical cooperation to support pilot studies using innovative methods. The technical advisory group on entomology in public health and vector control explicitly recommended to PAHO "Promoting rapid, robust and accelerated evaluation of new tools complementary to the control of *Aedes*, with particular attention to the use of mosquitoes infected with the bacteria *Wolbachia* and sterile and genetically modified insects."

Vector control programs do not use "single" methods. Innovations should be considered complementary tools to control programs, not substitutes. Traditional and/or new interventions of greater complexity can be implemented proactively using a risk stratification approach calling for different intensity and greater coverage in priority areas. However, we can anticipate complications on monitoring and evaluation, since there is little evidence and experience of multiple or combined interventions with intersectoral participation and IVM.

Traditional vector control has demonstrated limited impacts and transitory decreases in larval and adult mosquito populations. Monitoring of these traditional control programs is performed on an irregular basis throughout the year, without taking into account that there are important seasonal effects on vector populations. Furthermore, these evaluations are unstructured and usually not conduced at the time intervals necessary in order to estimate the magnitude and longevity of the effects on vector populations. In the case of GMM-BCMW, in addition to performing entomological monitoring to estimate the effects of suppression on target populations, in the case of substitution or population replacement strategies, it is necessary to include measurements of the reproductive and biological performance of the introduced populations.

Estimates of the effect of traditional actions (larval density) do not imply impacts on disease transmission (incidence). The IVM strategies share these limitations, although they diversify the indicators due to the multidisciplinary nature of their interventions. In the case of GMM-BCMW, the evaluations ought to incorporate continuous monitoring of adult mosquito populations (wild and introduced): their survival, performance (or *fitness*), competence as vectors or capacity to transmit the infectious agents, reproductive capacities, flight range, dispersal, and so on. The indicators should purvey information relevant to measuring the effects on reproductive capacity; reduction in infection and other entomological, epidemiological and even ecological parameters that describe the dynamics of adaptation of introduced populations.

Despite intense research on *Ae. aegypti*, we still do not have entomological parameters linking vector density to risk of transmission. It is also still difficult to define the transmission risk's direct impact on human populations and its duration (days, weeks and months) in mosquito populations—and even more difficult to count on indicators that allow for efficient evaluation of the effects of different vector control interventions on the impact of the illness within the community (infection, severity of clinical cases, mortality, etc.). These limitations are the same for GMM-BCMW, and we still need indicators that will correlate efficacy in terms of entomological parameters (reduction or substitution of mosquito populations) to effects on transmission of the illness.

Entomological surveillance is indispensable in order to monitor vector populations and to count on the basic parameters that allow for evaluation of direct impact on affected populations. Larval densities are not sufficient for evaluating the effects expected with the inclusion of these innovations, since the introduced populations are competing adults; as a result, it is necessary to evaluate adult density (males and females) as well as vector survival, mating habits, reproductive capacities (fecundity) and so on.

Last but not least, the success of any control intervention should be measured ultimately in terms of resultant decrease in infection transmission and in the impact of the illness on the community. This process entails decreased herd immunity in human populations and would introduce the risk of greater epidemics if the intervention measures lost intensity or effectiveness or were no longer applied. Decreased immunity augments the population's susceptibility, which results in lower vector density thresholds for transmission or risk of transmission.

Here, we have exposed some of the major challenges for the introduction, implementation and evaluation of innovative *Aedes aegypti* control strategies based on GMM/BCMW. Nowadays, they are still being evaluated to gauge their entomological impact; and evidence of epidemiological impact is desirable in the near future.

Other basic requirements for the adoption of technological innovations include a regulatory and legislative framework for their use in public health (Environmental, Biosecurity and Bioethics); following a set of Protocols & Portfolio having to do with safety, quality control, efficacy, and so on; and necessary integration with local vector control programs including agreement/acceptance by institutions and communities. In terms of administrative and financial requirements, we still need to resolve whether these technological innovations can be acquired under the current budget structure (as a product or service). In order to more quickly implement these new technologies, we need to develop a medium to long-term implementation and financing plan; production, distribution, monitoring and evaluation logistics and private-public partnerships.

Acknowledgements

To the Canadian Institutes of Health Research (CIHR) and IDRC (Preventing Zika disease with novel vector control approaches Project 108412) and Fondo Mixto CONACYT–Gobierno del Estado De Yucatán (Project YUC-2017-03-01-556). Abdiel Martin-Park is supported by the Cátedras–CONACYT program. Special thanks to Ana García-Moreno Malcolm for grammar corrections.

Author details

Héctor Gómez-Dantés[1], Norma Pavía-Ruz[2], Fabián Correa-Morales[3], Abdiel Martín-Park[4], Gonzalo Vázquez-Prokopec[5] and Pablo Manrique-Saide[4*]

*Address all correspondence to: msaide@correo.uady.mx

1 Instituto Nacional de Salud Pública, Cuernavaca, Morelos, México

2 Universidad Autónoma de Yucatán, Mérida, Yucatán, México

3 Centro Nacional de Programas Preventivos y Control de Enfermedades (CENAPRECE), Secretaria de Salud, México

4 Unidad Colaborativa para Bioensayos Entomológicos (UCBE), Campus Ciencias Biológicas y Agropecuarias, Universidad Autónoma de Yucatán, México

5 Emory University, Atlanta, USA

References

[1] Achee NL, Gould F, Perkins TA, Reiner RC Jr, Morrison AC, Ritchie SA, Gubler DJ, Teyssou R, Scott TW. A critical assessment of vector control for dengue prevention. PLoS Neglected Tropical Diseases. 2015;**9**(5):e0003655. DOI: 10.1371/journal.pntd.0003655

[2] Morrison A, Zielinski-Gutierrez E, Scott T, Rosenberg R. Defining challenges and proposing solutions for control of the virus vector *Aedes aegypti*. PLoS Medicine. 2008;**5**(3):e68. DOI: 10.1371/journal.pmed.0050068

[3] https://www.paho.org/hq/index.php?option=com_content&view=article&id=12861%3A2016-zika-evolved-from-emergency-into-long-term-public-health-challenge&catid=740%3Apress-releases&Itemid=1926&lang=pt

[4] McGraw EA, O'Neill SL. Beyond insecticides: New thinking on an ancient problem. Nature Reviews, Microbiology. 2013;**11**:181-193

[5] WHO. WHO Position Statement on Integrated Vector Management. Geneva: World Health Organization; 2008. (WHO/HTM/NTD/VEM/2008.2)

[6] WHO. Global Strategic Framework for Integrated Vector Management. Geneva: World Health Organization; 2004. (WHO/CDS/CPE/PVC/2004.10)

[7] Salem RM, Bernstein J, Sullivan TM. Tools for Behavior Change Communication. INFO Reports, 16. Baltimore: Johns Hopkins Bloomberg School of Public Health; 2008. https://www.k4health.org/sites/default/files/BCCTools.pdf

[8] WHO. Communication for Behavioural Impact (COMBI). A Toolkit for Behavioural and Social Communication in Outbreak Response. Geneva, Switzerland: WHO Publications; 2012. http://www.who.int/ihr/publications/combi_toolkit_outbreaks/en/

[9] Parks W, Lloyd LS. Planificación de la movilización y comunicación social para la prevención y el control del dengue. Guía paso por paso. Ginebra: Organización Mundial de la Salud; 2004. http://www.paho.org/hq/index.php?option=com_content&view=article&id=4504%3A2010-comunicacion-impactar-conducta-combi&catid=901%3Adengue-content&Itemid=41040&lang=en

[10] San Martín JL, Brathwaite-Dick O. Integrated strategy for dengue prevention and control in the region of the Americas. Revista Panamericana de Salud Pública. 2007;**21**: 55-63

[11] Spiegel J, Bennett S, Hattersley L, Hayden MH, Kittayapong P, Nalim S, Wang DNC, Zielinski-Gutierrea E, Gubler D. Barriers and bridges to prevention and control of dengue: The need for a social–ecological approach. EcoHealth. 2005;**2**:1-18. DOI: 10.1007/s10393-005-8388-x

[12] Horstick O, Runge-Ranzinger S, Nathan MB, Kroeger A. Dengue vector-control services: How do they work? A systematic literature review and country case studies. Transactions of the Royal Society of Tropical Medicine and Hygiene. 2010;**104**(6):379-386

[13] Smith DL, Battle KE, Hay SI, Barker CM, Scott TW, McKenzie FE. Ross, Macdonald, and a theory for the dynamics and control of mosquito-transmitted pathogens. PLoS Pathogens. 2012;**8**(4):e1002588. DOI: 10.1371/journal.ppat.1002588

[14] Lloyd L, Winch P, Ortega-Canto J, Kendall C. Results of a community-based *Aedes aegypti* control program in Merida, Yucatan, Mexico. American Journal of Tropical Medicine and Hygiene. 1992;**46**:635-642

[15] Knox TB, Yen NT, Nam VS, et al. Critical evaluation of quantitative sampling methods for *Aedes aegypti* (Diptera: Culicidae) immatures in water storage containers in Vietnam. Journal of Medical Entomology. 2007;**44**:192-204

[16] Barrera R. Recomendaciones para la vigilancia de *Aedes aegypti*. Biomédica. 2016;**36**: 454-462. DOI: 10.7705/biomedica.v36i3.2892

[17] Focks DA, Brenner RJ, Hayes J, Daniels E. Transmission thresholds for dengue in terms of *Aedes aegypti* pupae per person with discussion of their utility in source reduction efforts. American Journal of Tropical Medicine and Hygiene. 2000;**62**:11-18

[18] Focks D. A Review of Entomological Sampling Methods and Indicators for Dengue Vectors. Geneva: World Health Organization; 2003. TDR/IDE/Den/03.1

[19] Focks DA, Chadee DD. Pupal survey: An epidemiologically significant surveillance method for *Aedes aegypti*: An example using data from Trinidad. American Journal of Tropical Medicine and Hygiene. 1997;**56**:159-167

[20] Lenhart AE, Castillo CE, Oviedo M, Villegas E. Use of the pupal/demographic-survey technique to identify the epidemiologically important types of containers producing *Aedes aegypti* (L.) in a dengue-endemic area of Venezuela. Annals of Tropical Medicine and Parasitology. 2006;**100**(Suppl 1):S53-S59

[21] Arredondo-Jiménez JI, Valdez-Delgado KM. *Aedes aegypti* pupal/demographic surveys in southern Mexico: Consistency and practicality. Annals of Tropical Medicine and Parasitology. 2006;**100**(Suppl 1):S17-S32

[22] Tun-Lin W, Kay B, Barnes A. The premise condition index: A tool for streamlining surveys of *Aedes aegypti*. American Journal of Tropical Medicine & Hygiene. 1995a;**53**(6):591-594

[23] Espinoza-Gomez F, Hernandez C, Coll R. Factors that modify the larval indices of *Aedes aegypti* in Colima, Mexico. Revista Panamericana de Salud Pública. 2001;**10**:6-12

[24] Guzmán M, Kouri G, Díaz M, Llop A, Vázquez S, González D, Castro O, Álvarez A, Fuentes O, Montada D, Padmanabha H, Sierra B, Pérez A, Rosario M, Pupo M, Dáz C, Sánchez L. Dengue, one of the great emerging health challenges of the 21st century. Expert Review of Vaccines. 2004;**3**:89-88

[25] Nogueira L, Gushi L, Miranda J, Madeira N, Ribolla P. Application of an alternative *Aedes* species (Diptera: Culicidae) surveillance method in Botucatu city, São Paulo, Brazil. American Journal of Tropical Medicine & Hygiene. 2005;**73**:309-311

[26] Bonet M, Spiegel J, Ibarra A, Kouri G, Pintre A, Yassi A. An integrated ecosystem approach for sustainable prevention and control of dengue in Central Havana. International Journal of Occupational and Environmenatl Health. 2007;**13**(2):188-194

[27] Manrique-Saide P, Che-Mendoza A, Coleman P, Davies C, Dzul-Manzanilla F, Rebollar-Téllez E, Reyes-Novelo E, Zapata-Peniche A. Estudio de los criaderos del vector del dengue *Aedes aegypti* en Mérida, Yucatán: Implicaciones para su vigilancia y control. In: Ramírez-Sierra MJ, Jiménez-Coello M, Heredia-Navarrete R, Moguel-Rodríguez W, editors. Investigación y Salud. Vol. 3. Mérida: Universidad Autónoma de Yucatán; 2008. pp. 57-79

[28] Morrison A, Zielinski-Gutierrez E, Scott T, Rosenberg R. Defining the challenges and proposing new solutions for *Aedes aegypti*-borne disease prevention. PLoS Medicine. 2008;**5**:362-366

[29] Scott T, Morrison A. Vector dynamics and transmission of dengue virus: Implications for dengue surveillance and prevention strategies: Vector dynamics and dengue prevention. Current Topics in Microbiology and Immunology. 2010;**338**:115-128

[30] Reiter P, Gubler D. Surveillance and control of urban dengue vectors. In: Gubler DJ, Kuno G, editors. Dengue and Dengue Hemorrhagic Fever. New York: CAB International University Press; 1997

[31] Bowman LR, Runge-Ranzinger S, McCall PJ. Assessing the relationship between vector indices and dengue transmission: A systematic review of the evidence. PLoS Neglected Tropical Diseases. 2014;**8**(5):e2848. DOI: 10.1371/journal.pntd.0002848

[32] Bangs MJ, Focks DA. Abridged pupa identification key to the common container-breeding mosquitoes in urban Southeast Asia. Journal of the American Mosquito Control Association. 2006;**22**:565-572. DOI: 10.2987/8756-971X(2006)22[565:APIKTT]2.0.CO;2

[33] Gómez-Dantés H, Willoquet JR. Dengue in the Americas: Challenges for prevention and control. Cad. Saúde Pública, Rio de Janeiro. 2009;**25**(Supp 1):S19-S31

[34] WHO. Dengue: Guidelines for Diagnosis, Treatment, Prevention and Control. Geneva, Switzerland: WHO; 2009. http://whqlibdoc.who.int/publications/2009/9789241547871_eng.pdf [Accessed: March 07, 2015]

[35] Undurraga EA, Halasa YA, Shepard DS. Use of expansion factors to estimate the burden of dengue in Southeast Asia: A systematic analysis. PLoS Neglected Tropical Diseases. 2013;**7**(2):e2056. DOI: 10.1371/journal.pntd.0002056

[36] Horstick O, Morrison AC. Dengue disease surveillance: Improving data for dengue control. PLoS Neglected Tropical Diseases. 2014;**8**(11):e3311. DOI: 10.1371/journal. pntd. 0003311

[37] Pan American Health Organization (PAHO). Dengue and Dengue Hemorrhagic Fever in the Americas: Guidelines for Prevention and Control. Washington, D.C: PAHO; 1994

Permissions

All chapters in this book were first published in DFARTFI, by InTech Open; hereby published with permission under the Creative Commons Attribution License or equivalent. Every chapter published in this book has been scrutinized by our experts. Their significance has been extensively debated. The topics covered herein carry significant findings which will fuel the growth of the discipline. They may even be implemented as practical applications or may be referred to as a beginning point for another development.

The contributors of this book come from diverse backgrounds, making this book a truly international effort. This book will bring forth new frontiers with its revolutionizing research information and detailed analysis of the nascent developments around the world.

We would like to thank all the contributing authors for lending their expertise to make the book truly unique. They have played a crucial role in the development of this book. Without their invaluable contributions this book wouldn't have been possible. They have made vital efforts to compile up to date information on the varied aspects of this subject to make this book a valuable addition to the collection of many professionals and students.

This book was conceptualized with the vision of imparting up-to-date information and advanced data in this field. To ensure the same, a matchless editorial board was set up. Every individual on the board went through rigorous rounds of assessment to prove their worth. After which they invested a large part of their time researching and compiling the most relevant data for our readers.

The editorial board has been involved in producing this book since its inception. They have spent rigorous hours researching and exploring the diverse topics which have resulted in the successful publishing of this book. They have passed on their knowledge of decades through this book. To expedite this challenging task, the publisher supported the team at every step. A small team of assistant editors was also appointed to further simplify the editing procedure and attain best results for the readers.

Apart from the editorial board, the designing team has also invested a significant amount of their time in understanding the subject and creating the most relevant covers. They scrutinized every image to scout for the most suitable representation of the subject and create an appropriate cover for the book.

The publishing team has been an ardent support to the editorial, designing and production team. Their endless efforts to recruit the best for this project, has resulted in the accomplishment of this book. They are a veteran in the field of academics and their pool of knowledge is as vast as their experience in printing. Their expertise and guidance has proved useful at every step. Their uncompromising quality standards have made this book an exceptional effort. Their encouragement from time to time has been an inspiration for everyone.

The publisher and the editorial board hope that this book will prove to be a valuable piece of knowledge for researchers, students, practitioners and scholars across the globe.

List of Contributors

Hirotaka Takahashi
Proteo-Science Center, Ehime University, Matsuyama, Japan

Youichi Suzuki
Department of Microbiology and Infection Control, Osaka Medical College, Takatsuki, Japan

Shamaraz Firdous and Shahzad Anwar
Biophotonics Laboratories, National Institute of Lasers and Optronics (NILOP), Islamabad, Pakistan

Eliningaya J. Kweka
School of Medicine, Department of Parasitology and Entomology, Catholic University of Health and Allied Health Sciences, Mwanza, Tanzania
Tropical Pesticides Research Institute, Arusha, Tanzania

Vito Baraka
National Institute for Medical Research, Tanga Centre, Tanzania

Leah Mathias
Ministry of Education Science and Technology, Mzumbe High School, Morogoro, Tanzania

Beda Mwang'onde
Sokoine University of Agriculture, Morogoro, Tanzania

Germana Baraka
College of Natural Sciences, University of Dar es Salaam, Dar es Salaam, Tanzania

Lucile Lyaruu
Tropical Pesticides Research Institute, Arusha, Tanzania

Aneth M. Mahande
Tropical Pesticides Research Institute, Mabogini Field Station, Moshi, Tanzania

Imran Shahid
Department of Pharmacology and Toxicology, College of Pharmacy, Umm-Al-Qura University, Makkah, Saudi Arabia
Applied and Functional Genomics Laboratory, Center of Excellence in Molecular Biology (CEMB), University of the Punjab, Lahore, Pakistan

Muhammad Kashif Zahoor, Azhar Rasul, Iqra Sarfraz, Muhammad Zulhussnain, Rizwan Rasool, Farhat Jabeen and Kanwal Ranian
Department of Zoology, Government College University Faisalabad, Pakistan

Muhammad Asif Zahoor
Department of Microbiology, Government College University Faisalabad, Pakistan

Humara Naz Majeed
Department of Biochemistry, Government College Women University, Faisalabad, Pakistan

Om Parkash, Sham Lal, Javed Ahmed Ujjan, Fateh Muhammad Soomro and Nisar Ahmed Kanhar
Institute of Microbiology, Shah Abdul Latif University, Khairpur, Pakistan

Punam Kumari and Vasu Deva
Liaqat Medical University of Health Sciences, Jamshoro, Pakistan

Syed Mehmood Qadir and Rani Faryal
Quaid-i-Azam University, Islamabad, Pakistan

Elizabeth Orozco-García and Juan Carlos Gallego-Gómez
Translational and Molecular Medicine Group, Medellín Medical Research Institute, Faculty of Medicine, Universidad de Antioquia, Medellín, Colombia

Andrea Trujillo-Correa
Institute of Biology, Faculty of Exact and Natural Sciences, Universidad de Antioquia, Medellín, Colombia

Raúl Castro Rodríguez, Jorge Armando Rueda-Gallardo and Manuel Felipe Avella-Niño
Department of Economics, Universidad de los Andes, Bogotá D.C., Colombia

Wladimir J. Alonso
Laboratory for Human Evolutionary and Ecological Studies, Department of Genetics and Evolutionary Biology, University of São Paulo, Brazil

Benjamin J.J. McCormick
Fogarty International Center, National Institutes of Health, Bethesda, MD, USA

Meksianis Z. Ndii
Department of Mathematics, Faculty of Sciences and Engineering, University of Nusa Cendana, Kupang NTT, Indonesia

Eti D. Wiraningsih
Department of Mathematics, Faculty of Mathematics and Natural Sciences, State University of Jakarta, Jakarta DKI, Indonesia

Nursanti Anggriani and Asep K. Supriatna
Department of Mathematics, Faculty of Mathematics and Natural Sciences, Padjadjaran University, Jawa Barat, Indonesia

Jhon Carlos Castaño-Osorio and Alejandra María Giraldo-Garcia
Quindio University, Armenia, Quindio, Colombia

Maria Isabel Giraldo
Department of Microbiology and Immunology, University of Texas Medical Branch, Galveston, TX, USA

Héctor Gómez-Dantés
Instituto Nacional de Salud Pública, Cuernavaca, Morelos, México

Norma Pavía-Ruz
Universidad Autónoma de Yucatán, Mérida, Yucatán, México

Fabián Correa-Morales
Centro Nacional de Programas Preventivos y Control de Enfermedades (CENAPRECE), Secretaria de Salud, México

Abdiel Martín-Park and Pablo Manrique-Saide
Unidad Colaborativa para Bioensayos Entomológicos (UCBE), Campus Ciencias Biológicas y Agropecuarias, Universidad Autónoma de Yucatán, México

Gonzalo Vázquez-Prokopec
Emory University, Atlanta, USA

Index

www.ingramcontent.com/pod-product-compliance
Lightning Source LLC
LaVergne TN
LVHW080610210926
848485LV00003B/132